Strategic Management of the Healthcare Supply Chain

Strategic Management of the Healthcare Supply Chain

Second Edition

Eugene Schneller
W. P. Carey School of Business, Arizona State University, Tempe, Arizona, USA

Yousef Abdulsalam
College of Business Administration, Kuwait University, Kuwait City, Kuwait

Karen Conway
Global Healthcare Exchange (GHX), Louisville, Colorado, USA

Jim Eckler
W. P. Carey School of Business, Arizona State University, Tempe, Arizona, USA

WILEY

Copyright © 2023 by John Wiley & Sons Inc. All rights reserved.

Published by John Wiley & Sons, Inc., Hoboken, New Jersey.
Published simultaneously in Canada.

Edition History: John Wiley & Sons, Inc. (1e, 2006)

No part of this publication may be reproduced, stored in a retrieval system, or transmitted in any
form or by any means, electronic, mechanical, photocopying, recording, scanning, or otherwise,
except as permitted under Section 107 or 108 of the 1976 United States Copyright Act, without either
the prior written permission of the Publisher, or authorization through payment of the appropriate
per-copy fee to the Copyright Clearance Center, Inc., 222 Rosewood Drive, Danvers, MA 01923, (978)
750-8400, fax (978) 750-4470, or on the web at www.copyright.com. Requests to the Publisher for
permission should be addressed to the Permissions Department, John Wiley & Sons, Inc., 111 River
Street, Hoboken, NJ 07030, (201) 748-6011, fax (201) 748-6008, or online at http://www.wiley
.com/go/permission.

Trademarks: Wiley and the Wiley logo are trademarks or registered trademarks of John Wiley
& Sons, Inc. and/or its affiliates in the United States and other countries and may not be used
without written permission. All other trademarks are the property of their respective owners. John
Wiley & Sons, Inc. is not associated with any product or vendor mentioned in this book.

Limit of Liability/Disclaimer of Warranty: While the publisher and author have used their best efforts
in preparing this book, they make no representations or warranties with respect to the accuracy
or completeness of the contents of this book and specifically disclaim any implied warranties of
merchantability or fitness for a particular purpose. No warranty may be created or extended by
sales representatives or written sales materials. The advice and strategies contained herein may not
be suitable for your situation. You should consult with a professional where appropriate. Further,
readers should be aware that websites listed in this work may have changed or disappeared between
when this work was written and when it is read. Neither the publisher nor authors shall be liable for
any loss of profit or any other commercial damages, including but not limited to special, incidental,
consequential, or other damages.

For general information on our other products and services or for technical support, please contact
our Customer Care Department within the United States at (800) 762-2974, outside the United States
at (317) 572-3993 or fax (317) 572-4002.

Wiley also publishes its books in a variety of electronic formats. Some content that appears in print
may not be available in electronic formats. For more information about Wiley products, visit our web
site at www.wiley.com.

Library of Congress Cataloging-in-Publication Data applied for

Paperback ISBN: 9781119908449

Cover image(s): © zf L/Getty Images
Cover design: Wiley

Set in 11.5/13.5 pts and STIXTwoText by Straive
SKY10057142_100623

Comment on *Strategic Management of the Healthcare Supply Chain*
By Eugene Schneller, Yousef Abdulsalam, Karen Conway, Jim Eckler

Supply chain in healthcare is fundamental. And until the pandemic it was taken for granted. The pandemic raised supply chain skills to the level of a national security issue. Supply chain in its broadest sense is a fundamental strategic tool for all aspects of emergency preparedness and healthcare delivery in times of crisis. Objectives are to have ready materials, supplies, PPE, medications, warehouse management, and backup workforce reserves are all required to assure readiness, the ability to sustain a prolonged response, maintain core business activities, and manage surges.

—Denis A. Cortese, MD
Emeritus Professor, President/CEO Mayo Clinic
Professor and director of Arizona State University Center for Healthcare
Delivery and Policy

- This book goes beyond the lessons of the pandemic for emergency preparedness. It also makes clear the role of the CQO, cost-quality-outcomes. The value engineering triad, of which 2 out of the 3 won't do.
- As healthcare gets serious about value-based care this book clarifies the importance of the role supply chain managers and supply chain thinking brings to key strategic and tactical discussions, planning and implementation.
- As the authors wisely say, "Integration between supply chain practice and clinical practice is the hallmark of a high performing health care supply chain organization." I would rephrase this to say it is the hallmark of a high performing and resilient organization. This book is a fundamental guide for success.

—Doug Bowen
Senior Vice President
Banner Health

I am confident this updated edition of *Strategic Management of the Healthcare Supply Chain*, will prove valuable to all audiences. It is an orienting read for new entrants and practitioners to the field of supply chain. It is also an excellent core text for graduate courses, and a must-read for seasoned supply chain leaders.

Pay special attention to the information shared on product standardization, value analysis, and clinical integration—this is the gift that keeps on giving as it will pay dividends now and in the future. Also, I am especially excited about the Fully Integrated Supply Chain Organization (FISCO) model, which has the potential to transform and elevate healthcare supply chain practice.

As a leading healthcare supply chain practitioner and life-long supply chain student, I can attest that this dream team of collaborators—Dr. Schneller, Yousef, Jim, and Karen—have included all the required topics and insights needed to create and operate a more successful healthcare supply chain!

—Lawton Robert Burns, PhD, MBA,
James Joo-Jin Kim Professor, a Professor of Health Care Management
Professor of Management
Wharton School at the University of Pennsylvania.
Director of the Wharton Center for Health Management & Economics

Supply chain management is, at once, the most important source of potential cost savings and the least understood area in healthcare. Maybe that is why we, as a country, have failed to make a dent in lowering healthcare costs. Schneller and colleagues have come to the rescue, offering a comprehensive framework and holistic approach. Their book should be required reading for healthcare academics (and their students), executives, and clinicians. It is time for everyone to step up to the plate.

—Robert Handfield Bank of America University Distinguished Professor
of Supply Chain Management Executive Director, Supply Chain
Resource Cooperative North Carolina State University

An important update to this leading textbook on healthcare supply chains. The new book provides important insights into how hospitals and organizations in their supply chains will need to develop more resilient and agile approaches to managing the many disruptions and challenges that exist in a globally outsourced healthcare environment. These approaches are based on firsthand experience by the authors as well as ongoing discussions and interviews with healthcare executives. They are not theoretical, but rather provide important practical insights for any student of healthcare to understand and adopt. I have no doubt this book will have an enormous impact on the practice of healthcare supply chain management.

Strategic Management of the Healthcare Supply Chain is an eye-opener on how to make an effective, efficient supply chain happen in the health sector.

We do not know how many of the million-plus COVID-19 deaths were associated with the lack of protective and therapeutic supplies, but ironically, many of the products were available. They were not visible, however, in our fragmented supply chain system with its woesome transparency.

COVID-19 was not a Black Swan event. Supply chain preparedness explicated in *Strategic Management of the Healthcare Supply Chain* is critical for our future.

This is no ho-hum, hortative manual—but a terrific, easy-to-read, pragmatic book that:

- Demonstrates how to implement a fully integrated supply chain organization—a turn-of-mind program for health sector supply chain management—through an impressive team composed of an industry strategic leader, a seasoned supply chain practitioner and two highly regarded scholars.
- Provides academics, students, and practitioners guidance for the management of the supply chain not only in "normal times," but also incorporates key lessons from COVID-19 to help bullet-proof us against future disruptions.

Strategic Management of the Healthcare Supply Chain shows how to create the supply chain management that is so essential to an efficient and resilient healthcare system.

—Regina E. Herzlinger
Nancy R. McPherson Professor of Business Administration
Harvard Business School

Contents

Acknowledgments

The authors are grateful:

- For the support (okay, tolerance) by their spouses for the time away from family activities.
- To the W.P. Carey School of Business at ASU for its solid and unwavering commitment to education in healthcare supply chain management.
- To the W.P. Carey School of Business at ASU for supporting the fall 2022 sabbatical for Gene, which allowed for extensive time to be devoted to the text.
- To the ASU College of Health Solutions, which tolerated Karen Conway relating the importance of the supply chain to nearly every aspect of her graduate studies in the Science of Healthcare Delivery.
- To GHX and the many supply chain professionals at both healthcare delivery and supplier organizations for reinventing how they conduct business together.
- To Kuwait University for allowing Yousef the autonomy and flexibility to pursue an interdisciplinary research agenda in healthcare supply chains.
- To the thousands of healthcare professionals we have influenced in the past 15 years since the first edition of this book was published (and those who have influenced us in this rewrite). May our messages and advice on modern supply chain management practices continue to guide you through your careers and help you to improve the performance of global healthcare supply chains.
- To Zoom for providing the technology that allowed for a team located in the United States, Canada, and Kuwait to meet frequently to discuss the key factors constituting and influencing supply chain management in the health sector.
- To the many healthcare clinicians and administrators who responded to the COVID-19 pandemic and brought the term *supply chain management* (SCM) to the forefront of the public mind and for the recognition and respect that SCM has gained.

About the Authors

Eugene Schneller, PhD
Professor and Dean's Council of 100 Distinguished Scholar
Department of Supply Chain Management
Arizona State University

Eugene Schneller earned his PhD at New York University (Sociology). He was awarded an honorary Physician Associate (PA) degree from Duke University and an honorary Doctor of Humane Letters from the A.T. Still University. He has held faculty and research scholar positions at Duke University, Union College (New York), and Columbia University. His consulting and research focus on healthcare policy, best practice adoption, supply chain purchasing strategy design and governance, human resource development, and supply chain integration. He is a former director at Vomaris and the Barrow Neurological Institute, and has served on advisory boards for both device manufacturers and information technology companies. He was on the Expert Advisory Council for SCAN health and serves in an advisory capacity to W. L. Gore Associates. He was Principal Investigator for the U.S. Department of Defense efforts to integrate the medical supply chains for the three services. He is the former Chair of the Board of the Association of University Programs in Health Administration and the former Western Network for Health Care Management. He is co-founder of Healthcare Supply Chain Excellence and Principal at Health Care Sector Advances. In 2022, he was appointed as Co-Director for the design and management of the Resilience Initiative at the W.P. Carey School of Business. He is a frequent speaker at academic and corporate conferences, and has facilitated strategic planning retreats, focus groups, and scenario planning exercises for medical device companies, group purchasing organizations, and universities.

Yousef Abdulsalam, PhD
Associate Professor of Operations and Supply Chain Management
College of Business Administration
Kuwait University

Yousef Abdulsalam is an Assistant Professor of Operations & Supply Chain Management at Kuwait University's College of Business Administration. He earned his PhD in Supply Chain Management from the W.P. Carey School of Business at Arizona State University under the supervision of Professor Gene Schneller. His academic research relates to supply management in the health sector, including supply chain integration, purchasing alliances, and the physicians' influence on supplier selection. The research has been published in both supply chain management journals (*Journal of Business Logistics, Journal of Operations Management*) and healthcare management journals (*Health Care Management Review, Medical Care Research & Review*). He teaches undergraduate courses in supply chain management, business analytics, and operations research. Prior to his academic career, Yousef was a certified Project Management Professional (PMP) working at Ernst & Young's Advisory Services division in the Information Technology, Project Management, and Business Process Reengineering domains.

Karen Conway, MSc, CMRP, CLSSGB
Healthcare Delivery Scientist/Supply Chain Evangelist
Vice President, Healthcare Value; Head of ESG
Global Healthcare Exchange (GHX)

Trained as a healthcare delivery scientist, Karen Conway applies extensive knowledge of supply chain operations and systems thinking to align processes and data across the healthcare ecosystem to generate evidence on what improves the health of people and populations, and the performance of organizations upon which an effective healthcare system depends In 2017, she completed a Capstone research project for the U.S. FDA, exploring the importance of trading partner collaboration in successful implementation of the agency's unique device identification (UDI) rule. She has also consulted internationally on the value of data standardization in the healthcare supply chain. During the Covid-19 pandemic, she led the supply chain curricula for national summits on health system recovery and health equity and delivered closing remarks on leadership to support sustainability in the health sector at a G20 Summit pre-event. She has served as elected national chair of AHRMM, the supply chain association for the American Hospital Association, as board secretary for Strategic Marketplace Initiative (SMI) and as a member of the GS1 Global Healthcare Leadership Team, the healthcare advisory board for CAPS Research, and the expert advisory council for SCAN Health. She co-wrote a best-selling book on global leadership, Leading from the Edge, and was a contributing author to the Springer publication, eBusiness in Healthcare. Her monthly column on the supply chain and value-based healthcare has been one of the most well read in Healthcare Purchasing News for more than a decade. She holds a masters in the Science of Healthcare Delivery from Arizona State University and a bachelor's degree from The Colorado College.

Jim Eckler, B. Math, MS, CMC, ICD.D
Clinical Faculty, Department of Supply Chain Management
W.P. Carey School of Business
Arizona State University

Jim Eckler is a graduate in Mathematics from the University of Waterloo and in Management Science from the Wharton School of the University of Pennsylvania. He is a past chair of the Supply Chain and Logistics Association of Canada. As well, he is a Certified Management Consultant (CMC). Over the past 45 years, he has authored numerous articles and regularly speaks on a broad range of supply chain topics. Professionally, Jim provides advisory services in the supply chain management field delivering practical strategic and operational advice to his clients. He focuses exclusively on supply chain management, outsourcing, business strategy, corporate governance, and operations. He has a particular specialty in the healthcare field, advising hospital systems and other healthcare organizations toward the achievement of supply chain excellence.

To support this focus, Jim co-founded Healthcare Supply Chain Excellence (www.hscxi.com), a consulting firm focused on strategy, cost management, improved patient outcomes, and quality improvement, all driven to improve supply chain management performance. He is also the cofounder of Physicians for Supply Chain Excellence, an organization to help physician leaders gain clinical alignment on supply chain matters, particularly toward rationalizing high-cost physician preference items. For 18 years, Jim held senior executive roles in operating companies, including Health Shared Services BC, a provider of shared services for the healthcare system across British Columbia, and as President and CEO of SCI Group Inc., a leading supply chain management outsourcing services company, providing logistics services for major technology, healthcare, and retail companies such as Xerox, Bell Canada, Amazon, Wal-Mart, Siemens, and Lowes.

In addition to operational roles, Jim has served on six boards with roles including chair, executive committees, finance, and pensions. He also holds the ICD.D designation from the Institute of Corporate Directors. Prior to his senior executive positions, Jim was a supply chain management consultant for 18 years with Booz Allen and KPMG.

Remembering

Larry R. Smeltzer

The first edition of this book was based on work I carried out with Larry Smeltzer, beginning in 2002. Larry passed away in 2004, at the young age of 57, after co-writing but just prior to the publication of the first edition of this book. He was my dear friend and collaborator, and is greatly missed.

Larry was a pioneer in the field of supply chain management. He was significantly shocked by the extent to which healthcare supply chain practice lagged so significantly behind supply chain practice in other industries. He was equally shocked by the absence of supply chain education for senior healthcare organization leaders, and perhaps, most shocked by my ignorance and the ignorance of most health services researchers about the supply chain's centrality for operations and patient care. How could we train future health sector CEOs without ever hearing about the healthcare supply chain?

Larry started me on a supply chain journey. While I think he failed to convince me that inventory was interesting—he did convince me that it was (and still is) important. If one needs any confirmation of this, just consider the value of inventory during the COVID-19 pandemic's early days. In our travels to healthcare systems across the nation, Larry dared to ask tough and challenging questions—especially around the failure of supply chain managers to see themselves and be seen as both the agent of a healthcare organization's important assets, materials, and processes, and as influencers to improve value to healthcare business professionals, clinicians, and ultimately, patients. He was appropriately puzzled by the strong influence of physicians and the gaps in incentives between buyers and sellers in the health sector. He said, "Gene, we need to write about this!" While the influence of the first edition has been considerable for both undergraduate and graduate students, it has also been, curiously, influential in helping to shape managers from nonhealth sectors transitioning into health and physicians who have grown into roles that interface with supply chain. Hopefully, this new edition will continue to provide that influence. Healthcare needs talent that will improve the practice of supply chain management, and in turn, the delivery of healthcare.

If Larry is looking down from a heavenly perch, he is surely smiling. Terms in this new edition would excite him—value-based purchasing, clinician integration, and evidence-based practice,"....

Perhaps, most importantly, Larry was a great mentor. He changed the focus of so many undergraduate and graduate students, and unknowingly, sent me on a trajectory I had never even known existed. We thus dedicate this recasting of *Strategic Management of the Healthcare Sector* to Larry Smeltzer.

—*Gene Schneller, PhD*
Dean's Council of 100 Distinguished Scholar
Arizona State University

About the Companion Website

This book is accompanied by a companion website:

www.wiley.com/go/schneller/health_care_supply_chain2e

To assist students and other readers to fully benefit from this textbook, we have prepared supplemental material in the form of web-based references, discussion questions for groups, and short answer questions which are interactive in design. These resources will help to extend the learning from the text and, resulting from the web-based capability, it will be updated frequently to keep the students and other readers current on this topic.

The website includes:

- Listing of Key Associations, Trade Organizations, Trade Magazines & Journals, Peer-Reviewed Journals, and Websites
    - Associations and Research Centers for advancing supply chain
    - Trade Organizations
- Key Concepts
- Discussion Questions
- Short Answer Questions
- Selected Readings
- Case studies and Supplemental Materials

List of Exhibits

List of Acronyms

3PL	Third-party Logistics
ACA	Patient Protection and Affordable Care Act
AHC	Academic Health Center
AHRMM	Association for Healthcare Resources & Materials Management
AHRQ	Agency for Healthcare Research and Quality
AI	Artificial Intelligence
AP	Accounts Payable
ASC	Ambulatory Surgery Center
ASU	Arizona State University
ASU/CHMR	A 2004 research study carried out by Larry Smeltzer and Gene Schneller
AVAP	Association of Value Analysis Professionals
B2B	Business-to-Business
BATNA	Best Alternative to a Negotiated Agreement
C2SHIP	Center to Stream Healthcare in Place
CAM	Complementary and Alternative Medicine
CAPS Research	Center for Advanced Purchasing Studies
CATH Lab	Interventional Cardiology Laboratory
CHMR	Center for Health Management Research
CIPS	Cloud Infrastructure and Platform Services
CMS	U.S. Centers for Medicare and Medicaid Services
COE	Center of Excellence
COVID-19	Coronavirus Disease Pandemic
CQO	Cost, Quality, and Outcomes
CRM	Customer Relationship Management
CSC	Consolidated Service Center

DOD	U.S. Department of Defense
DHA	Defense Health Agency
DRG	Diagnostic-related Group
DRP	Distribution Requirements Plan
DES	Drug-eluting Stent
EDI	Electronic Data Interchange
EHCR	Efficient Healthcare Consumer Response
EHR	Electronic Health Record
EMA	European Medicines Agency
EMR	Electronic Medical Record
EOQ	Economic Order Quantity
ERP	Enterprise Resource Planning
FDA/U.S. FDA	U.S. Food and Drug Administration
FFS	Fee-for-Service
FISCO	Fully Integrated Supply Chain Organization
FTC	Federal Trade Commission
FTE	Full-time Equivalent
HIGPII	Healthcare Group Purchasing Industry Initiative
GPO	Group Purchasing Organization
HCSA	Healthcare Supply Chain Association
IBP	Industry Best Practice
IDC	International Data Corporation
HMO	Health Maintenance Organization
HMPI	Health Management, Policy & Innovation
ICU	Intensive Care Unit
IDN	Integrated Delivery Network
IoT	Internet of Things
ISM	Internal Supply Management
IT	Information Technology

JIT	Just-in-Time
KPI	Key Performance Indicator
LGBTQ	Lesbian, Gay, Bisexual, and Transgender
ML	Machine Learning
MRI	Magnetic Resonance Imaging
NEST	National Evaluation System for Health Technology
NLP	Natural Language Processing
NHS	National Health Service
NPI	New Product Introduction
NSF	National Science Foundation
ONC	Office of the National Coordinator
OR	Operating Room
PBM	Pharmacy Benefit Manager
PO	Purchase Order
RFI	Request for Information
RFP	Request for Proposal
RFQ	Request for Quote
P2P	Procure-to-Pay
PCORI	Patient-centered Outcomes Research Institute
PO	Purchase Order
PPE	Personal Protective Equipment
PPI	Physician Preference Item
PPM	Purchasing Partner Management
PPO	Preferred Provider Organization
PSO	Point of Service Organization
ROA	Return on Assets
RPA	Robotic Process Automation
RWE	Real World Evidence
SaaS	Software-as-a-Service

SCM	Supply Chain Management
SCOR	Supply Chain Operations Reference
SCRM	Supply Chain Risk Management
SDOH	Social Determinants of Health
SKU	Stock Keeping Unit
SMART	Specific, Measurable, Achievable, Relevant and Time-based
SMI	Strategic Marketplace Initiative
SNS	Strategic National Stockpile
SOW	Statement of Work
SRM	Supplier Relationship Management
TCO	Total Cost of Ownership
TKA	Total Knee Arthroplasty
TQM	Total Quality Management
TQO	Total Cost of Ownership
UDI	Unique Device Identification
U.K.	United Kingdom
VA	Veterans Administration
VAT	Value Analysis Team
VMI	Vendor Managed Inventory
VMO	Vendor Management Office
VOI	Vendor Owned Inventory
WCC	Weighted Cost of Capital
WMS	Warehouse Management System

Preface

1 Addressing the Needs of an Evolving Healthcare Industry

This edition of the book was substantially revised in consideration of the evolution of health sector supply chain research and practice over the past decade and a half. This includes the critical learnings that arose out of the COVID-19 pandemic, especially as it relates to a heightened appreciation of the need for preparedness and resiliency. Most importantly, the book incorporates the substantive changes in the supply chain necessitated by the fundamental shift to a value-based healthcare system. Foremost, as hospitals, healthcare systems, and clinicians are increasingly compensated based on their ability to create value in relation to money spent and resources consumed, healthcare institutions have greater dependencies on the ability of the supply chain to source, secure and deliver products and services that support the delivery of high-quality care at an affordable cost. The centrality of the physician as the predominant decision-maker as to what is needed and what is prescribed remains intact, but changing value-based payment methodologies and incentives are increasing interest in the cost of care and fostering more collaboration with supply chain leaders.

Supply chain management teams are also important contributors to broader initiatives that seek to integrate the delivery of both clinical and social resources. For example, food, transportation, and housing are products and services necessary to optimize the health and well-being of entire communities and populations of patients. An expanding role for supply chain is to manage the sourcing, procurement and delivery of products and services associated with the so-called social determinants of health (SDOH).[1] This is driven in large part by the increasing number of value-based reimbursement programs that are tied to improving the health of entire populations, especially among the poor and communities of color that have historically lacked access to these resources, which have been proven to enhance health status and longevity.

Governments, commercial payors, and health systems are also using reimbursement policies to shift some of the care that has traditionally or frequently been delivered in the acute care hospital setting to community locations, such as ambulatory surgery centers and the home, where the same quality of care can be delivered at a lower cost.[2,3] The U.S. Centers for Medicare and Medicaid Services (CMS) have also expanded the list of procedures that can be performed in the non-acute setting, while commercial insurers have begun to deny coverage for certain services, for example, imaging, unless handled outside the hospital.[4]

The first edition of this book had been based on research conducted from 2001 to 2004 by its authors, Eugene Schneller and Larry Smeltzer.[5] At that time, there was relatively little written about supply chain management in the health sector from a strategic perspective. Gene and Larry each brought a unique perspective to the evolving field — one through a lens grounded in health management, policy research, and education, and the other substantiated by a practitioner's knowledge of the fundamentals of supply chain management and how the field had developed in other industries. Gene's teaching had been principally to students, including physicians, in health management programs, where supply chain was infrequently mentioned. Larry, on the other hand, spent his career teaching supply chain management students and consulting with multinational companies, such as Motorola and John Deere. Thus, he brought to the project an in-depth understanding of how the non-health sector had utilized the supply chain for competitive advantage. Larry, who passed away in 2004, was also a pioneer in the area of supply chain management research and education at Arizona State University and served as a chair of the Department of Supply Chain Management. From his perspective from multiple roles in supply chain, Larry observed that hospitals and healthcare systems failed to recognize both supplies and the supply chain itself as strategic assets. In the first edition, the authors challenged supply chain researchers and practitioners to foster a vision for the field that would drive benefits similar to what other industries had achieved, noting at the time that a few progressive organizations had begun to do so.

For the second edition, Gene is joined by three new authors to support this broader and more impactful role for supply chain. Yousef Abdulsalam brings an additional academic perspective steeped in healthcare supply chain research, while both Karen Conway and Jim Eckler offer decades of practical experience in the practice of healthcare delivery, technology, and supply chain. All four authors also have substantial knowledge of healthcare supply chain operations and performance across global markets.

This breadth of experience and perspectives also supports the revised volume's approach to the supply chain as a system of systems, operating in the larger context of the overarching healthcare ecosystem. A systems-based approach takes into consideration how overall performance of the supply chain is closely linked to the interdependencies among myriad stakeholders, including manufacturers, distributors, healthcare delivery organizations, clinicians, group purchasing organizations, technology partners, and regulators, among others. Together with a foundational understanding of the shifts in both the market and regulatory environment, applying systems thinking uniquely positions the revised edition to support the needs of a broad array of learners.

2 A New Framework: The Fully Integrated Supply Chain Organization (FISCO)

This volume incorporates a new framework, elaborated upon within the text and Appendix 1, for a Fully Integrated Supply Chain Organization (FISCO) as the desired destination for those seeking to develop a mature supply chain. The FISCO concept, developed at Arizona State University, takes emphasis off any one supply chain function, allowing for a more holistic assessment of current status and realization of a vision that supports improved clinical, financial, and operational performance.

3 The Audience: Who Will Benefit from the Revised Edition

While supply chain management has occupied a pivotal position for change in other industry sectors, leading to a proliferation of interest in this topic in both undergraduate and graduate-level business management education in the United States, supply chain management strategy remains almost non-existent in comparable graduate-level programs in healthcare. For this reason, a primary audience for the revised edition are graduate students in health sector and/or supply chain management programs. Those exploring and advancing their careers as practitioners in the healthcare field will benefit from a better understanding of supply chain's potential to not only manage the spiraling increases in the costs of the supply chain and healthcare delivery, but also to improve the ability to meet the evolving demands of value-based healthcare. Those in supply chain programs, in turn, will appreciate the unique and broad-reaching opportunities in healthcare that can have significant implications for individuals, organizations and society as a whole. Identifying progressive practices will assist managers to meet the challenges posed in designing, managing, and monitoring an effective supply strategy, understanding the roles and inter-relationships between multiple business, clinical and technical partners, hiring competent supply managers, and assuring accountability, all which are critical competencies for the modern healthcare supply chain professional.

Similarly, the book will serve programs in executive education for clinicians, with much of the research and framing "tested" across cohorts of students at Arizona State University and the University of

Colorado's executive program in health sector management, as well as in physician-specific MBA and business in medicine programs. Both clinicians and practicing supply chain leaders will learn the importance of collaborating in the redesign of care for specific patient cohorts based on evidence as to the impact of products and services on the quality and cost of care. In this regard, supply chain leaders can support the clinician's need for evidence on product performance, while clinicians can gain a new understanding of the factors that drive costs, affordability and value for health systems and most importantly patients.

The book can also assist senior hospital and health system executives, given heightened recognition of the critical importance of supply chain made evident during the global pandemic and their need to adapt systems and processes in the move to value-based healthcare. It supports the transition of managerial understanding of the supply function beyond what many have seen as an organizationally bound and narrow "purchasing" or "procurement" function to what is quickly evolving into a mission-critical, multi-enterprise business network operation.

Chief supply chain officers, along with their vice presidents, directors, and managers, will value the lessons to be learned from progressive supply chain organizations both in healthcare and other industries. By focusing on the fundamentals, but with thoughtful consideration of critical issues in healthcare, the revised edition provides guidance to those seeking to transform the supply chain function to support both a wider and higher-level range of strategic organizational goals. The aforementioned FISCO model has been utilized to assess and improve supply chain performance for organizations in the process of undergoing change. It has also been applied to the evolution of the Defense Health Agency, which brought together the healthcare systems operated independently by the U.S. Army, Navy and Air Force, and represented a merger of entities with very different needs, cultures, and mission.

This book will also benefit those organizations that serve healthcare delivery organizations. The move to value is creating fundamental disruption in the marketplace, and companies seeking to survive, if not thrive, during this transition will require a deep understanding of their customers' journeys, including those of the myriad new players entering the market, and what they need from their business, clinical and technology partners. Those who fully understand the business, clinical, market and regulatory needs of the healthcare client will be best positioned to bring value to their respective organizations and customers.

Finally, the revised edition provides critical insights for public policy makers as they seek to create a more resilient healthcare supply chain that can support the health and well-being of the population, as well as both national security and global competitiveness. By understanding how the system operates and its critical interdependencies, legislators and regulators can target their actions to achieve the intended results while avoiding taking well-intentioned steps that too often result in unintended consequences and system suboptimization.

4 Persisting Questions

The first edition of this book was supported by the National Science Foundation (NSF) and the Center for Health Management Research (CHMR), an industry-university cooperative research center supported and governed by health systems from across the United States. Focus group sessions and interviews with provider organizations revealed an overwhelming consensus that, at the time, (a) the supply chain was one of the more ignored aspects of management, (b) clinician preference was a major barrier to supply chain progress, (c) supplier "power" was an overwhelming obstacle and (d) the costs of operating the supply chain were expected to continue to increase. When the authors for this volume revisited the original research, it became obvious that although there has been great progress, the principal questions for concern, derived from focus groups with leading U.S. hospitals during the earlier study, remain relevant for driving an analysis of the strategies being employed (Sidebar P1). See these persistent questions in the sidebar.

This volume addresses these key issues by a team with extensive experience in research, education, consulting, strategy, and design for supply chains in the health sector. It is also a team that has experience in assessing supply chains from other industries — and thus able to assess health sector supply chain strategies and processes within the context of supply chain practices that have progressed, for all sectors, over the last decade and a half.

5 Organization of the Book

The book is organized to reflect the three hospital and health system supply chain macro processes that Chopra and Meindl, authors of one of the most influential texts in the area of supply chain management, identified as (a) customer relationship management (CRM), (b) internal supply management (ISM), and (c) supplier relationship management (SRM),[6] as well as a key issue that we believe is critical to understanding and managing the health sector supply chain—purchasing partner management (PPM). Finally, the book is systematically attentive to the principal aspects of the FISCO functions—supply chain management

Sidebar P1

Persistent Healthcare Supply Chain Management Questions for Concern Across 2+ Decades

1. What are the characteristics of the more progressive hospital and hospital systems in managing supply chain?

2. How do the business strategy, organizational structure, personnel capabilities, and environmental/competitive forces of the organizations with more progressive supply chain practices differ from the organizations with less progressive supply chain practices?

3. What is the role of leadership by clinicians and non-clinicians in organizations characterized by progressive supply chains?

4. What conditions predisposed these organizations to have leading-edge supply chain structures and practices?

5. What are the enablers and barriers to progressive supply chain management practices in hospitals and hospital systems?

6. What guidelines will lead to progressive supply chain practices?

7. What progressive supply chain practices can hospital and system managers best adopt from leading practices in manufacturing and retail supply chains?

processes, technology tools, and organization support. This disciplined approach is packaged into each of the following chapters.

- *Chapter 1 Healthcare's Supply Chain Environment—Here's the Big Picture.*
- *Chapter 2 Building a Strategy for Healthcare Supply Chain Management—Creating the Vision*
- *Chapter 3 Risk Management Strategies—Healthcare Is Risky, So Is Supply Chain Management*
- *Chapter 4 Product Preference, Standardization, Value, and Clinical Integration—You Can't Just Buy Anything*
- *Chapter 5 Purchasing Strategies and Alliances—Success Requires Good Partnerships*

- *Chapter 6 Logistics Strategies and Alliances—The Devil Is in the Details*
- *Chapter 7 Performance and Maturity—You Only Get What You Measure.*
- *Chapter 8 Organization Design for Managing the Supply Chain—A Well-designed Organization Makes It Easier to Succeed*
- *Chapter 9 Information Technology (IT) Strategies—Information is the Glue that Binds*
- *Chapter 10 The Fully Integrated Supply Chain Organization (FISCO)—Tying It Together and Looking Forward*

Notes

1. Healthy People 2030. U.S. Department of Health and Human Services, Office of Disease Prevention and Health Promotion. Retrieved [date graphic was accessed] from https://health.gov/healthypeople/objectives-and-data/social-determinants-health
2. Hospital for Special Surgery. (2019, March 14). No increased risk of complications for joint replacement in ambulatory surgery setting. Hospital for Special Surgery, News Release. https://www.eurekalert.org/news-releases/517261
3. Levine, D. M., Ouchi, K., Blanchfield, B., Diamond, K., Licurse, A., Pu, C. T., & Schnipper, J. L. (2018). Hospital-level care at home for acutely ill adults: a pilot randomized controlled trial. *Journal of General Internal Medicine*, *33*(5), 729-736. https://www.acpjournals.org/doi/10.7326/M19-0600
4. Butcher, L. (2018). (2018, Jan. 31). What anthem's imaging policy means for hospitals. Healthcare Financial Management Association. https://www.hfma.org/topics/article/59296.html
5. Schneller, E. S., & Smeltzer, L. R. (2006). Strategic management of the health care supply chain. Jossey-Bass.
6. Chopra, S., & Meindl, P. (2021). *Supply chain management strategy, planning, & operations*, 7. Pearson.

1 The Healthcare Supply Chain Environment— *Here's the Big Picture*

1.1 The Healthcare Supply Chain: Evolving Recognition and Importance

After years of being ignored by the general public and even by many in the healthcare sector, the supply chain became a regular news item during the early days of the COVID-19 pandemic as hospitals in the United States and around the world faced critical shortages of personal protective equipment (PPE) and ventilators. This marked a pivotal moment for supply chain practitioners, who had heretofore been recognized as performing a core supporting function, but not one generally considered to have strategic influence beyond the ability to support expense reduction. As the pandemic exposed the frailties and fragmentation of a highly resource-dependent system that had been designed for efficiency over resilience, many began to question longstanding cost containment initiatives such as just-in-time (JIT) inventory management and reliance on offshore production to secure the lowest possible per unit price. The experience of the pandemic demands a broader set of competencies among supply chain professionals who must simultaneously be able to achieve daily performance metrics while preparing for future disruptions and creating the capacity to quickly recover from such circumstances. Despite this, as healthcare spending and the costs to deliver care continue to escalate without commensurate increases in revenue, financial executives will likely persist with their view of supply chain as a source of expense reduction.

A more fundamental shift impacting healthcare, and in turn the strategic role of the supply chain, is the overarching march to create a value-based healthcare system (Exhibit 1.1).[1]

The move to value is in response to the fundamental deficiencies in a fee-for-service (FFS) reimbursement environment, in which hospitals and physicians are paid based on the volume of services provided, as opposed to the value of their services. When multiple providers caring for the same patients are paid under a FFS arrangement, as has been the case in the United States for more than 50 years, care is often not well coordinated, resulting in overutilization and duplication of services, less than satisfactory patient outcomes, and higher overall expenditures, which in turn, leave less money available to reimburse providers.[2] The move to a value-based healthcare system requires excellence in management and innovation to achieve an accountable care healthcare system.[3]

In the healthcare context, *value* is defined as the "health outcomes achieved that matter to patients relative to the cost of achieving those outcomes."[4] In the broadest sense, the value equation (Exhibit 1.2) itself

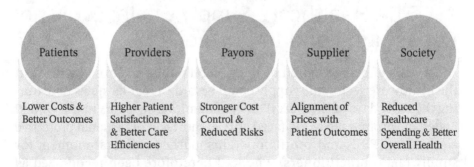

Patients	Providers	Payors	Supplier	Society
Lower Costs & Better Outcomes	Higher Patient Satisfaction Rates & Better Care Efficiencies	Stronger Cost Control & Reduced Risks	Alignment of Prices with Patient Outcomes	Reduced Healthcare Spending & Better Overall Health

Exhibit 1.1: Value-based healthcare benefits.
Adopted from NEJM Catalyst.

$$Value = \frac{Quality + Outcomes + Patient\ Experience}{All\ Resources\ Consumed\ in\ Care\ Delivery}$$

Exhibit 1.2: The formula for value in healthcare.

takes into account multiple factors: the quality of care delivered, the outcomes achieved, and the patient experience of care, divided by all of the resources (fixed and variable) used in the delivery of care, including the physical and technological infrastructure as well as all personnel, products, and services involved in support of care delivery.[5,6]

A variety of terms have been used to describe the move to value as well as the mechanisms (mostly financial) being developed to drive the transition. See Sidebar 1.1 for clarification of how those terms are used throughout this book.

In the United States, the cornerstone of the value-based healthcare movement is the Affordable Care Act (ACA), which included numerous mechanisms to tie reimbursement to the value delivered as opposed to the volume of services performed. Increasing patient value requires greater coordination among members of care teams, and ultimately, between supply chain and clinicians. To support many of these new payment models, along with the fundamental need to deliver quality care at an optimum price, supply chain has become a more strategic partner to clinicians as they seek to acquire the products and services that will deliver the most value to patients, a topic discussed further in Chapter 5.

Shortly after the passage of the ACA in 2010, the Association for Health Care Resource & Materials Management (AHRMM), the professional supply chain association for the American Hospital Association (AHA), launched the Cost, Quality, Outcomes Movement (CQO) to increase awareness of the "critical role supply chain professionals play in driving high-quality care, at a more affordable cost, to deliver greater value to patients."[7] At its foundation, the CQO Movement taught that any consequential exploration of healthcare supply chain management from a strategic perspective must begin with an understanding of its role in supporting the evolving objectives of the healthcare ecosystem as a whole.[8] Chapter 4 provides a further discussion of CQO and its larger implications on value and what is referred to as the clinically integrated supply chain.

Clearly, through the efforts of the CQO Movement, the ACA, and experiences drawn from the COVID-19 pandemic, the management of the supply chain has become much more critical and more substantial within healthcare organizations. The driver of this growth is the fundamental value proposition brought by the practices of professional supply chain management, which encompasses both the parties and processes needed to fulfill a customer request, and when performed successfully, enhances customer satisfaction.[9]

Side Bar 1.1

Making Valuable Sense

A concept related to utility, productivity, effectiveness, efficiency, and many others, *value* is often used in terms that describe business paradigms and operating models focusing on value. Sidebar 1.1 provides some clarification and distinctions around common and inter-related concepts associated with value, some used exclusively in the healthcare context, while others recognized more generally in supply chain management.

More Healthcare Specific

- *Value-based healthcare*—"a healthcare delivery model in which providers, including hospitals and physicians, are paid based on patient health outcomes" (https://catalyst.nejm.org/doi/full/10.1056/CAT.17.0558).
- *Value-based purchasing*—"linking provider payments to improved performance by health care providers. This form of payment holds health care providers accountable for both the cost and quality of care they provide. It attempts to reduce inappropriate care and to identify and reward the best-performing providers." (https://www.healthcare.gov/glossary/value-based-purchasing-vbp).
- *Healthcare value analysis*—"contributes to optimal patient outcomes through an evidenced-based systematic approach to review healthcare products, equipment, technology, and services. Using recognized practices, organizational resources collaborate to evaluate clinical efficacy, appropriate use and safety for the greatest financial value" (https://www.ahvap.org/overview).

More Generic

- *The value chain*—"the process in which businesses receive raw materials, add value to them through production, manufacturing, and other processes to create a finished product, and then sell the finished product. . .and to create a competitive advantage" (What's the Difference Between Value Chain vs. Supply Chain? [http://investopedia.com]).
- *Value engineering*—"a systematic, organized approach to providing necessary functions in a project at the lowest cost [that]. . .promotes the substitution of materials and methods with less expensive alternatives, without sacrificing functionality. . .also called value analysis" (What's the Difference Between Value Chain vs. Supply Chain? [http://investopedia.com])

1.2 Healthcare System Challenges and Strategies

The healthcare system faces a multitude of challenges, including the increasing needs of an aging population, the expectations of more discerning healthcare consumers, and disparities in health status and outcomes among poor and marginalized populations due to lack of access to both health and social services, all of which put pressure on the system.

The fundamental challenge for supply chain managers is to assure that on a day-to-day basis their organizations are prepared to provide patients and customers with the most appropriate products, at the best price, in the right location, at the right time, and in the right condition in order to achieve the best outcomes. Given the critical role physicians play in the delivery of healthcare services, this requires supply chain professionals to collaborate with clinicians in the redesign of care (including what kind of care is delivered, with which resources, where, at what cost, and for which kinds of patients). Supply chain plays an important role in meeting clinicians' needs for evidence on product performance, as well as their growing interest in the costs of the care they prescribe for their patients.[10,11]

In an attempt to lower the total cost of healthcare and to meet consumer demands for greater convenience, many hospitals and healthcare systems are moving healthcare delivery to less expensive locations than the acute care hospital, including ambulatory surgery centers (ASCs) and patients' homes. Studies have found that procedures performed in ASCs are more than 40% less expensive than the acute care hospital,[12] while treating acute level patients in their own homes can save nearly as much,[13] without reducing quality in either scenario. Insurers, too, are driving the move to non-acute locations as a result of their coverage decisions.[14] As the geographic footprint and locations of care broaden, so, too, does the complexity of the supply chain.

Technology advancements are supporting both the move to non-acute settings as well as the overall performance and maturation of the supply chain. For example, the ability to deliver hospital-level care in the home is significantly improved through use of remote patient monitoring technology that enables clinicians to observe and direct patient care virtually. Healthcare supply chain professionals are also investing in technologies that have been proven to be transformational in other industry sectors. The Center to Stream Healthcare In Place (C2SHIP), a National Science Foundation (NSF) Industry/University Cooperative Research Center, is an example of the robust investment and commitment to this transformation.[15] Success of this effort, engaging academic and industrial partners in joint efforts that develop healthcare technologies for in-place care and accelerate innovation through multi-specialty collaborations, will ultimately rest on the ability to provide the supplies needed for newly crafted settings of care.

The move to more cloud-based systems has advanced the ability to manage data about the multitude of products used by healthcare delivery organizations in multiple settings, for both clinical care and to keep their operations going. These technologies also support the ability to share data across disparate systems, most notably between enterprise resource planning (ERP) systems, which support key supply chain functions, and electronic health records (EHRs) in which products used in patient care are documented. Clinical supply documentation in EHRs also supports the analysis of data to understand what contributes to better patient outcomes. The application of artificial intelligence and machine learning offers a range of opportunities for supply chain, from automating repetitive tasks through robotic process automation (RPA) to the application of predictive and prescriptive analytics to guide clinical and supply chain purchasing decisions. The use and associated value of supply chain technologies will be discussed in greater detail in Chapter 9.

Healthcare systems have sought growth in order to have more negotiating power with payors, to achieve market penetration, and to improve performance. An uptick in merger and acquisition activity has led to more hospitals within single healthcare systems. It has also created systems with a breadth of healthcare delivery options and settings beyond the hospital, from telemedicine and hospital-level care in the home to the use of micro-hospitals and Ambulatory Surgical Centers (ASCs). As these organization have changed in both size and structure through both horizontal and vertical acquisitions and as they incorporate both clinicians and operating units, they are frequently described as integrated delivery networks (IDNs).[16,17]

Meanwhile, as healthcare systems have grown, so too has the operating focus of the supply chain management function, from serving individual hospitals to meeting the varied resource needs of the entire enterprise for integration.[18] And while one of the goals for consolidation has been to support more standardization in products and processes to advance both cost and quality initiatives, research has found mixed results from such efforts.[19] Levels of true integration within and across systems are variable. Thus, throughout the book, we generally refer specifically to hospitals and systems—unless the idea of their adherence to the broader meaning of an IDN is relevant. And, of note, our focus is on supply chain integration, which while influenced by integration with clinicians and other aspects of the organization, is an area for distinction.

1.3 Supply Chain as a System of Systems within Healthcare as a System

From a societal and public policy perspective, healthcare as a "system" is intended to advance the health of individuals and populations in an equitable, accessible and affordable manner.[20] Despite this relatively straightforward objective, healthcare is a highly complex socioeconomic system,[21] as reflected by "the number, variety, and fragmentation of producers involved in the delivery of healthcare: patients, professionals, provider organizations, buyer organizations. . .insurers or payors, and suppliers"[22] as well as supporting actors that include group purchasing organizations (GPOs), third-party logistics companies (3PLs), technology vendors, and consultancies. Regulatory agencies are also impactful participants given the extent to which healthcare, including the supply chain, must comply with numerous policies and regulations that shape priorities, drive funding decisions and can both hinder and foster innovation. These many agents each operate within a variety of subsystems, with different and at times competing objectives and incentives.

In his book *The U.S. Healthcare Ecosystem: Payers, Providers, Producers*, Lawton Burns expands on a previously developed healthcare model that highlights the major players[23] (see Exhibit 1.3), many of which are influential in the performance of the supply chain and described in greater detail later in this chapter. While this book does not detail the role of every item in Exhibit 1.3 (such as the payors and insurers), the model is

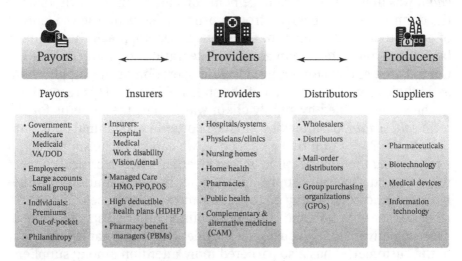

Exhibit 1.3: The healthcare ecosystem.
Adopted from Burns.[17]

presented in recognition that supply chain management and its stake-holders are embedded in an even larger ecosystem.

The supply chain itself is also a system comprised of multiple subsystems, each with specific purposes (e.g., sourcing, purchasing, production, logistics, etc.) and dependent on numerous stakeholders. Beyond providing an overview of the primary players and processes that make up the healthcare supply chain, the content and structure of this book relies heavily on an understanding of the characteristics of highly mature supply chain organizations, which we depict as "Fully Integrated Supply Chain Organizations" or FISCOs. Developed at Arizona State University, the FISCO framework, discussed in the following text and throughout the book, builds upon the concept of the supply chain as a complex system, delineating how some organizations have been able to optimize the totality of their supply chain performance, as opposed to simply focusing on the performance of individual parts. Further exploration of the FISCO framework (fully detailed in Appendix 1) first requires a foundational understanding of healthcare supply chain management, the various processes, and the primary actors.

1.4 What Is (Healthcare) Supply Chain Management?

There is significant variation in the literature as to the definition of *supply chain management*, with the differences often reflecting the approaches and priorities of different industries.[24] In the years since the term *supply chain* was first coined by management consultants in the early 1980s,[25] the definitions have evolved from a primary focus on the movement of goods to market to more of a systems-based approach that requires both intra- and inter-organizational integration to produce value for not only the end customer, but also the operation of the supply chain as a whole as well as for each of the stakeholders.[26,27] This recognition of the value enabled by supply chain was in part the impetus for the term *value chain*, promoted by Michael Porter in his seminal book published in 1985.[28] From this perspective, we can view the supply chain as managing the flow of value within an enterprise—a critical concept when considering the supply chain's potential contribution to value-based healthcare. Building on this, Ford and Scanlon[29] speak to the criticality of coordination and cooperation among myriad stakeholders in order to deliver value to customers. Understanding what is important to the customer(s) has also garnered more attention among suppliers, particularly in relation to the total cost to serve.[30] This topic is further discussed in the Chapter 4 discourse around the clinically integrated supply chain and the degree to which an organization strategically brings together internal functions and external supply chain members to manage the intra- and inter-organizational processes. Integration between supply chain practice and clinical practice is the hallmark of a high-performing healthcare supply chain organization.

Beyond the physical supply chain, research has underscored the importance of coordinating the flow of corresponding funds and information (the financial and digital supply chains) along with the movement of goods.[31,32] Supply chain financial data supports the flow of payments, but it can also be used as an important input in an effort to calculate the actual costs to deliver care. Calculating the cost of care has been a challenge in healthcare given traditional reimbursement methodologies that historically are set by external parties (both government and commercial payors) and are tied to the average price of a procedure versus actual costs. With the move to a value-based payment methodology and the introduction of price transparency regulations, designed to help patients shop for services,[33] healthcare delivery organizations need to better understand their actual costs, both fixed and variable. From a supply chain lens, this is particularly important for common healthcare procedures, such as hip, and knee replacements, in which the price paid for the implants can make up a significant percentage of the total costs.[34,35]

More recent definitions of supply chain management specific to healthcare have also incorporated expanding viewpoints on the importance of integration across inter- and intra-organization processes and systems, which is foundational to measuring value defined in terms of both cost and quality.[36] Some definitions focus on the coordination of both the physical and digital (data) aspects of the supply chain, while others consider the investments needed to deliver greater customer value, for example, through both better clinical outcomes and cost control.

Finally, the appropriateness of the term *supply chain* has come into question in that it suggests a linear process focused on physical "supplies," when the healthcare supply chain, in reality, is more of a network supporting the provision of numerous products and services used in the delivery of healthcare services, the operation of the facilities in which care is delivered, and increasingly helping patients with access to nonclinical products and services. Examples of nonclinical product and services include nutritious food, transportation, and housing, all which are considered to be social determinants of health that have proven to have more of an impact on a person's health status than much of the clinical care received. Indeed, much academic research has pushed toward shifting the paradigm from "chains" to "networks" of products and services.[37,38]

1.5 Supply Chain Processes and Functions

From both an operational and strategic perspective, supply chain management includes a range of functions and activities to support "the acquisition and movement of goods and services from the supplier to the end user in order to enhance clinical outcomes while controlling costs."[39] Three process groups, involving stakeholders both internal and external to the buying organization, are identified in classic supply chain textbooks.[40]

- Internal supply management (ISM);
- Customer relationship management (CRM); and
- Supplier relationship management (SRM).

The FISCO framework (Appendix 1) purports that supply chain maturity (discussed below and in Chapter 10) results from the ability to integrate and optimize the performance and experience of these players and processes.

Given the complexity of the healthcare supply chain, a fourth process group—for managing intermediary players involved in purchasing—is included in the mix. Intermediaries include GPOs, information management firms, technology companies and other players that support sourcing and procurement. We identify this additional process group (detailed later in this book) as *Purchasing partner management (PPM)*.

The supply chain begins with the identification of a need (for a product or service) and the evaluation and selection of the resources that best meet those requirements, continuing through to the timely delivery and use of those products and/or services. Following are high-level descriptions of key supply chain functions, viewed primarily from the perspective of the buying organization, that is, the hospital or other healthcare delivery organization. Each of these will be discussed in more detail and in the context of the FISCO framework in subsequent chapters.

Value analysis. Value analysis is an evidence-based and systematic approach to evaluating alternative products and services to identify which best meet clinical or other performance needs and provide the most value in terms of cost and quality. Value analysis teams often focus on new product introductions to the system at the request of a physician or other clinician. The output of these teams can provide important guidance for the FISCO function strategic sourcing.

Strategic sourcing. Strategic sourcing is a multi-step process designed to reduce both costs and risks in the acquisition of products and services, often conducted within categories of similar products. In healthcare, these categories are numerous and varied, given advances in medical science and continued innovation in the resources used to promote health and prevent and treat illness, as well as the myriad of products and services used to support the operation of the healthcare delivery organization itself. While the steps are similar, the strategic sourcing process (as described in Chapter 5) varies based on the cost and risk of each category of product. The process includes identification of the resources that can meet a specified need and an analysis of the performance of those organizations that can supply the needed product or service. The latter lays the groundwork for contract negotiations and agreement to purchase.

Contract management. Following the sourcing and selection process, contract management constructs and executes contractual relationships with suppliers, often with price tied to the volume of business. More recently, hospitals and suppliers have explored more risk-sharing through outcomes-based contracts in which the price of the product is dependent on its ability to achieve marketed results. Following the COVID-19 pandemic, contract language increasingly includes terms and conditions related to supply continuity.

Purchasing. Purchasing involves the transactional steps related to the execution of a purchase order pursuant to the terms of the agreed-on contract terms, specifying the product, manufacturer, vendor, quantity, and contract price. Purchase orders may be preceded by a requisition from an internal customer. Upon receipt of a purchase order, a supplier typically confirms the order, including the product, the quantity, and the unit price.

Sourcing, value analysis, contract management, and purchasing are described in further detail in Chapter 5.

Distribution. Distribution, at its core, is the logistics process by which a manufacturer gets its product to a customer. Manufacturers and third-party distributors play a large role here. A typical hospital purchases around 35,000 SKUs (stock-keeping units) with only 6,000–8,000 of these physically stored on the hospital's premises at any given time.[41] For relatively expensive and sophisticated products, distribution is often handled by the product's manufacturer or through designated specialty distributors. High-volume, low-cost supplies (and pharmaceuticals) are typically handled by third-party distributors, as well as manufacturers themselves, which often offer additional inventory management services. Within a healthcare system, products are also distributed among central warehouses, storerooms, and patient care delivery locations, such as the operating room, nursing ward, or patient bedside.

Shipping/receiving. Upon receipt of a purchase order, a vendor may provide detailed information about shipping status/timing, along with notification of any backorders. Upon arrival of the products, the receiving organization (e.g., a hospital) documents receipt of the items purchased, which supports downstream payment and inventory processes.

Inventory management. Within a healthcare delivery environment, inventory management involves both the physical management of products as well as the data associated with the products on hand, their location, expiration dates, and use or consumption. The documented use of a product supports replenishment and billing processes. Effective management helps ensure adequate supplies are on hand, while avoiding waste, such as when products expire before use, and the ability to effectively respond to product recalls.

Demand planning. Data sharing between buying and selling organizations supports demand planning—the ability of buyers to purchase the right quantity of product and for suppliers to be prepared to meet those needs. Using data from hospitals and health systems on anticipated demand, inventory levels, and consumption rates, manufacturers can better plan production output. Hospitals, in turn, can reduce risks of stockouts and/or not having necessary supplies to deliver care. Demand planning, distribution, shipping, and inventory management are described in further detail in Chapter 6.

Accounts Payable. While not always included in the scope of some hospital or healthcare system's supply chain, accounts payable is highly dependent on effective upstream supply chain data and operational management. Proper documentation and matching among purchase orders, product receipts, and invoices is often a prerequisite for payment for products received.

While many of these functions involve multiple internal and external stakeholders, there is generally one leader at the hospital or health system charged with optimizing the processes "from a total system viewpoint rather than the viewpoint of the individual functions or activities."[42] Having this systems-level leadership perspective is core to becoming a FISCO, given that a more holistic view of the supply chain enables the leader to balance numerous objectives across the system and make the inevitable trade-offs.[43]

Historically, there has been limited executive appreciation for not only the complexity of the supply chain itself, but also the breadth and variety of competencies required by the supply chain leader. In addition to strong operational skills, the leader must also be able to shift to the more strategic aspects of supply chain management rapidly and easily, while being adept in interpersonal relations, informatics, and finance.[44] Growing recognition of the criticality and degree of difficulty in strategic supply chain management in healthcare is demonstrated by the growing number of leaders holding the title "chief supply chain officer" or "vice president for supply chain management." Supply chain leadership roles are detailed further in Chapters 8 and 10.

1.6 The Supply Chain Stakeholders

The stakeholders in the healthcare supply chain are wide-ranging, each associated with the various functions that support, finance, and regulate the acquisition and movement of goods, funds, and data from supplier to the end user. The following is a representative (although not exhaustive) list of those actors and the roles they play.

1.6.1 Primary Actors: Buying and Selling Organizations

Manufacturers and other suppliers of products and services used in the delivery and administration of healthcare are the primary players on the sell side of the supply chain. This includes upstream suppliers of raw materials and components, and contract manufacturers to which a supplier may outsource production. It is upon these organizations that the healthcare delivery system is dependent for carrying out its everyday mission.

Healthcare delivery organizations, both public and private, purchase and consume supplies and services in the delivery of care to support the health of the patient as the end consumer. The majority of healthcare supply chain research and practice has focused on the hospital as buyer, although that is broadening as care is increasingly being delivered outside the acute care hospital. These locations include ASCs; urgent care and retail clinics; work, school and even the home; along with pharmacies, labs, and those used by other allied service providers, such as physical therapy offices and imaging centers.

Distributors play both roles, often buying products from manufacturers and reselling them to healthcare delivery organizations. Distributors also provide critical logistical functions, delivering products and managing inventory levels, especially for lower-cost, high-volume commodity products. Some distributors specialize in the delivery of products (i.e., consignment products) that are not purchased until after their use in a particular procedure.

1.6.2 Supporting Actors

Group purchasing organizations (GPOs). GPOs were originally created to aggregate purchasing across a multitude of healthcare delivery organizations in order to secure better volume pricing from suppliers. As healthcare systems have grown larger through mergers and acquisitions, some have created their own GPOs and/or partnered with their peers to create regional purchasing collaboratives. GPOs, meanwhile, have expanded their business and revenue models beyond sourcing and contracting to provide more services to support both clinical and operational performance.[45]

Technology partners. Technology has advanced, both in terms of the number and types of vendors. Such firms now offer a wide variety of resources, from more traditional materials management information or ERP systems and inventory and warehouse management software to business-to-business (B2B) exchanges that automate and standardize the procure-to-pay process between a multitude of buying and selling organizations across a single platform. With greater appreciation for the value of the data associated with the supply chain, there has been a marked increase in the type and number of companies that help buyers and sellers cleanse, normalize, and manage their own supply chain data, while others specialize in clinical supply documentation and analytics, from descriptive to predictive, if not prescriptive, to support clinical, operational, and/or financial decision-making.

1.6.3 Influencers

Patients and the surrogates historically have been more passive participants in healthcare delivery, generally following the lead of trained clinicians. As those accessing healthcare services become more informed as active consumers and are responsible for an increasingly large share of their healthcare expenditures, patients are having more of a say as to where they receive care and by whom, although much of healthcare spending is still largely driven by what payors will reimburse. Patient preferences (e.g., level of risk) and feedback on their experience of care are increasingly being used to inform sourcing decisions.

Clinicians, and in particular physicians, have historically had the most influence on the selection of products, based on their medical knowledge, understanding of patient needs, and professional training around the use of specific products. As clinicians have more access to data on the efficacy and costs of products, personal preference is playing less of a role in product selection in favor of evidence as to which products work best for specific patient populations.

Regulatory agencies impact supply chain in a number of ways. It begins with manufacturers gaining approval by organizations such as the U.S. Food and Drug Administration (FDA) or comparable agencies in other countries for manufacturers to market their products for specific uses. Regulators are also involved in ongoing post-market surveillance to address adverse events, improve recall management, prevent the introduction of counterfeit devices, and gather data on how products perform in routine clinical practice. Other federal agencies, such as the Office of the National Coordinator for Health IT (ONC) and the U.S. Centers for Medicare & Medicaid Services (CMS), dictate the kind of data that must be collected and shared by parties across the supply chain, often as a requirement for reimbursement. The Federal Trade Commission (FTC) works to assure that healthcare markets are competitive—for providers, suppliers, and intermediaries. These are only a few examples of the regulatory environment in which the supply chain resides.

Payors/purchasers include those organizations and individuals responsible for the purchase and payment of healthcare services. These have typically included commercial insurers, self-insured employers, and government agencies, such as the CMS in the United States or the National Health Service (NHS) in the United Kingdom. Payors can influence the types of services, and in turn, products used in the delivery of care as the result of decisions as to what they will cover or reimburse.

1.6.4 Fusion Organizations

As the healthcare system continues to evolve, so, too, have the players, with the emergence of hybrid organizations that are either part of or have influence on the supply chain. With hospitals and healthcare systems seeking the most efficient and effective operational structures for supply chain, it is not uncommon for them to experiment with different approaches. Some have insourced functions typically handled by external players, such as contracting and distribution, while others are outsourcing more of their supply chain activities to third parties.

Examples of more disruptive trends include a hospital becoming a manufacturer by utilizing 3D printing to manufacture custom implants for patients[46] or a manufacturer taking responsibility for various aspects of care delivery.[47] Given the considerable impact of payor-provider contract negotiations on financial performance, a new entity referred to as *payviders* is emerging, either as health systems owning their own health plan or when insurers get more involved in directing if not delivering care.[48] Major retailers and technology companies have also tried their hand (but not all successfully) in providing patient care. With each of these innovations, there will be corresponding impacts on the operation and design of the supply chain, which is discussed further in Chapter 10.

1.7 FISCO Functions and Supply Chain Maturity

The preceding listed issues and actors are common to many healthcare supply chains. What distinguishes highly mature organizations is their ability to integrate the various activities and players, both internally and externally, in a manner that provides maximum value to customers. As mentioned previously, these organizations are FISCOs. The FISCO framework focuses on a set of supply chain management processes, technologies, tools and support functions that together (as discussed throughout the book and elaborated upon in Appendix 1) optimize an organization's supply chain capabilities as a system (Exhibit 1.4).

As such, the framework can help organizations assess and advance the degree to which they are able to optimize intra- and inter-organizational

Exhibit 1.4: Key FISCO functions

SCM processes	Technology	Organizational support
Product sourcing	System integration and architecture	Organization structure
Product selection and standardization		System training
	Key performance indicators and metrics	Governance of the supply chain
Contracting		
Supplier relationship management	Item master management	
Order processing	Electronic health record	
Inventory management	Integration	
Receiving	Emergency preparedness	
Accounts payable (AP)		
Asset management		
Supply chain risk management		

processes. Advanced FISCO organizations are able to reduce complexity, leverage respective competencies and capabilities, standardize approaches to improve patient outcomes, and innovate at the enterprise if not the system level. The benefits include reduced risk, improved predictability, increased capacity, reduced cost, and the ability to better identify and act on opportunities for systemic improvement. The dimensions and journey to a FISCO are described in more detail in Appendix 1. Performance measurement systems that define and assess supply chain maturity models, such as the FISCO framework, are discussed in Chapter 7.

1.8 From Cost Center to Strategic Asset

Both the pandemic and the move to value have elevated the role of the supply chain in numerous organizations, but there remains considerable variation in the cost of the supply chain and its ability to support overall hospital performance, even when controlled for geographic region, case mix, and so on.[49] This is likely due, in part, to historic underinvestment in the management of the supply chain by hospitals given it has only recently started to gain strategic status. The performance of many purchasing agents, and even their managers, is still principally measured by their ability to lower acquisition costs.

Management of the healthcare supply chain first began to attract executive-level attention in the late 1990s and early 2000s following publication of research that identified the opportunity for billions of dollars in annual savings in the United States alone.[50] According to the research, the savings would result from the application of supply chain practices proven successful in other industries and for which large, well-known consumer brands have attributed their competitive advantage.[51] In other industries (including automotive, electronics, and consumer packaged goods), a scrutiny of a more strategic approach to supply chain management has been correlated not only with greater efficiencies, but also overall organizational performance made possible through improved supplier-customer relationships, the sharing of quality information, and lower costs to serve.[52,53] The research reveals considerable supply chain savings, leading to a significant uptick in adoption of both e-commerce and ERP systems in healthcare,[54] although decisions regarding the latter are still primarily driven by finance and human resources. Many hospitals have achieved more efficient and less costly operations as a result of the enhanced automation and the data management capabilities of these respective technologies. Still, the managerial mandate for supply chain executives largely remained the same: negotiate the lowest per unit pricing possible with suppliers.[55] The nearly singular focus on product acquisition price stems from a longstanding belief that the introduction of increasingly sophisticated, and in turn, more expensive medical devices is a primary driver behind rising healthcare expenditures.[56] Historically, these more sophisticated new technologies have been marketed directly to physicians as surrogate buyers. This unique aspect of the healthcare sector is discussed throughout the book.

1.8.1 Clinician Centrality and the Customer

Clinicians drive a great deal of what happens in the course of day-to-day hospital activities. Physicians, in particular, diagnose illness and decide, within the context of acceptable parameters, how to care for their patients. These decisions impact the length of stay and the resources consumed over the course of patient care. To the extent that clinicians are central decision-makers, their influence on the hospital supply chain is profound. With the dual imperative of addressing both quality and cost of care, any substantive effort to manage the rising cost and proliferation of new products requires close coordination and collaboration between physicians and the supply chain. The COVID-19 pandemic laid the groundwork for such collaboration, which was required to quickly identify clinically acceptable alternatives when the originally preferred product was no longer available.

As clinicians and the supply chain become more integrated and utilize data on both cost and quality, they can make decisions that deliver the best care for specific populations, often at a lower cost. As a result of the pandemic and critical supply shortages, data on product availability and a supplier's efforts to minimize disruptions is also being considered in sourcing decisions, including the proactive identification of clinically acceptable alternatives. When products are not available or not acceptable for the designated purpose, the organization and its patients can face risk; the procedure may not be able to be performed optimally, if at all. Both can lead to a loss of revenue, poor patient outcomes, and a negative clinician and patient experience.

Specific physicians often prefer one product over another. These items are often referred to as *physician preference items* (PPIs), reflecting the products on which physicians were initially trained or with which they have the most experience. Notably, preferences may also extend from physician relationships with suppliers that provide continuing education and technical support. Others have commercial relationships with suppliers, working as advisors on new product development and/or generation of real-world evidence on product performance. How evidence can be used to influence clinician decision-making and advance standardization is revealed in the case of the Plymouth Trust, "Clinician, Supplier, and Buyer Working as One to Improve Patient Outcomes" (Appendix 2). Notably this case of a system of hospitals in the United Kingdom, reveals that the challenges associated with achieving clinical collaboration are not unique to the United States.

From the perspective of supply chain maturity, more clinical-supply chain integration (discussed further in Chapter 4) has begun to erode some of the influence of suppliers over physicians in sourcing decisions, while increasing the use of evidence garnered from both clinical trials and post-market performance studies. As discussed in later chapters, clinical preference, in the absence of evidence, can hinder product standardization efforts designed to increase safety, reduce unnecessary variation in care, and support efforts to reduce acquisition price by aggregating spend with certain suppliers on specific product categories.

1.8.2 Who Is the Customer?

A leading supply chain management text proffers a straightforward and customer-focused definition of supply chain as the "parties involved, directly or indirectly, in fulfilling a customer request."[57] Applying this definition to healthcare has raised a number of critical questions, beginning with "Who is the customer?" Historically, the answer has been dependent on the perspective of the specific stakeholder and the corresponding position in the supply chain. For example, a manufacturer or distributor might consider the customer to be the hospital or healthcare delivery organization that purchases its products or services, while a hospital supply chain executive might consider the customer to be the internal clinician or other professional buyer for whom a product or service is procured. Both of these answers are correct, but only at the subsystem level, and as a result, can lead to sub-optimization that can negatively impact another part of the system, and in turn, the output of the system as a whole and its ability to deliver value to the end customer, the patient. For example, if a hospital supply chain overprioritizes the product preferences of a specific physician, the result could be a lack of overall compliance with purchasing contracts and higher supply expenses for the hospital. The physician as a customer might be satisfied but not necessarily the hospital or the purchaser of healthcare services, be that an insurance company, an employer, and/or the patient. On the other hand, if the supply chain is viewed as a system operating within and in support of the larger healthcare system and its ability to optimize the health of people and populations, then a more appropriate definition is one that considers the breadth of stakeholders involved in upstream and downstream processes that ultimately procure value for patients.[58]

1.8.3 Advancing Capabilities

With the move to value-based healthcare, increasing financial pressures on hospitals and health systems, and advances in analytical capabilities, greater attention is paid to collecting and analyzing data to measure and advance the role of supply chain in improving clinical, financial, and operational performance. Analytics range from evaluating whether the products selected achieved the intended and expected results in order to inform future sourcing decisions to measuring the performance of supply chain operations and suppliers.

The experience of the COVID-19 pandemic has forced a further upstream view, as healthcare delivery organizations and suppliers seek to minimize risk to supply continuity and support demand planning. With more executive-level recognition of the dependencies on the upstream supply chain and the ability of manufacturers and distributors to support dynamic downstream demand, there is more interest and investment being made not only to improve upstream visibility, but also to more accurately document and share information on supply utilization. The consumer-packaged goods industry has long benefitted from collaborative planning, forecasting, and replenishment, which has remained largely non-existent in the healthcare industry.[59] Risk management in the healthcare supply chain is discussed further in Chapter 3.

An emerging area of supply chain maturation speaks to its ability to support numerous social agendas, from reducing health disparities to addressing climate change. For years, many hospitals have measured and reported on the percentage of their overall spend with certified diverse suppliers. More recently, with the move to value-based healthcare, hospitals and health systems are interested in reducing the social, economic, and environmental factors that have more of an impact on a patient's health status and longevity than the clinical care they receive.[60,61] Accordingly, they are expanding their supplier diversity initiatives to direct more of their spend toward local businesses that hire and train individuals from the most disadvantaged communities, the same neighborhoods that generate frequent and repeat patient visits often for otherwise avoidable healthcare conditions. By creating economic opportunity, hospitals and healthcare systems collaborate with other community resources to advance economic well-being and address the social determinants of health (SDOH).

The healthcare supply chain is also the growing focus of national and international efforts to stem climate change. Globally, healthcare operations contribute 4% of total greenhouse gas emissions, but U.S. operations account for 8.5% of the total U.S. carbon footprint.[62] Eighty percent of the greenhouse gas emissions associated with healthcare operations are linked to the supply chain and the impact of products across their entire lifecycles, including production, packaging, transportation, use, and disposal. The idea of a "circular economy," as relates to devices in the healthcare industry, is of increased importance.[63]

COVID-19 pandemic-related shortages also illuminated another critical social problem: the proliferation of forced labor in supply chains. Glove shortages experienced during the early days of the pandemic were often tied to import restrictions on manufacturers and countries known to violate human trafficking regulations. Meanwhile significant increases in the utilization of healthcare services globally, often driven by an aging population and the growth of the ability to support services in evolving economies, has expanded demand for surgical instruments, PPE, and other products that are sometimes manufactured by individuals, including children, forced into labor to help pay off debt to human traffickers.[64]

1.8.4 Lessons from Other Industries

The complexity and evolving nature of the healthcare system continues to distinguish the structure and operation of the supply chain compared to other industries. At the same time, there are also important similarities that can inform and advance the performance of the healthcare supply chain and in turn the organizations and patients it supports. Given that scant attention has been paid to the healthcare supply chain in both general supply chain and healthcare management textbooks, it is important to spend some time considering where there are commonalities in approach, where aspects of supply chain in general need to be adjusted to meet the demands of healthcare, and where the differences are so significant that a completely different approach to the same task or function is required.

Beyond the topics discussed previously, for example, the centrality of the clinician, the following are a few key differences, which have been described as health sector exceptionalism.[65]

- **Mission:** The majority of healthcare delivery organizations in the United States are not-for-profit, with a stated mission to improve and save lives. This is in contrast with suppliers, many of which are global in scope, publicly traded, and operate at much higher profit margins than providers to satisfy shareholders.
- **Intermediation:** While supply chains in general involve multiple parties, the complexity of healthcare operations and finance depends on effective interaction among an even greater number of players, including patients, clinicians, healthcare delivery sites, GPOs, distributors, and manufacturers.

- **Breadth, criticality and complexity of supplies:** Given the wide range of clinical specialties and patient needs, hospitals and other healthcare delivery organizations require a wide breadth of products. In some cases, there are limited options for the kinds of products needed to treat a particular patient, and in such cases, stockouts could lead to disability or death. Many medical products are also highly complex, expensive, and require special handling, for example, cold chain, sterilization before use, and so on.
- **Regulatory approval:** Medical products must be approved by regulatory bodies, such as the FDA, before they can be marketed for use and often only for specific indications.

1.8.5 Clockspeed

Key differences in the health sector, as well as some of the nuances, require the supply chain manager to systematically and analytically consider the unique aspects of the healthcare system. Charles H. Fine advanced the concept of "clockspeed" to help explain different rates of change and maturation in different industries, which provides a robust framework for such analysis.[66] He refers to the extraordinary rapid clockspeed of the entertainment business, where talent and programs were rapidly changing, compared to the slower clockspeed of the aviation industry, where the life of an aircraft model carries over for several decades. Each industry, Fine explains, is subject to changes within its respective environment, leading to a different organizational design, structure, and set of strategies associated with its supply chains. His elaboration on the impact of clockspeed associated with products, technology, processes, and organizations themselves provides insight into the healthcare sector. Using a patient ailment (identified need) as the focal point for a specific healthcare product, Fine considers the overall design of the healthcare industry (except for emergency services) as dispersed, modular, and slow in both time and space.[67] Within the hospital itself, clockspeeds vary by departments and specialties, the products used, and the relationship between products and stakeholders. For example, the clockspeed for a psychiatry ward may be very slow compared to spine surgery where the proliferation of new products and processes continually impacts both the organization and the individual players. The supply organization itself, which must cater to the needs of multiple and varied stakeholders, has a very different clockspeed than an information technology function that more often makes decisions for the enterprise as a whole.

The introduction of new technologies can impact the clockspeed of several aspects of healthcare delivery. For example, consider a hospital-based physician with a desktop specimen analyzer. He or she can conduct a test and move ahead with treatment during the same visit, versus the more traditional approach where the patient is seen and sent to a lab for a test, after which the patient must wait until the results are back and then schedule treatment if needed. Such a change may not only disrupt the relationship between the hospital and the laboratory, but also necessitate that the hospital has the necessary inventory on hand to provide the treatment. The ripple of such an innovation can change many things. What was once very modular and required several visits to many different specialists is now tight and integral, requiring a more highly coordinated supply chain process. Similarly, as patient care is increasingly provided outside the acute care hospital, the technologies and logistics required, from telemedicine to a larger geographic distribution footprint, will change, necessitating further supply chain adaptations. As care previously performed primarily by physicians is handled by a wider range of practitioners, such as physician assistants, nurse practitioners, and pharmacists, the customer base for supply chain further expands and diversifies.

1.9 Chapter Summary

This chapter provided a high-level overview of the healthcare supply chain, its primary functions, and stakeholders, and most importantly, its expanding role in supporting the strategic objectives of an evolving healthcare industry. Revealed is the need for balance, trade-offs, and collaborative efforts by supply chain managers. In order to achieve industry best practice, FISCO-related functions require not just great management, but also effective orchestration. This is especially critical given the objective of a supply chain: "To synchronize the requirements of the customer with the flow of materials from suppliers in order to effect a balance between what are often seen as conflicting goals of high customer service, low inventory management, and low unit cost."[68] Balancing costs with value for money takes on greater significance in healthcare given that the goods delivered, for example, medical devices and pharmaceuticals, are primarily used in the delivery of a clinical service as opposed to holding intrinsic value on their own. Achieving strategic fit first requires an understanding of the needs of various customers[69] and the ability of the supply chain to meet those needs given the inherent unpredictability in both supply and demand. The remaining chapters in this book provide the insights and tools for those aspiring to become managers and leaders in the health sector.

Notes

1. NEJM Catalyst. (2017). What is value-based healthcare? *NEJM Catalyst*, *3*(1).
2. Center for Medicare and Medicaid Services. (2020, June 11). The fundamental shift to value-based care. Volume 1. VIDEO from HHS. https://www.youtube.com/watch?v=Yz4VO2s01cs (accessed April 14, 2023).
3. Fisher, E. S., Shortell, S. M., & Savitz, L. A. (2016). Implementation science: A potential catalyst for delivery system reform. *Jama*, *315*(4), 339–340.
4. Porter, M., & Lee, T. (2013, Dec.). The strategy that will fix healthcare. Harvard Business Review. https://hbr.org/2013/10/the-strategy-that-will-fix-health-care
5. Teisberg, E., Wallace, S., & O'Hara, S. (May, 2020). Defining and implementing value-based health care: A strategic framework. *Academic Medicine*, *95*(5), 682–685. http://dx.doi.org/10.1097/ACM.0000000000003122. PMID: 31833857; PMCID: PMC7185050
6. Smith, T.M. (2020, Jan. 10). What is value-based care? These are the key elements. AMA Delivery and Payment Models. https://www.ama-assn.org/practice-management/payment-delivery-models/what-value-based-care-these-are-key-elements
7. AHRMM. (2020). CQO movement. https://www.ahrmm.org/cqo-movement, https://www.ahrmm.org/cqo-movement
8. AHRMM. (2018). Cost, Quality, and Outcomes (CQO) Report on the Clinically Integrated Supply Chain.
9. Tarver E. (2022, Nov. 12). Value chain vs. supply chain: What's the difference? Investopedia. Retrieved February 21, 2023, from https://www.investopedia.com/ask/answers/043015/what-difference-between-value-chain-and-supply-chain.asp
10. Falk S, Cherf J, Schulz J, Huo A. (2019, Jan. 23). Cost and outcomes in value-based care. *Physician Leadership Journal*. Retrieved June 7, 2019, from https://www.physicianleaders.org/news/research-costs-outcomes-value-based-care.
11. Deloitte Insights Study. (2018, Oct. 11). Volume to value-based care: Physicians willing to manage cost by lack data and tools. Retrieved July 5, 2019, from https://www2.deloitte.com/insights/us/en/industry/health-care/volume-to-value-based-care.html
12. Hospital for Special Surgery. (2019, Mar. 14). No increased risk of complications for joint replacement in ambulatory surgery setting. Hospital for Special Surgery News Release. https://www.eurekalert.org/news-releases/517261
13. Leff, B., Burton, L., Mader, S. L., Naughton, B., Burl, J., Inouye, S. K., Greenough III, W. B., Guido, S., Langston, C., Frick, K. D., Steinwachs, D., & Burton, J. R. (2005). Hospital at home: Feasibility and outcomes of a program to provide hospital-level care at home for acutely ill older patients. *Annals of Internal Medicine*, *143*(11), 798–808. https://www.acpjournals.org/doi/abs/10.7326/0003-4819-143-11-200512060-00008

14. Condon, A. (2022, Feb. 7). Commercial payors driving cases to ASCs; orthopedics most primed for growth. Becker's ASC. `https://www.beckersasc.com/asc-coding-billing-and-collections/commercial-payors-driving-cases-to-ascs-orthopedics-most-primed-for-growth.html?utm_medium=email&utm_content=newsletter`

15. Center to Stream Healthcare in Place. Our Mission. Center to Stream Healthcare in Place. `https://c2ship.org/about-2`

16. Furukawa, M. F., Machta, R. M., Barrett, K. A., Jones, D. J., Shortell, S. M., Scanlon, D. P., Lewis, V. A., O'Malley, A. J., Meara, E. R., & Rich, E. C. (2020). Landscape of health systems in the United States. *Medical Care Research and Review, 77*(4), 357–366.

17. Burns, L. R., & Pauly, M. V. (2002). Integrated delivery networks: A detour on the road to integrated health care? *Health Affairs, 21,* 128–143.

18. Bazzoli, G. J., Shortell, S. M., Dubbs, N., Chan, C., & Kralovec, P. (1999). A taxonomy of health networks and systems: bringing order out of chaos. *Health services research, 33*(6), 1683.

19. Fulton, B. D., King, J. S., Arnold, D. R., Montague, A. D., Chang, S. M., Greaney, T. L., & Scheffler, R. M. (2021). States' merger review authority is associated with states challenging hospital mergers, but prices continue to increase: Study examines the association of state merger review author with challenges to hospital mergers. *Health Affairs, 40*(12), 1836–1845.

20. Donev, D., Kovacic, L., Laaser, U. (2013) The role and organization of health care systems.

21. Uzsoy, R. (2005). Supply-chain management and health care delivery: Pursuing a system-level understanding. `https://www.ncbi.nlm.nih.gov/books/NBK22867`

22. Begun, J.W., Zimmerman, B., Dooley, K. (2002). Health care organizations as complex adaptive systems. Adapt Knowledge. `http://adaptknowledge.com/wp-content/uploads/rapidintake/PI_CL/media/Begun_Zimmerman_Dooley.pdf`

23. Burns, L. R. (2021). *The U.S. Healthcare Ecosystem: Payers, providers, producers* (1st ed.). McGraw Hill/Medical.

24. Sweeney, E. (2011). Towards a unified definition of supply chain management: The four fundamentals. *International Journal of Applied Logistics, 2*(3), 30–48.

25. Oliver, R. K., & Webber, M. D. (1992). Supply-chain management: Logistics catches up with strategy. In M. Christopher (Ed.), *Logistics: The strategic issues* (pp. 63–75). Chapman & Hall..

26. Lambert, D. M., & Cooper, M. C. (2000). Issues in supply chain management. *Industrial Marketing Management, 29*(1), 65–83.

27. Mentzer, J. T., DeWitt, W., Keebler, J. S., Min, S., Nix, N. W., Smith, C. D., & Zacharia, Z. G. (2001). Defining supply chain management. *Journal of Business Logistics, 22*(2), 1–25.

28. Porter, M. E. (1985). *Competitive advantage: Creating and sustaining superior performance* (pp. 1985). Simon and Schuster..

29. Ford, Eric W., & Dennis P. Scanlon. (2006). Promise and problems with supply chain management approaches to health care purchasing. *Academy of Management Proceedings, 2006* (1. Briarcliff Manor, NY 10510: Academy of Management.

30. Christopher, M. (2005). *Logistics and supply chain management: Creating value adding networks* (3rd ed.). FT Prentice Hall.

31. Op. cit. Sweeney.

32. Luke, R. D., Walston, S. L., & Plummer, P. (2004). *Healthcare strategy: In pursuit of competitive advantage.* Association of University Programs in Health Administration/Health Administration Press.

33. Centers for Medicare and Medicaid Services. (2022, June 8). Hospital price transparency. CMS. https://www.cms.gov/hospital-price-transparency

34. Abdulsalam, Y., & Schneller, E. (2019). Hospital supply expenses: An important ingredient in health services research. *Medical Care Research and Review, 76*(2), 240–252.

35. Schneller, E. S., & Wilson, N. A. (2009). Professionalism in 21st century professional practice: Autonomy and accountability in orthopaedic surgery. *Clinical Orthopaedics and Related Research, 467*(10), 2561–2569.

36. Nyaga, G. N., Young, C. J., & Zepeda, D. E. (2015). An analysis of the effects of intra- and interorganizational arrangements on hospital supply chain efficiency. *Journal of Business Logistics, 36*(4), 340–354.

37. Carter, C. R., Rogers, D. S., & Choi, T. Y. (2015). Toward the theory of the supply chain. *Journal of Supply Chain Management, 51*(2), 89–97.

38. Choi, T. Y., & Dooley, K. J. (July 1, 2009). Supply networks: Theories and models*. *Journal of Supply Chain Management, 45*(3), 25–27.

39. Beitler, B. G., Abraham, P. F., Glennon, A. R., Tommasini, S. M., Lattanza, L. L., Morris, J. M., & Wiznia, D. H. (2022). Interpretation of regulatory factors for 3D printing at hospitals and medical centers, or at the point of care. *3D Printing in Medicine, 8*(1), 1–7. https://link.springer.com/article/10.1186/s41205-022-00134-y

40. Chopra, S., & Meindl, P. (2021). *Supply chain management. Strategy, planning & operation* (7th ed.). Pearson.

41. Darling, M., & Wise, S. (April, 2010). Not your father's supply chain. Following best practices to manage inventory can help you save big. *Materials Management in Health Care, 19*(4), 30–33.

42. Monczka, R. M., Handfield, R. B., Giunipero, L. C., & Patterson, J. L. (2020). *Purchasing and supply chain management* (7th ed.). Cengage Learning.

43. Sweeney, op. cit.

44. Schneller, E. S., & Smeltzer, L. R. (2006). *Strategic management of the health care supply chain.* Jossey-bass.

45. Burns, L. R. (2022). *The healthcare value chain: Demystifying the role of GPOs and PBMs.* Springer International Publisher.

46. Beitler, Abraham, Glennon, Tommasini, Lattanza, Morris, & Wiznia, op. cit. Point of care*3D Printing in Medicine, 8*(1), 1–7. https://link.springer.com/article/10.1186/s41205-022-00134-y

47. Biospace. (2016, Nov. 29). Medtonic to send up to 10 employees to help run labs in Cleveland Medical Center: New agreement focuses on Improved

System Efficiency at University Hospitals Cleveland Medical Center. https://www.biospace.com/article/releases/medtronic-to-send-up-to-10-employees-to-help-run-labs-in-cleveland-medical-center-/

48. Goldberg, Z. N., & Nash, D. B. (2021). The payvider: An evolving model. *Population Health Management, 24*(5), 528–530.
49. Abdulsalam, & Schneller, op. cit.
50. Ibid.
51. Li, S., Ragu-Nathan, B., Ragu-Nathan, T. S., & Rao, S. S. (2006). The impact of supply chain management practices on competitive advantage and organizational performance. *Omega, 34*(2), 107–124.
52. Yanamandra, R. (2018). Development of an integrated healthcare supply chain model. *Supply Chain Forum: An International Journal, 19*(2), 111–121. http://dx.doi.org/10.1080/16258312.2018.1475823
53. Zhou, H., & Benton, W. C. (2007). Supply chain practice and information sharing. *Journal of Operations Management, 25*(6), 1348–1365. http://dx.doi.org/10.1016/j.jom.2007.01.009
54. Conway, K., & Perrin, R. (2006). The evolution of eBusiness in healthcare. In U. Hübner & M. A. Elmhorst (Eds.), *eBusiness in healthcare. eProcurement to supply chain management* (pp. 157–176). Springer.
55. Rahmani, K., Karimi, S., Rezayatmand, R., & Raeisi, A. R. (2021). Value-based procurement for medical devices: A scoping review. *Medical Journal of the Islamic Republic of Iran, 35*, 134. http://dx.doi.org/10.47176/mjiri.35.134
56. Congressional Budget Office Blog. (2008, Jan. 31). Technological change and the growth of health care spending. https://www.cbo.gov/publication/24748
57. Chopra, & Meindl, op. cit..
58. Christopher, M. (2005). *Logistics and supply chain management: Creating value adding networks* (3rd ed.). FT Prentice Hall.
59. Conway, K. (2020). Demand planning and forecasting: Healthcare's time has come. *Healthcare Purchasing News.* https://www.hpnonline.com/sourcing-logistics/article/21150785/demand-planning-and-forecasting-healthcares-time-has-come
60. Pronk, N. P., Kleinman, D. V., & Richmond, T. S. (2021). Healthy People 2030: Moving toward equitable health and well-being in the United States. *EClinicalMedicine, 33*. Accessed April 14, 2023
61. Hasbrouck, L. (2021). Healthy people 2030: An improved framework. *Health Education & Behavior, 48*(2), 113–114. Accessed April 14, 2023. Retrieved April 21, 2023, https://pubmed.ncbi.nlm.nih.gov/33650451/
62. Commonwealth Fund. (2022, Apr. 19). How the U.S. health care system contributes to climate change. Commonwealth Fund. Retrieved February. 21, 2023, from https://www.commonwealthfund.org/publications/explainer/2022/apr/how-us-health-care-system-contributes-climate-change
63. MacNeill, A. J., Hopf, H., Khanuja, A., Alizamir, S., Bilec, M., Eckelman, M. J., Hernandez, L., McGain, F., Simonsen, K., Thiel, C., Young, S.,

Lagasse, R., & Sherman, J. D. (2020). Transforming the medical device industry: Road map to a circular economy. *Health Affairs*, *39*(12), 2088–2097.

64. Conway. K. (2022, Aug. 24). Building the moral and business case for supply chain visibility. *Healthcare Purchasing News.* https://www.hpnonline.com/sourcing-logistics/article/21277991/building-the-moral-and-business-case-for-supply-chain-visibility

65. Abdulsalam, Y., Gopalakrishnan, M., Maltz, A., & Schneller, E. (2015). Health care matters: Supply chains in and of the health sector. *Journal of Business Logistics*, *36*(4), 335–339. http://dx.doi.org/10.1111/jbl.12111

66. Fine, C. H. (1998). *Cloclspped: Winning industry control in the age of temporary advantage*. Basic Books.

67. Fine. Op. cit., 1998 p. 144.

68. Stevens, G. C. (1989). Integrating the supply chain. *International Journal of Physical Distribution and Materials Management*, *19*, 3–8.

69. Chopra, & Meindl, op. cit.

2

Building a Strategy for Healthcare Supply Chain Management— *Creating the Vision*

2.1 Introduction

Strategy sets an organization's direction for interacting with the environment to achieve its goals. Goals will define where the organization wants to go. Action strategies will define how it will get there. For example, the goal might be to achieve a net income of 5%, while the associated strategy might be to reduce materials costs, improve operational efficiency, and improve employee productivity. Strategies can include any number of tactics to achieve the goal.

All organizations, including supply chain management departments, need a strategy to guide the decisions they make to further their respective enterprise's objectives. Without a strategy, an organization drifts without purpose nor with a viable end game. Perhaps baseball legend Yogi Berra said it best, "If you don't know where you're going, you might end up someplace else." Accordingly, organizations need strategies to direct their actions in a consistent and synchronized way to achieve their goals.

For most organizations, strategies emerge through the process of creating a strategic plan. This is a fundamental set of statements and commitments to align the organization in a specific direction. The planning process must begin with a clear statement of purpose. As stated by renowned organization theorist, Russell Ackoff, "Planning is the design of a desired future and of effective ways of bringing it about."[1] This is the essence of planning. When we refer specifically to strategic planning, the process is more precisely defined, as stated by Peter Drucker, "Strategic planning is the continuous process of making present entrepreneurial (risk-taking) decisions systematically and with the greatest knowledge of their futurity; organizing systematically the efforts needed to carry out these decisions; and measuring the results of these decisions against the expectations through organized, systematic feedback."[2]

A strategy begins with an articulation of the intended end game of the organization, typically called a "vision" statement. Accompanying the vision is an action-oriented statement defining the mission of the organization—how it intends to perform. Completing the articulation of organizational intentions is a set of objectives that the organization intends to achieve. This sets out the foundation for the organization to define its purpose.

Within a healthcare organization, which is typically clinically focused, the healthcare supply chain management organization acts as a business. Hence, in describing the strategic framework for a supply chain management organization, we draw from the learnings and experiences of business organizations. At a minimum, all organizational strategies comprise these fundamental components:

1. Statements of vision, mission, and objectives;
2. An understanding of the needs of stakeholders;
3. A situational understanding of the environment around the enterprise;
4. Structures to manage the enterprise that are either operated internally or outsourced to an outside (third-party) organization;
5. Organization structures;
6. Business processes;
7. Technology frameworks and plans;
8. Distribution network structures;
9. Human resources plans to ensure that the organization has the talent it needs and the means to retain it;
10. Action initiatives (strategies) designed to deliver results in accordance with the organization's mission;

11. Identification of risks and associated mitigation steps; and
12. Performance expectations and measurable targets.

Amongst all organizations, healthcare organizations are typically very complex and have many interrelated components that must work harmoniously. Since supply chain management activities interface with many functions within a provider organization, the role and the activities of the supply chain organization must be clearly articulated and understood by all. Consequently, for healthcare supply chain management organizations, while the corporate entity will have an overall strategy, the supply chain department or division should have its own strategy formed along the preceding lines. This will ensure that within the complex healthcare provider organization that the supply chain organization is recognized and supported as it undertakes its activities.

In a healthcare organization, the strategies that the supply chain management team undertakes address business processes, technology, and organization design within the context of the supply chain functions. In Chapter 1, we described supply chain design functions in what we call a Fully Integrated Supply Chain Organization (FISCO). Strategies for this will inform decisions including:

1. Supply chain organization structure and the activities each stage of the supply chain will perform;
2. Products that are to be sourced or made and where they need to be stored;
3. Supply chain management processes to be conducted by the supply chain organization and whether other processes, such as accounts payable, are led and operated by other departments within the provider organization;
4. Supply chain processes to be operated internally or that will be outsourced, such as contracting through a group purchasing organization (GPO) or sourcing products on a Just-in-Time (JIT) basis through a distributor;
5. Location and capacities of facilities;
6. Modes of transportation and the location from where the products are shipped; and
7. Design of information management solutions for the supply chain management team to enable them to conduct their work efficiently and effectively.

In this chapter, we briefly describe several components of a typical supply chain management strategy. Other sections of this book help the reader understand the remaining components of the strategy. Chapter 8 focuses on how organizational strategy and design are related.

2.2 Vision Statements

Vision statements express the desired future of the organization. In fact, such expressions reflect an ideal situation—one that is always sought, but never fully attained. By having this elusive goal, the organization always focuses on and makes great efforts toward achieving it. Such progress toward a desired end state provides a powerful way to direct and manage an organization's efforts toward successful outcomes.

Two examples of vision statements are provided to offer a sense of the content and aspiratory nature of a vision statement. These statements are highly personal to each organization. There is no formula for drafting them. They should simply state in the words of the organization's leadership team, their ideal for the outcomes of the organization's undertakings. The first example is the vision statement of the supply chain management organization of the U.K. National Health Service (NHS).

> *Through our passion and excellence we improve lives as the supply chain partner of choice for the NHS.*

The statement is simple and to the point in identifying how and what the supply chain management team does for its partner, the NHS.

In this second vision statement example, the organization specifically identifies the stakeholders and references the role of sourcing products and services.

> *Our vision is to surpass the expectancies of our customers, coworkers, suppliers, and stakeholders so that the supply chain area is recognized as the most important source for products and services.*

Both examples are succinct, yet powerful aspirational statements of the intent and expected outcomes of the organization's efforts.

2.3 Mission Statements

The mission statement of an organization expresses how and in what form the organization conducts its business. It provides spatial (geographic) context, reference tools, and resources that are used to achieve the desired outcomes. Examples of mission statements for supply chain management organizations are provided here:

> *To provide a globally integrated supply chain solution that leverages standard business processes and tools, optimizes organizational capability, minimizes waste, improves predictability, and delivers comprehensive value to the customer.*

*To create a competitive advantage for ABC through pur-
chasing, manufacturing, and distributing products and services which provide superior value to our customers.*

*To enable clinicians to deliver great medicine with supplies,
devices, and equipment available when and where they need
them and sourced at a competitive cost.*

A mission statement worthy of reflection is that from the U.S. Defense
Health Agency (DHA), with its special mission on reliability and readiness.[3]

*We support the National Defense Strategy and service military
departments by leading the Military Health System as an
integrated, highly reliable system of readiness, medical
training, and health.*

2.4 Corporate Objectives

As suggested earlier, and discussed in greater detail in Chapter 8,
design and structure must be consistent with strategy. The question that
must be addressed is: "How can the supply chain management organizational design make the greatest contribution to the system's goals
and strategy?" How to balance cost, quality, and outcomes remains a
challenge. The importance of linking the supply chain organizational
design to the strategy cannot be overstated. How does one accommodate the demands of an academic health center's (AHC) goals to expose
students to a wide range of products in concert with the goal of standardization? If the decision regards the supply chain design for a large
system, and the individual units within the system, what are the system
goals for the entity as a whole and how do each of the delivery points of
service fit into that goal?

A first step is to ensure that the system is clear on its goals and strategy.
Confusion may exist between the focus on both low-cost and service
differentiation strategies. When strategies are developed to meet multiple
goals concurrently, the organization may attempt to achieve satisfactory
goals rather than a maximum level of performance with a single goal.
As cost, quality, and outcomes become more transparent to patients, in
response to requirements to make procedural pricing and quality data
more available, there will be increased pressure on hospitals to control
supply costs in order to be seen as a high-quality/low-cost provider.

The best way to meet customer needs is to thoroughly understand the
goals and strategies of each hospital or unit within the system and the
system itself. Therefore, the next question is: "What are the goals and
strategies of each unit within the system and how, through organization
design, can they be integrated?" Integration of strategies is extremely

difficult, but supply chain management may be able to maximize integration opportunities much better than other functions. Seeking to accommodate clinician choice, a health system supply chain may choose a dual sourcing strategy, while allowing its regions to make the individual decisions regarding which two contenders for a product to choose.

Alfred Chandler, in the late 1960s, coined the phrase "structure should follow strategy."[4] A significant element of the structural framework of a business is its organizational design, which is discussed in greater detail in Chapter 8. If the design does not achieve strategic goals, it will probably be the wrong decision. Strategy should trigger consideration of how work will be achieved including choice decisions regarding the seven areas listed earlier. Three areas where supply chain decisions must be especially aligned with strategy are (a) business process, (b) technology framework, and (c) distribution network.

2.5 Business Process Strategies

Knowing the overall mission of an organization is an important foundational step, but there is still a need for strategic thinking supported through a process by which decisions will be made from various options.

Business operations adhere to formalized processes to provide a consistent and high-quality outcome. In supply chain management, these processes range from product sourcing to order management to inventory management. In developing the process design, organizations require a thorough mapping process often with the support of the technology solution chosen for their enterprise resource planning (ERP) system. The map that results from process analysis should provide an indication of the level to which supply chain is supporting the organization's mission.

It is particularly important to consider the difference between organizational units and the inter-organizational processes within the system. Understanding strategy will inform how the integration of goals could be better supported through supply chain design. In addition, it is important to assess the extent to which information technologies are present to support supply chain performance, and thus, influence design. This is especially the case as more and more systems have automated supply functions, including sourcing and contracting. The Institute for Supply Management, working in collaboration with the Association for Health Care Resources & Materials Management (AHRMM) and the Strategic Marketplace Initiative (SMI) has established an economic index for the healthcare supply chain to identify trends and to assist supply chain and business leaders in making important decisions.[5]

Process mapping may also indicate where communication and operational linkages are deficient. For instance, it may be found that supply waste is occurring because one unit does not realize that excess supplies can be transported to another unit. Or it may be that one unit is not aware of the standardization processes that occurred in another unit.

Supply chain strategy will inform how an organization should work with external suppliers and markets to deliver value to the organization and to operationally engage with clinicians and other internal customers to "provide internal functions with external supply market intelligence and actionable opportunities."[6] As discussed in detail in Chapter 5, many healthcare systems' supply chains are designed around the use of intermediaries, such as group purchasing organizations (GPOs) and distributors for sourcing, contracting, and distributing. Others have built their capabilities around many of these functions in the form of consolidated service centers or shared service organizations.[7] Other so-called "hybrid organizations" are expanding their own competencies and capabilities as they evolve. Before providing more insight into these hybrid designs, it is important to consider the questions and challenges that organizational designers need to address. One academic health center, having clearly articulated its goals and mission, decided to fully outsource its sourcing and distribution to a major supply chain intermediary—defining supply chain management as a competency and capability beyond its vision. This is a dramatic, although infrequent, example of strategic choice exercised by a prominent healthcare provider.

Any one of the FISCO business processes mentioned in Chapter 1 and elaborated on in Appendix 1 is a candidate for outsourcing. Organizations must carefully assess the business requirements and the availability of appropriate service providers. For example, supply chain organizations may outsource some or all of their sourcing programs to GPOs and their warehouse and transportation services to third-party logistics providers. A strategic decision is to make or buy the service. Appropriately, this is an important strategic decision that must consider the competitive value of the market and the organization's competitive performance. Exhibit 2.1 illustrates the decision factors in outsourcing.

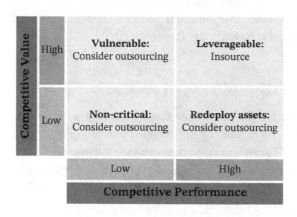

Exhibit 2.1: Outsourcing decision-making considerations.

As portrayed in Exhibit 2.1, if either the business process competitive performance or its competitive value to the business is low, outsourcing the process should be considered. However, if the business process' competitive value is high and its performance in the market is considered high, then the process is a strong candidate to be insourced.

The decision to outsource is complex and has a profound impact on the overall strategy of the organization. This is discussed in much further detail in Chapter 6. Decisions such as these need to be regularly reviewed.

2.6 Technology Framework Strategies

Accompanying the business processes are strategies regarding the technology framework of applications and systems that support it. It consists of policies, plans, and procedures for acquiring knowledge and ability, managing that knowledge and ability within the company and exploiting them.[8] Succinctly, it is the overall plan that consists of tactics relating to the use of technologies within the organization.

Many supply chain applications are incorporated within organizational technology, particularly ERP software solutions. However, a few specialized solutions (e.g., warehouse operations and product standardization processes) are often independent and may rely on interfaces with the core systems. Since supply chain management involves the management of thousands of transactions, the strategy regarding the design of the technology architecture is important from both a comprehensiveness and accuracy point of view and will impact the choice of solutions. Careful design and implementation are keys to success. Much more detail of the considerations for technology design is provided in Chapter 9. It is critical to recognize that the ongoing transformation within the healthcare sector toward greater integration and more process-oriented healthcare chains requires a shift in strategy, structure, and control mechanisms. Accordingly, supply chain orientation within the healthcare sector can be regarded as a complex social change process with the potential to improve performance.[9]

2.7 Distribution Network Strategy

Supply chain managers oversee the movements of products from acquisition to the patient. As such, facilities are needed to affect these movements. These facilities are used to store, process, and transport the products. For a healthcare organization these facilities could include:

- Warehouses with pallet racks and shelving;
- Material handling equipment;

- Cold storage areas;
- Storage lockers and cabinets in patient wards;
- Storage carts and bins; and
- Truck and loading/receiving docks.

In some cases, these facilities are not owned or operated by the health-care organization but are contracted to external organizations, such as major distributors. While the day-to-day operating responsibility is not held by the healthcare organization, the supply chain organization must focus on the performance expectations and the operating results of the contractor. The decision, for example, to develop a consolidated service center, as discussed in Chapter 6, is an important strategic decision, defining and impacting the design of the organization's distribution network.[10]

2.8 Action Initiatives/Strategies

It is important for designers to understand the role of supply chain strategies, and articulated goals and their relationship to design and tactics.

Exhibit 2.2: Common organizational strategies and their tactics.

Strategy	Tactics
Low-cost leadership: increase market share by achieving lower costs compared to competitors **Hospital example/goal:** community hospital that competes by being the lower-cost, higher-quality alternative	- Tight cost control - Process engineering skills across departments - Intense supervision of employees, including professional staff - Frequent and detailed control reports - Intense efforts to reduce costs of product and service delivery
Differentiation: attempt to distinguish their products or services from others in the industry **Hospital example/goal:** a hospital promoting its oncology services	- Strong marketing emphasis - Attempt to develop unique capabilities - Purchase of high-quality capital equipment and development of unique specialties - Emphasize research
Focus: the organization concentrates on a specific regional market or buyer group **Hospital example**: a hospital system focuses on obtaining dominant market share in a focused geographic region	- Combine the above tactics but focus on a unique market - Attempt to promote one specialty over the others

A supply chain strategy is a plan for interacting with the environment to achieve goals. Goals define where the organization wants to go and strategies define how it will get there. For example, as we had indicated above, the goal might be to achieve 5% net income while the strategy might be to reduce materials costs, improve operational efficiency, and improve employee productivity. Strategies can include any number of tactics to achieve the goal. Michael Porter[11] developed a popular method for categorizing organizational strategies. Each of the strategies and tactics (Exhibit 2.2) attempts to maximize the organization's strengths in order to develop a competitive advantage within its environment; in order to accomplish its goals, different organizational designs are required.

2.9 Chapter Summary

The supply chain management strategy for healthcare organizations drives decisions for all parts of the many supply chain management processes. The strategy forces managers to ask and answer fundamental questions about the way that they wish the supply chain to perform. The strategy becomes the statement by which the supply chain is designed and operates. Strategy also informs how an organization will approach each of the FISCO functions, which in turn, will impact approaches to cost, risk management, organizational intentions for growth and opportunity. Consequently, it is one of the first areas we examine in the management of a healthcare supply chain. Throughout the balance of this book, we build on the components of the supply chain strategy, providing a thorough guide to the best practices for supply chain management.

Notes

1. Ackoff, R. L. (1970). *A concept of corporate planning.* Wiley.
2. Drucker, P. F. (2006). *The practice of management* (Reissue edition). Harper Business.
3. Interestingly, no civilian healthcare system has the idea of readiness or preparedness as a core system statement. This serves the system well during both times of peace and military actions, but also served well during the COVID-19 pandemic.
4. Chandler, A. D., Jr. (1969). *Strategy and structure: Chapters in the history of the American industrial enterprise* (Vol. 120). MIT Press.
5. Derry, T. (2020). Shaping the health care field: ISM Hospital Report on Business. https://www.ahrmm.org/resource-repository-ahrmm/ahrmm-and-ismshaping-the-healthcare-field-through-the-hospital-report-on-business-1
6. Rodgers, S. (2004). Supply management: Six elements of superior design. *Supply Chain Management Review, 19*(3), 48–54.

7. Abdulsalam, Y., Gopalakrishnan, M., Maltz, A., & Schneller, E. (2015). The emergence of consolidated service centers in health care. *Journal of Business Logistics*, *36*(4), 321–334.
8. Ford, D. (1988). Develop your technology strategy. *Long Range Planning*, *21*(5), 85–95.
9. De Vries, J., & Huijsman, R. (2011). Supply chain management in health services: An overview. *Supply Chain Management: An International Journal*.
10. Abdulsalam, et al., op. cit.
11. Porter, M. E. (1980). *Competitive strategy: Techniques for analyzing industries and competitors*. Free Press.

3

Risk Management Strategies— *Healthcare Is Risky, So Is Supply Chain Management*

3.1 Introduction

Management in the health sector has been shown to make a significant difference in cost, quality, and outcomes.[1] Supply chain risk management (SCRM) is a critical function for healthcare provider organizations. Risk exists when (a) outcomes are uncertain, (b) goals are challenging to achieve, and (c) there is potential for extreme consequences.[2] Another way to look at risk is the potential inability of supply chain activities to meet system objectives. SCRM is a cross-functional process to identify, assess, mitigate, and monitor relevant risks that can disrupt an organization's supply chain.[3,4]

SCRM is a critical function of a Fully Integrated Supply Chain Organization (FISCO) with a strong association with other FISCO functions such as inventory management, asset management, and recall management (a very specific type of risk). Importantly, it is a function to identify, assess, mitigate, and monitor relevant risks (e.g., natural disasters, accidents, sabotage, or production problems, and product-related problems such as recalls) that can disrupt an organization's supply chain operations. When carried out effectively, well-managed supply chain risk leads to improved predictability for resource utilization, increased capacity, reduced cost, greater certainty in clinical performance, and the ability to capitalize on opportunities. Exhibit 3.1 lays out the core SCRM functions.

Supply risk can be formally defined as "*the probability of an incident (event) associated with inbound supply from individual supplier failures or the supply market occurring, in which its outcomes result in the inability of the purchasing firm to meet customer demand or cause threats to customer life and safety.*"[5] First, a healthcare provider's supply chain contains multiple risks emanating from the upstream manufacturing supply chain. These include disruptions to a manufacturer's suppliers of ingredients/components and transportation risks associated with moving goods downstream to their customers. Recent research suggests that lower-tier suppliers of multinational corporations carry higher risks in terms of probability and impact, and it is difficult for these corporations to screen or audit their suppliers' suppliers.[6] Risks are also associated with a health organization's choices, such as implementing lean or just-in-time (JIT) inventory strategies without accounting for the upstream partners' ability to provide the needed resources consistently. During the COVID-19 pandemic, organizations across the healthcare ecosystem (including providers, intermediaries, and manufacturers) experienced many risks associated with dramatic interruptions of the upstream supply chain to support manufacturers and downstream supply chains from manufacturers to distributors and the point of use. For many U.S. industries, including the healthcare sector, the interruption in simple yet critical supplies from abroad, such as protective equipment, led to unprecedented shortages—resulting in downstream risks to patients, such as procedure postponement and risks to healthcare workers.

Broadly, supply risk refers to the potential to be deprived of use (either because of long lead time, non-delivery, or unacceptable quality), not satisfying end-users or customers,[7] and increasing threats to the organization's financial viability due to cost escalation. In the health sector, the impact of such disruptions on products needed for patient care is a top-of-mind risk requiring close attention. This chapter scrutinizes how progressive systems manage risk associated with the supply chain, emphasizing sourcing of products, purchasing, cost reduction, and

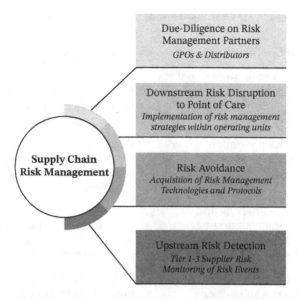

Exhibit 3.1: The primary components of a risk management strategy.

resilience. Chapter 10 addresses an essential aspect of risk: a lack of attention to preparedness for major disruptions.

The initial edition of this book looked principally at risk due to cost and for good reasons. As hospital and outpatient settings became "supply-intensive," supplies accounted for an increasingly large proportion of costs.[8,9] Medical and surgical supply costs accounted for over half of total supply expenses, approximately 57% in 2020. Between 2016 and 2020, total supply chain costs increased by 5% each year on average.[10] As of 2020, the average total supply costs were $30 million per hospital.[11]

The first two years of the COVID-19 pandemic accelerated the cost increases for supplies in many areas. For intensive care units (ICUs) and respiratory care departments, especially those treating COVID-19 patients, medical supply expenses increased by 31.5% and 22.3% for those in respiratory care departments, respectively. Furthermore, drug expenses increased by 36.9% compared to pre-pandemic levels.[12] While such costs diminished, the pandemic raised awareness of the supply chain's vulnerability and costs. Exhibit 3.2 identifies some of the important risk management practices before and after the height of the COVID-19 pandemic.[13]

Other types of risk are important to consider. Many risks, such as drug and medical device stockouts and recalls, occur regularly; beyond the potential safety issues associated with recalled products, these issues deprive the provider organization and patients of products necessary for care. Interestingly, factory fires are consistently the number one disruption reported globally, with over one thousand fires impacting the

Exhibit 3.2: Changes in risk management practices stemming from the COVID-19 pandemic.

Before COVID-19	After COVID-19
Risk evaluations of first-tier suppliers at the time of onboarding	Use of Supply Chain Risk Management (SCRM) tools that continually and proactively evaluate supply chain risks
Supply chain risk mitigation strategies induced by specific triggers	Ongoing risk evaluation of the extended supply chain network, including second and third-tier suppliers
Visibility into the financial and operational viability of first-tier suppliers, with annual or semi-annual reviews of the supplier network	Activation of business continuity plans to secure critical inventories and activate alternate suppliers when necessary
Existence of standard business continuity plans with revisions triggered by specific events	Redevelopment and upgrading of business continuity plan to support ongoing and anticipated supply chain disruptions

Note. Adapted from: Hung, S. Kannan V. Malhotra, B. Future-proofing Supply Chain Management: Building Resilience and Agility through Digital Transformation. Everest Group. 2020. `https://www.capgemini.com/wp-content/uploads/2021/10/Everest_Group_Future-proofing_Supply_Chain_Management.pdf`[19]

healthcare industry in 2021.[14] Others are less common (e.g., disruptions due to extreme weather), yet others are extremely rare or considered high-risk but low-probability events, such as a pandemic.[15] Suppliers and commercial firms specializing in disruption identification and mitigation track systematic risks for such natural disaster disruptions.[16] At no time have the risks associated with disruptions been more pronounced than during the COVID-19 pandemic, where the absence of supplies posed risks to patients and providers of care as well as to access to care and the integrity of care processes. These shortages included demand shock resulting from increased hospitalizations, reduced ability of inventory buffers such as the Strategic National Stockpile (SNS) to supply, delayed deliveries, supplier allocation failures, and reduced shipping lines from global suppliers.[17] Shortages resulted in shipment delays and difficulties in finding alternative products, resulting in rationing of care.[18]

Uncertainties regarding the depth of disruptions (how many were impacted and the ability to respond), the period associated with the COVID-19 disruption (days, weeks, months, and beyond), and the shape of the recovery (gradual, cyclical, many plateaus, and starts) led to great difficulties is managing supply chain risks in the health sector.

3.2 The Nature of Supply Risk

Risk, an essential element in supply management, is not easy to see and quantify.[20] When assessing cost-related risks, surgical masks, gowns, and other protective equipment have traditionally been classified as relatively low risk and frequently categorized as commodities and not of strategic importance. However, if we consider the risk to healthcare workers, patients, and organizational sustainability, many of these items became critical for provider organizations to carry out their clinical missions safely during the COVID-19 pandemic. Types of risk for different products may, indeed, be situational and transitory.

The level of risk is generally estimated using two components: (a) the probability of the risk event occurring, and (b) the consequences or impact of the risk (Exhibit 3.3). Each quadrant in Exhibit 3.3 requires a strategy, including risk avoidance, reduction, transfer, and response.[21]

Catastrophic events (high impact, low probability risks) are complex, making it difficult for supply chain managers to develop mitigation strategies. Such difficulties were extensive during the early days of COVID-19 as we experienced an unprecedented number of patients within hospital ICUs, requiring respirators, ventilators, and pharmaceuticals in volumes not previously anticipated by providers nor the manufacturers of these products. Cyber-attacks are increasing in healthcare, often at a higher cost and with longer resolution time than other industries.[22] While these high-impact, low-probability items are frequently related to risks associated with an organization's strategy (discussed later), arriving at an appropriate strategy can be difficult. Insurance plans can provide a means to mitigate some risks where impact and probability can be reasonably quantified (such as facility damage from natural disasters). Other risks, like the COVID-19 pandemic or other "unknown unknowns," are much

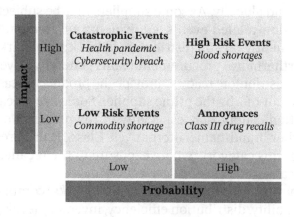

Exhibit 3.3: Event probability and its consequences.

harder to anticipate, let alone estimate a related insurance premium. Sometimes simply striving for overall business resilience and preparing a robust disaster recovery plan is the best any business can do in anticipation of these risks.

High-risk events (high-impact and high-probability risks) include drug shortages, of which there are over 1,200 annually in the United States,[23] can result in severe health complications. In healthcare supply chains, a recall refers to the removal or correction of a marketed product (e.g., pharmaceutical or medical device) to address a problem with that product that violates the laws administered by the U.S. FDA. Class I drug recalls (when there is a reasonable probability that the use of or exposure to a violative product will cause serious adverse health consequences or death as defined by the FDA) also constitute high-impact risks and need to be traced and withdrawn from the points of use quickly. Mitigating such risk is also tricky, especially when no substitute products exist. When a recall may impact one of several manufacturers, purchasing professionals attempt to reduce such risks by ensuring that multiple suppliers are accessible should one supplier experience a recall. Blood is another example of a product where shortages can be life-threatening. Providers transfer the risk for blood availability to blood banks, which are accomplished by anticipating patterns for donations and periods where demand exceeds supply. However, outsourcing the risk does not guarantee that the risk will be fully mitigated. Chapter 4 discusses physician preference for high-impact products, especially implantable devices. Given that such items are also subject to recalls, equivalent products are frequently available, and many are related to elective procedures. Group purchasing organizations (GPOs) and providers of care refrain from single-sourcing such items, providing a buffer from risk.

Annoyances (low impact with a high probability risk) include many low-impact products that healthcare organizations use while providing care, most of which are commodities provided by multiple suppliers, domestically and globally. As some suppliers may be subject to weather or transportation-related events, equivalents are frequently pursued. Hospitals frequently rely on distributors to track such markets and disruptions. Furthermore, procurement teams generally have alternative suppliers and distributors ready to provide the products in case of unforeseen delays or cut-offs by the prime supplier. Some drug recalls may also have less patient safety risk, especially in the presence of numerous generic or other brand-name alternatives. Class III drug recalls can be considered in this category, where exposure to the recalled product is not likely to cause adverse effects.

Low-risk events (low-impact, low-probability risks) commonly arise in product availability, distribution efficiency, inventory levels, etc. Supply managers will likely accept many of these risks that result in minor disruptions and price fluctuations and manage them as they arise. Nonetheless, the probabilities and impact of risks should be frequently assessed, and managers need to be ready to act when simply accepting certain risks becomes costly. Low-impact, low-probability risks may be placed on a watch list, such as cotton balls used in many healthcare settings for various applications. Cotton is produced domestically and in many nations across the globe. The cotton market may be impacted by weather-related and transportation-related events that may impact market conditions related to cost and availability. Again, supply managers may not concern themselves with such fluctuations and depend on their distributors and GPOs to set appropriate forecasts and mitigate these risks on their behalf.

3.3 Risk Categories

Managing risk can be further understood by dividing risk into five categories that consider both cause and consequences: (a) strategy risk, (b) market risk, (c) demand risk, (d) implementation risk, and (e) cost risk.[24] Each type of risk has very different characteristics and can be attributable to various causal factors (Exhibit 3.4).

3.3.1 Strategy Risk

Inappropriate strategy for hospital goods or services is frequently related to the lack of knowledge by supply chain managers about the availability of a product in the marketplace and the nature of the product in its contribution to care. This risk occurs due to supplier manufacturing difficulties, breakdown in distribution channels, and the internal handling and communication related to products. Shelf-life issues are critical for many health-related products (e.g., pharmaceuticals and infusion products). For such products, strategy risk must revolve around the ability for timely and frequent movement of fresh supplies to the proper location and monitoring of product availability at the point of use. Strategy risk can also be related to the supply chain manager not correctly understanding how a product will be used in the hospital and whether there are preferences for specific brands and different versions of a product by clinicians. Products have a lifecycle, and different products have a short lifecycle due to continuous innovation. As discussed in Chapter 1, spine surgery, where there is a proliferation of new products and multiple versions of products, is an excellent example of risk in an area with rapid new product clockspeed. In 2021, orthopedic device manufacturers received almost 200 FDA spine clearances and over 100 joint replacement clearances.[25] Managing strategy risk can be especially difficult in areas with fast clockspeed in product development and introduction.

Exhibit 3.4: Types of risk: Causes and consequences.

Type of risk	Cause of risk	Consequences of risk
Strategy risk *Inappropriate supply strategy for product or service*	▪ Inappropriate match between product and supply strategy ▪ Poor knowledge of supply strategies	▪ Product not delivered at the right place at the right time at the best price
Market risk *Inappropriate strategy for market conditions*	▪ Lack of knowledge about cost trends within the market	▪ Purchase incorrect goods or service ▪ Pay too much for goods or services ▪ Use inferior goods
Demand risk *Buying too much or too little of the good or service*	▪ Volatility of customer demand ▪ Over or under specifying requirements	▪ Incorrect inventory levels ▪ Overpay for unnecessary product specifications ▪ Use of inappropriate materials ▪ Poor customer relationships
Implementation risk *The supply strategy is not implemented correctly*	▪ Poor information and communication within the hospital	▪ Too high of inventory costs ▪ Materials unavailable ▪ Unnecessary administrative costs
Cost risk *The total supply spend runs higher than budgeted*	▪ Excessive use, or need for, off-contract purchases ▪ Unforeseen fluctuations in product prices due to environmental or regulatory factors	▪ Seeking alternative, potentially inferior, products to meet budget requirements ▪ Lower profitability of supply-intensive services and procedures

Strategy risk can also emanate from not adequately vetting suppliers' risks and the risk of their suppliers' suppliers. Many of these risks are related to strategic sourcing deficiencies, as discussed later in this chapter. Monitoring strategy risk for products quickly changing in marketplace demand and utilization can be challenging. Industry best practice systems hedge against this risk by achieving a commitment from suppliers based on anticipated, if not guaranteed, volume and loyalty. This is done by developing a contracting system with well-developed terms and conditions containing escape clauses that specify the conditions under which contract conditions can be altered or canceled. While having trusting relationships, frequently developed over time, is an essential feature of risk reduction, solid contracts are highly supportive of risk reduction.[26] Both buyers and suppliers express frustration in negotiating product and service pricing, particularly concerning how the indirect "value-added" support services factor into the price. Suppliers frequently report that their clinical customers did not appreciate the value-added services bundled with the product's purchase but missed them when they were cut.

Clarity is important! Mini Case 3.1 provides insight into the challenges posed to the supply chain as a new product, characterized by uncertainty in its utilization, emerges and progresses in the market.

It is important that supply chain managers understand and develop action plans to mitigate risk. There are a variety of substantial costs associated with poor performance in this area—especially concerning purchase price and transaction costs. Hospitals can afford few stockouts. For example, when goods are unavailable for a surgical procedure, or a diagnostic test, the hospital or system is forced to take immediate action or suffer a loss of revenue to another facility. Also at risk is the loss of physicians whom hospitals rely on for admissions to competing organizations. Given the cost of lost revenue and the considerable effort of replacing a supplier, progressive systems think about "future-proofing" against their risks and those of their suppliers in the market. Thus, systems have an inherent vested interest in a supplier's financial weaknesses and vulnerabilities.[35]

The health sector supply chain has been characterized by a strategy of just-in-time (JIT) delivery in an attempt to reduce costs and increase productivity. JIT reduces the required space for inventory and can free up space for patient-centered activities. Inventory management involves more than purchasing supplies; it involves handling, storing, moving, and restocking supplies—at a cost often equal to the inventory's original purchase price.[36] JIT deals with goods, suppliers, and inventories and can impact risk if there is a low level of coordination or unexpected surges in demand with barriers to product availability. Interestingly, some systems envisioned JIT as a supply strategy while others recognized it as a lack of strategy. For some systems, deliveries by such carriers represent the hospital's deliberate strategy to secure a rarely used item and to avoid carrying inventory. Others report that the volume of JIT deliveries through the loading dock represents a breakdown in the ability of the supply chain management staff to anticipate the demand for specific products. Regardless of the reason for implementing JIT, few supply chain managers carefully monitor or manage such shipments nor understand the actual cost of "management" of risk in this manner.

Unfortunately, hospitals did not give more attention to risks related to JIT. In 2006, the *Wall Street Journal* published "Just-in-Time Inventories

MINI CASE 3.1 Risk and Uncertainty in Interventional Cardiology

Interventional cardiology is an example of an area with uncertainty in demand for a product, as a new product/technology impacted the market. In the early 1990s, bare metal stents, small tubes placed in coronary arteries to supply blood to the heart by keeping arteries open and reduce the chance of narrowing again, demonstrated superiority over previous procedures interventional procedures. These devices were approved for general use by the FDA in 1994, and while successful and beneficial to patients, stenting was associated with subsequent arterial closure (stenosis). Even with the risk of stenosis, bare metal stents continued to be significantly utilized. By 1995, stents were used in nearly 85% of procedures.[27]

Starting in 1999, research and subsequent clinical trials demonstrated that adding a substance/drug to the stent would reduce stenosis and the rate of clinical events and angiographic restenosis.[28] Introducing drug-eluting stents (DES) was considered another revolution in interventional cardiology. Exhibit 3.5 provides a timeline of the rapid evolution of DES. It is notable that there were, at inception and for some time to come, no clear standards on the mix of bare metal stents versus DES on a given patient. Thus, even when working closely with clinicians, supply chain staff was challenged by the high level of uncertainty when contracting such devices. Exhibit 3.5 provides the historical development of coronary heart stents.

Uncertainty contributes to risk management. For stents, how long it would be before new versions of stents would be introduced and how different clinicians would adopt new technologies, especially in the absence of reliable comparative data, increased uncertainty for purchasing strategies. Exhibit 3.6 demonstrates the variety in the design of platforms and associated drugs.

Noteworthy has been a movement toward risk- or outcomes-based contracting to align physicians with hospital objectives better (i.e., both physicians and hospitals assuming responsibility for cost and supply utilization). In practice, we are noticing more health institutions moving away from the fee-for-service model outcomes-based-based contract structures, such as gainsharing or making price dependent on the ability of a product to deliver on value.[29,30] The growth in risk-based structures,[31] where physicians and hospitals assume responsibility for cost and supply utilization, may well lead to significant changes in the triadic relationship.[32] This is especially the case under bundled payment scenarios where success depends on the physician

Exhibit 3.5: Historical development of coronary heart stents.

Time	Person(s)	Landmark events
1964	Dotter and Judkins	Conceptual description of coronary angioplasty using an implantable prosthetic device
May 1977	Gruntzig and Myler	First coronary angioplasty during coronary artery bypass graft surgery
September 1977	Andreas Gruntzig	First coronary angioplasty in an awake patient; a revolution in interventional cardiology
1979	Geoffrey Hartzler	First balloon angioplasty to treat acute myocardial infarction (AMI)
1986	Sigwart and Puel	The first implantation of a stent in human coronary arteries; second revolution in interventional cardiology
1991	Cannon and Roubin	First coronary stenting to treat AMI
1994	Serruys et al. and Fischman et al.	Publication of first two landmark (Benestent and STRESS) trials
1994	FDA	FDA-approved use of stents to treat acute and threatened vessel closure after failed balloon angioplasty
1999	Eduardo Sousa	The first drug-eluting (sirolimus) stent implanted in human coronary artery; third revolution in interventional cardiology
2002–2004	EMA* and FDA*	Approvals of Cypher and Taxus stents in Europe and United States
2011	EME	Approval of Absorb BVS (bioresorbable vascular scaffold) in Europe; fourth revolution in interventional cardiology

*FDA, Food and Drug Administration USA; EMA, European Medicines Agency.

working closely with the hospital to manage care and cost over an entire episode of care and physicians participating in accountable care organizations.[33]

In 2019, the coronary stent market revenue was over $15 billion, with a compound annual growth rate (CAGR) of 6.24% anticipated. With over 965,000 procedures each year to open blocked or narrowing arteries, there has been a concern about "over-stenting," with evidence that approximately 30% of all procedures were unnecessary. While unusual, an important study revealed a patient with 67 stents.[34] Uncertainty for both suppliers and providers was significant.

makes U.S. Vulnerable in a Pandemic," reflecting that low hospital stock-piles boost efficiency by leaving no extras for an outbreak.[37] Retaining a "just-in-case" strategy can make sense, as there are, increasingly, guidelines on how to best manage a JIT effort, including the mapping of the supply chain to understand JIT vulnerabilities, the identification of segments that can be best run by JIT, the creation of buffers at the points where such segments meet, and a better understanding of supplier relationships.[38] As a consequence of the challenges associated with COVID-19, there is a greater understanding of strategies in periods when there are significant uncertainties regarding when the next disruption and increased demand may occur, uncertainties regarding the nature of the disruption, and uncertainty in the resolve of how government and distributors may be prepared to support inventories and stockpiles.[39]

Exhibit 3.6: Coronary stent types.

	Cypher	Taxus-Express	Endeavor	Resolute	Xience-V	Promus Element	BioMatrix
Manufacturer	Cordis	Boston Scientific	Medtronic	Medtronic	Abbott Vascular	Boston Scientific	Biosensors
Platform	Bx-Velocity	Express	Driver	Driver	Vision	Omega	Gazelle
Design							
Material	SS	SS	MP35N® CoCr	MP35N® CoCr	L605® CoCr	PtCr	SS
Thickness of struts (μm)	140	132	91	91	81	81	112
Polymer	PEVA, PMBA	SIBS	PC	BioLinx	PBMA, PVDF-HFP	PBMA, PVDF-HFP	PLA
Polymer thickness (μm)	12.6	16	4.1	4.1	7.6	6	10
Drug	Sirolimus	Paclitaxel	Zotarolimus	Zotarolimus	Everolimus	Everolimus	Biolimus
Drug conc. (μg/cm²)	140	100	100	100	100	100	156
Drug release in 4 weeks	80%	<10%	100%	70%	80%	80%	45%
Late lumen loss (mm)[a]	0.17[19]	0.39[20]	0.61[37]	0.27[38]	0.16[39]	0.15[70]	0.13[42]

SS, stainless steel; CoCr, cobalt–chromium; PtCr, platinum–chromium; SIBS, Poly (styrene-b-isobutylene-b-styrene); PEVA, polyethylene-co-vinyl acetate; PMBA, poly (n-butyl methacrylate); PC, phosphorylcholine; PVDF, poly-vinylidene fluoride; HFP, hexafluoropropylene; PLA, polylactic acid.
[a]Late lumen loss varies depending on trial population, timing of angiography and study era. The values gives are indicative only, based on pivotal trials (referenced) of these stents.

Source: Javaid et al. (2013) with permission from Oxford University Press.

3.3.2 Market Risk

Market risk is associated with upstream supply availability and how such availability affects the willingness of suppliers to offer flexibility in their pricing. Notably, an excessive focus on price can lead to purchasing inferior products and increasing medical staff dissatisfaction.

Providers benchmark their prices with information from consulting firms and intelligence gained through networking discussions. As discussed in greater detail in Chapter 5, there is a great reliance on intermediaries, such as GPOs, to assist in understanding demand and cost trends. GPOs and other information providers provide cost data comparisons on a national basis. GPOs also benchmark their members, nationally and regionally, on metrics associated with utilization, price, cost, and other key outcome variables. Other commercial services allow their customers to compare their pricing to like organizations. While purchasing at an inappropriate price may not lead to purchasing inferior technology or goods, it can result in reduced operating margins—thus resulting in the inability to provide high-quality services.

One goal of mergers and acquisitions in the health sector is to gain efficiencies in operations, though mergers also introduce high-impact market risks.[40] Supply chain integration following mergers has sometimes proven challenging to the acquiring system due to suppliers' differences in culture, technologies, and intermediaries (i.e., GPOs and distributors). There are frequently significant costs associated with converting from one set of products to another, as well as dissatisfaction by clinicians who have, if not strong product preferences, then at least familiarity with the products being phased out. Physicians have been accustomed to demanding goods regardless of price and availability.[41] The result is a failure to manage market risk from higher purchasing prices and, as discussed later, inordinately high transaction costs due to the proliferation of suppliers and stock-keeping units (SKUs) that need to be managed within a system.

3.3.3 Demand Risk

Demand risk is related to the (a) uncertainty associated with disease patterns in a hospital or a system's population, (b) the supply manager's lack of understanding and poor anticipation of admissions trends, (c) failure to understand and manage clinician preferences, and (d) an inability to carry out value analysis effectively. When demand is poorly understood, disruptions occur, and there is an increased chance for costly supply shortages, obsolescence, and inefficient capability utilization.[42] Demand risk is exceptionally costly when there is a failure to manage medical staff expectations around physician preference items. The inability to manage demand risk also affects the customer relationship efforts carried out by supply chain managers. And when there is significant uncertainty about a clinician choosing a product, demand risk is firmly related to strategy risk. This is demonstrated in "Clinician, Supplier, and Buyer Working as One to Improve Patient Outcomes" (Appendix 2).

3.3.4 Implementation Risk

Hospitals are highly departmentalized organizations and frequently lack fundamental protocols to facilitate communication regarding materials that are utilized in an integrated fashion. In progressive systems, organizational redesign and increased centralization counter the risk that different departments will not collaborate. Knowledge management in the health sector provides the evidence required for clinicians and others to understand the impact of their decisions. When extended to the scrutiny of supplies, it begins to provide evidence for choice and foster the goal of value-based purchasing.[43,44,45] The value analysis process, detailed in Chapter 4, can provide critical support for the standardization and implementation of strategic programs. Artificial intelligence (AI) and machine learning (ML) have the potential for decision-makers to scrutinize product contribution to patient care and compare products based on outcomes and cost—thus reducing risk to both the organization and the ultimate client—the patient.[46] If the health sector is to capitalize on its information base adequately, continued investment and implementation in knowledge management and AI systems will be necessary.[47]

3.3.5 Cost Risk

Cost risk relates to adverse fluctuations in supply prices, potentially exceeding target budgets and impacting profitability metrics. Importantly, reimbursement rates to hospitals for supplies have not notably increased. As value-based purchasing has become more prevalent and supply expenses are part of an episode of care payment, such as diagnosis-related groups (DRG) and bundled payments, the impact of supply costs grows.[48] Notably, when reimbursement covers an entire episode of care, consideration of the quality of products and their contribution to outcomes concerning price is significant. It is not just about price! Risks associated with costs must be balanced with product performance.

It is increasingly recognized that risk management must be associated with "unusual circumstances." During COVID-19, medical supply costs hit new highs with significant price increases across various medical supplies. Between 2019 and 2021, medical supply prices increased by 46%, with much of the increase in products that were formerly considered commodities, such as surgical masks and gowns.[49] This was an essential lesson to buyers about how prices can be in flux in many unexpected ways.

It is noteworthy that supply expenses vary considerably across hospitals due to ownership, patient mix, and different goals (e.g., teaching hospitals).[50,51] The following discussion first reviews the type of costs that can be reduced and managed—purchase, transaction, and administrative costs. This is important as not all costs can be treated the same. Next, the meaning and types of supply risk and the costs associated with each risk type are reviewed. Lastly, a strategic sourcing process derived from the numerous case studies is presented and discussed in the context of cost and risk.

Purchase Costs

Purchase cost represents the price of the good or the service being acquired. By far, this is the most frequent cost mentioned by hospital supply managers. It is common for managers to refer to cost when only considering the purchase price. The other types of costs, including total delivered costs and total cost of ownership, discussed in some detail later, are only sidebar conversations by many managers in discussions of their roles in pricing strategies and risk reduction. However, more progressive supply chain managers differentiate among the types of costs when making supply chain decisions.

Transaction Costs

Transaction cost[52] is incurred with the exchange of goods between the buyer and seller.[53] Transaction costs include costs associated with the search for vendors, bargaining/negotiating, contracting, and compliance. And like purchase price, transaction costs can fluctuate and carry risks. Because transaction cost is much more challenging to measure than purchase price, it is less frequently mentioned or included in annual supply management goals and infrequently monitored as part of the cost of ownership. A goal of any purchasing organization is to reduce such costs. Transaction costs range from high-cost efforts by staff to manually prepare and transmit an order instead of low-cost electronic ordering to costs associated with purchasing partner fees and commissions (e.g., distributors) and the monitoring of order fulfillment. An essential aspect of risk management is the avoidance of transaction cost risks. Technologies can be deployed to manage transaction costs.

Blockchain is a good example of a technology (Chapter 9), which can be employed to track prescription drug routing and allow wholesalers of pharmaceutical companies to increase information sharing to improve patient safety. The time spent assessing such products adds to the cost of the secured supplies. Such costs can be averted with track-and-trace technology to certify the authenticity of products. During the COVID-19 pandemic, many previously unknown suppliers of products offered off-brand personal equipment such as masks to healthcare systems. Supply chain managers were challenged to vet the authenticity of products. Lacking were technology applications, especially for high-value/high-impact items, to:

- Track supply shipments in real-time;
- Assess utilization/demand;
- Support inventory management;
- Minimize transportation costs;

- Identify issues faster along the supply chain; and
- Reduce ordering, receiving, and processing errors.[54]

Firms that work together over long periods develop trust and can frequently reduce transaction costs by developing inter-organizational mechanisms for reducing conflict and adapting to each other's cultures.[55] As discussed throughout this book, selecting highly effective purchasing partners represents an important process in reducing the price paid for goods, potential costs associated with ownership of goods over time, and value-adding services received from suppliers.

Administrative Costs

Administrative cost is the internal cost incurred by the buyer for such items as accounts payable and receivables and the costs of typical errors in these processes. Many administrative costs are affected by the hospital's or system's direct transactions. This cost is also problematic to measure, so quantifying the cost and assessing its risks is challenging.

Prices for goods and services are frequently attributable to contracts negotiated by GPOs for their members and by health systems, with pricing based on the level of committed spending on a supplier's product. Hospitals and hospital systems have variability in meeting contractual price targets. Large systems are characterized by different degrees of independence of each hospital to comply with preferences.[56] Progressive systems have strategies to reduce implementation risk through product standardization to gain commitment. However, managing the preferences of physicians and other clinicians and gaining commitment from clinicians remains a challenge.[57] "Clinician, Supplier, and Buyer Working as One to Improve Patient Outcomes" (Appendix 2) demonstrates how multiple parties can support supply chain management in cost-related risk reduction to meet organizational goals.

In the most progressive systems, supply chain executives identify risk management as an essential, if not defining, characteristic of their job. Perhaps this should be no surprise as the metrics associated with cost frequently constitute how they are evaluated. And while cost reduction may be a principal value-added outcome emanating from a purchasing department, there are other value-added consequences, such as increases in the value of a product for an internal customer. Further cost-related consequences of purchasing include cost avoidance, the reduction or elimination of a future cost as the result of contractually agreed-on reductions in price in the future.[58] Side Bar 3.1 provides a list of actions that can lead to cost savings and cost avoidance.[59] "Best Practices within the Context of Non-governmental Fully Integrated Supply Chain Organization (FISCO)" (Appendix 1) include (a) the presence of formal and cross-functional risk assessment processes and mitigation programs;

Side Bar 3.1

Cost Savings versus Cost Avoidance

Cost Savings

- Reduced Baseline Appropriation—A reduction in available resources based on targeted cuts in certain areas.
- Reduction from Budgeted Spend—A reduction in the projected/budgeted resources (e.g., staff time, materials, and equipment) used for an activity or business process, as a result of a Savings Project.
- Volume Reductions—Reducing the amount of a good or service used. Savings captured in this category include projects that intentionally seek volume reductions through direct action (e.g., demand management).
- Refunds/Credits/Rebates—Payments made to the state by vendors as a result of a Savings Project.
- New Revenue—New streams of revenue payors, and so on.
- Enhanced Reimbursement—Improvements in the accuracy or completeness of a business process that generates a higher rate of recovery of funds from external organizations. This activity may be generally associated with business process re-engineering.

Cost Avoidance

- Cost Avoidance—A cost reduction opportunity that results from an intentional action, negotiation, or intervention.
- Procurement Cost Avoidance—A cost reduction opportunity that is generated from the competitive bidding process.
- Negotiated Cost Avoidance—An avoided cost as a result of the issuance of Best and Final Offers, Sole-Source negotiations, or post-procurement/post-award negotiations.
- In-Contract Cost Avoidance—A cost reduction opportunity produced as a result of the intervention of a purchasing official in responding to contractor requests for increases in prices, market fluctuations, indices' upward alterations, etc. or Rate Reductions—Obtaining lower rates or prices for purchased goods or services.

Source: National Association of State Procurement Officials. (2007, Sept.) Benchmarking cost savings and cost avoidance. Research Brief.

(b) collaboration with supply chain partners; (c) continuous improvement of SCRM programs; and (d) the presence of risk metrics in scorecards, and the alignment of risk management with the organization's objectives and embedded in the organization's culture.

3.4 Response and Resilience to Risks

Two equally important aspects of SCRM, and much brought to the forefront during the COVID-19 pandemic, are supply chain response and resilience, especially in the face of disruptions. Yossi Sheffi[60] has identified the critical aspects of risk-related resilience as a network of suppliers, lower-tier suppliers, and service providers. To be considered in the assessment of products are:

- The parts that go into a company's products;
- The identities of the networks of suppliers that make those parts;
- The locations where parts and products are made, assembled, and distributed;
- The flows of parts and products (including the transportation links that move materials, information, and cash); and
- The inventories of materials, parts, and finished goods stored or being handled in various stages of the chain.

Whereas resilience strongly focuses on the prophylactic measures taken by a supply chain to avoid disruption and/or minimize the impacts, response relies on capacity and quick recovery, attributes highly aligned to the ideas of flexibility and agility.[61] Supply chain response is the "capacity of the organization to successfully react to a disturbing event while keeping the continuity of the supply chain flow."[62] Notably, the disruptions in the manufacturing and transport of personal protective equipment (PPE), much of which is manufactured in Asia, brought U.S. healthcare systems face-to-face with global supply chain risks.[63]

3.4.1 Mitigating Risks

A research team at Arizona State University (ASU)[64,65] summarized the steps associated with SCRM, including:

1. *Risk identification.* Discovery of all relevant risks that can influence an enterprise's operations (e.g., natural disasters, sabotage, supplier production problems, or quality defects).
2. *Risk assessment.* Estimating the probability of occurrence and severity of impact for the relevant risks identified in Step 1 and prioritizing such risks according to the enterprise's risk tolerance.

The impact on patients and staff (e.g., the potential for injury or death) is important for healthcare provision and the likelihood of postponing needed procedures. Risk assessment is also attentive to monetary loss, damage to the environment, and time to recover.

3. *Risk management.* Identifying and developing strategies to reduce the probability or severity of the risks. Risk management includes risk acceptance, avoidance, transfer, or mitigation. In the health sector, risk management is frequently carried out by GPOs and distributors who serve as intermediaries for sourcing, contracting, and monitoring the supply chain environment.

4. *Risk monitoring.* Evaluation of the efficacy of the risk-management strategies developed in Step 3. Identification of improvement opportunities and updating the SCRM process. This can also involve identifying opportunities for improvement and updating the SCRM plan based on changes in regulations, suppliers, or processes and performance evaluation.

3.4.2 Reducing Risk Through Technology

Over the last decade, there have been major advances in purchasing automation (Chapter 9). These include cloud-based systems that catalog and categorize products, automate the procure-to-pay (P2P) process, manage inventory, document product receipts, and automate payments. A feature of these systems is the redundancy reduction in the procure-to-pay process. Such systems increasingly utilize ML and AI to support not just the transactional aspects of ordering and fulfillment but also the revenue cycle management process and integration of processes. Using automation reduces risk by identifying and decreasing purchasing backlogs, providing accuracy in inventory management, and supporting the management of supplies through to the point of care. Automatic replenishment systems prevent over- or understocking to support Periodic Automatic Replenishment (PAR) levels, determined by calculating weekly inventory use and safety stock/deliveries per week.

While one would think that such automation dominates the industry, a survey by Cardinal in 2016 revealed that:[66]

- 78% manually count inventory in some parts of their supply chain, and only 17% have implemented an automated technology system to track inventory in real-time.
- Frontline clinicians spend an average of 17% of their workweek dealing with inventory—taking valuable time away from patients.

While one would hope that insight into supply presence would have significantly increased, the inadequacy of inventory systems was revealed in the early days of the COVID-19 pandemic as hospitals had little knowledge of inventory levels for PPE and their locations. Automation in the supply chain has a solid relationship with reducing risks to the patient and the organization. A 2017 survey by Cardinal Health, the large distributor, revealed that:[67]

- 40% of the respondents canceled cases due to missing supplies;
- 69% delayed cases; and
- 27% heard of an expired product being used on a patient.

3.5 Chapter Summary

This chapter considers potential risks in the healthcare supply chain and provides a strategic sourcing model observed in several integrated delivery networks (IDNs) to manage risks and reduce costs. Excellence in managing risk depends on balancing *"downward cost pressures and the need for efficiency with effective means to manage market-driven service requirements and the known risks of routine supply chain failures."*[68] Risk management is critical to achieving a FISCO organization. Industry best practices, as identified in FISCO (Appendix 1), are critical, including:

- Providing information to end users in formats that are conducive to efficient tracking of products—including serial numbers, lot numbers, and/or unique identification;
- Having a "full court press" with a focus on a broad range of supply disruptions. The feed for such information is frequently a commercially available technology;
- Utilizing ML/AI for early identification of defective products;
- Utilize third-party provider to engage in the monitoring and providing alerts regarding disruptions due to natural disasters and other events by providing supply node; and
- Mapping, event monitoring, supplier monitoring.

It is important for managers to assess how the various strategies can be applied to manage and buffer different types of risk (Exhibit 3.4). Strategy risk can be buffered and averted by systematically and rigorously implementing the seven steps of the sourcing and market analysis processes discussed in Chapter 5. Many managers also indicate that cross-functional teams and value analysis teams significantly help manage demand risk, as discussed in Chapter 4. Risk is also averted by developing effective information systems and engaging purchasing partners who comprehensively understand supply and demand. Managers are required to learn from a broad base group of clients about the factors contributing to and providing relief from risk. Supplier analysis, inventory analysis, and outstanding operational staff provide necessary buffers for averting implementation risk.

Concern for managing risk is heightened in the post–COVID-19 environment, where there was a recognition of the inadequacy of ongoing management strategies for dealing with significant periods of uncertainty.[69] While a number of states have taken on some risk strategies related to disruptions, such as requiring multi-month inventories and pools for supply backup, these raise new questions for provider organizations about the cost and management of implementing and sustaining such mandates. In short, risk management is an ever-present concern across FISCO functions and a defining attribute of health sector supply management as a business role impacting care delivery and organizational sustainability.

Notes

1. McConnell, K. J., Lindrooth, R. C., Wholey, D. R., Maddox, T. M., & Bloom, N. (2013). Management practices and the quality of care in cardiac units. *JAMA Internal Medicine, 173*(8), 684–692.
2. Smeltzer, L. R., & Sifred, S. (1998). Proactive supply management: The management of risk. *International Journal of Purchasing and Materials Management* Winter, *34*(1), 38–45.
3. Schneller, E. ASU-MEDLOG. (2019, June). Recommendations for defense medical logistics in the context of a Fully Integrated Supply Chain Organization (FISCO). Report presented as ASU-MEDLOG Project, submitted to Advanced Technology International, Summerville, SC. Under Contract Number: W81XWH-15-9-0001
4. Ho, W., Zheng, T., Yildiz, H., & Talluri, S. (2015). Supply chain risk management: A literature review. *International Journal of Production Research, 53*(16), 5031–5069.
5. Zsidisin, G. A. (2003). A grounded definition of supply risk. *Journal of Purchasing and Supply Management, 9*(5–6), 217–224.
6. Villena, V. H., & Gioia, D. A. (2020). A more sustainable supply chain. *Harvard Business Review, 98*(2), 84–93.
7. Young, R.D. Knowledge management in supply, Business Briefing, Pharmatech p. 4,
8. U.S. Government Accountability Office. (2014, Feb.). Drug shortages: Public health threat continues, despite efforts to help ensure product availability. Retrieved April 20, 2019, from https://www.gao.gov/products/GAO-14-194
9. Abdulsalam, Y., & Schneller, E. (2019). Hospital supply expenses: An important ingredient in health services research. *Medical Care Research and Review, 76*(2), 240–252.

10. Definitive Healthcare. (2022, April). Annual changes in hospital supply costs. `https://www.definitivehc.com/resources/ healthcare-insights/changes-in-supply-costs-year-to- year#:~:text=Total%20supply%20expense%20averages%20over% 20%2430%20million&text=Between%202016%20and%202020%2C% 20total,are%20%2430%20million%20per%20hospital`

11. Ibid.

12. American Hospital Association. (2022, April). Massive growth in expenses * Rising inflation fuel financial challenges for America's hospitals & health systems. `https://www.aha.org/system/files/media/ file/2022/04/2022-Hospital-Expenses-Increase-Report- One-Pager.pdf`

13. Hung, S., Kannan, V., Malhotra, B., & Kahn, A. (2020). *Future-proofing supply chain management: Building resilience and agility through digital transformation.* Everest Global, Inc. `https://www.capgemini.com/ wp-content/uploads/2021/10/Everest_Group_Future-proofing_ Supply_Chain_Management.pdf`

14. Resilinc. EventWatch data and analysis: Factory fire. chrome-extension:// efaidnbmnnnibpcajpcglclefindmkaj/`https://resource.resilinc .com/rs/863-OTG-034/images/white-papers-reports-factory- fires-the-top-supply-chain-disruption.pdf`

15. Resilinc. Resilinc annual report 2020. Carpe Diem. chrome-extension:// efaidnbmnnnibpcajpcglclefindmkaj/`https://resource.resilinc.com/ rs/863-OTG-034/images/Resilinc_2020_Annual_Supply_Chain_ Risk_Report.pdf`

16. See, for example, Event Watch that continually streams data on disruptions at `https://www.everstream.ai/ppc-2021-supply-chain-risk- report/?utm_medium=ppc&utm_source=google&utm_campaign= competitor&gclid=Cj0KCQjws4aKBhDPARIsAIWH0JW8QX7p13TgWYMK gYVitb8tvbBDbpaI2GQ_GKV5qOsiJEgTkHlBuAQaAmXGEALw_wcB`

17. Bovit, J and Vaikil, B. (2020, April 230. COVID-19 pandemic: Adapting to supply chain's new normal, 5th (series of conference calls. Resilinc at `http://Resilinc.com`; Interos at `http://interos.com` and Supply Wisdom at `http://supplywisdom.com`

18. U.S. Government Accountability Office. (2014, Feb.). *Drug shortages: Public health threat continues, despite efforts to help ensure product availability.* Retrieved April 20, 2019, from `https://www.gao.gov/products/ GAO-14-194`

19. Hung, S., op. cit.

20. Zsidisin, G. A., & Ellram, L. M. (2003). An agency theory investigation of supply risk management. *The Journal of Supply Chain Management, 39*(3), 15–29.

21. Sheffi, Y. (2005). *The resilient enterprise: Overcoming vulnerability for competitive advantage.* MIT Press Books.

22. Eddy. N. (2022). Healthcare breach costs hit record high. Healthcare IT News website. HIMMS. Healthcare IT News July 27. `https://www.healthcareitnews .com/news/healthcare-breach-costs-hit-record-high?mkt_tok =NDIwLVlOQS0yOTIAAAGF99IhHbpfzmdRPdt1PMwS7xGPZNnp75D`

f3J9sgD_Soi0uJnA–ngpZCUm2u43yyKjVIKGH1QPFvYfPPfhC3y6lnSoFI
0XKxmDprMDdUzU

23. U.S. Food and Drug Administration. Data Dashboard. (2020). https://
    datadashboard.fda.gov/ora/cd/recalls.htm
24. Clouse, M. and Busch, J. (2003). How to identify and manage
    supply risk. October. http://www.supplychainplanet.com/
    e_article000195015.cfm
25. Bonezone Editors. (2022, Jan. 25). Orthopedic FDA 510 (k)s: A look at 2021
    Clearances. https://bonezonepub.com/2022/01/25/orthopedic-
    fda-510ks-a-look-at-2021-clearances
26. Abdulsalam, Y. J., & Schneller, E. S. (2021). Of barriers and bridges: Buyer-
    supplier relationships in health care. *Health Care Management Review*,
    46(4), 358–366.
27. Iqbal, J., Gunn, J., & Serruys, P. W. (2013). Coronary stents: Historical
    development, current status and future directions. *British Medical Bulletin*,
    106(1), 193–211. https://doi.org/10.1093/bmb/ldt009
28. Tang, L., et al. (2019). The number of stents was an independent risk
    of stent restenosis in patients undergoing percutaneous coronary inter-
    vention. *Medicine, 98*(50), e18312. http://dx.doi.org/10.1097/
    MD.0000000000018312
29. Ketcham, J. D., & Furukawa, M. F. (2008). Hospital-physician gainsharing
    in cardiology. *Health Affairs, 27*(3), 803–812.
30. Stankiewscz, M. (2018). Researchers back outcomes-based payments for
    medical devices as industry braces for a shift. Fierce Healthcare web-
    site. Fierce Healthcare. Retrieved November 7, 2022, from https://www
    .fiercehealthcare.com/payer/value-based-payment-way-future-
    for-device-makers
31. Conrad, D. A. (2015). The theory of value-based payment incentives and
    their application to health care. *Health Services Research, 50*, 2057–2089.
32. Miller, H. D. (2009). From volume to value: Better ways to pay for health
    care. *Health Affairs, 28*(5), 1418–1428.
33. Rana, A. J., & Bozic, K. J. (2015). Bundled payments in orthopaedics.
    Clinical Orthopaedics and Related Research, 473(2), 422–425.
34. Khouzam, R. N., Dahiya, R., & Schwartz, R. (2010). A heart with 67 stents.
    Journal of the American College of Cardiology, 56(19), 1605 http://
    dx.doi.org/10.1016/j.jacc.2010.02.0771605. https://www
    .jacc.org/doi/abs/10.1016/j.jacc.2010.02.077
35. Carter, C. R., Rogers, D. S., & Choi, T. Y. (2015). Toward the theory of the
    supply chain. *Journal of Supply Chain Management, 51*(2), 89–97.
36. Dennision, R., Kathawala, Y., & Elmuti, D. (1993). Just-in-time: Implica-
    tions for the hospital industry. *Journal of Hospital Marketing, 8*(1), 131–141.
37. Wysocki, B., & Lueck, S. (2006). *Wall Street Journal.*
38. Sodhi, M., & Choi, T. (2022). Don't abandon your just-in-time supply
    chain, revamp it. *Harvard Business Review.* https://hbr.org/2022/10/
    dont-abandon-your-just-in-time-supply-chain-revamp-it
39. Barocas, J., Gounder, C., & Madad, S. (2021). Just-in-time versus just-in-case
    pandemic preparedness. *Health Affairs.* Blog https://www.healthaf-
    fairs.org/do/10.1377/hblog20210208.534836/full

40. Harris, J., Ozgen, H., & Ozcan, Y. (2000). Do mergers enhance the performance of hospital efficiency? *Journal of the Operational Research Society, 51*(7), 801–811.

41. Burns, L. R., Housman, M. G., Booth, R. E., Jr., & Koenig, A. (2009). Implant vendors and hospitals: Competing influences over product choice by orthopedic surgeons. *Health Care Management Review, 34*(1), 2–18.

42. Mäkimattila, J. (2022). Supply base strategies and supply chain resilience driven by COVID-19 [Master's Thesis, Lappeenranta-Lahti University of Technology].

43. Medium. (2016, Oct. 24). How to use knowledge management in the healthcare industry. https://medium.com/@itsquiz15/how-to-use-knowledge-management-in-the-healthcare-industry-8d2749722f30

44. Collins, J. D., Worthington, W. J., Reyes, P. M., & Romero, M. (2010). Knowledge management, supply chain technologies, and firm performance. *Management Research Review, 33*(10), 947–960. https://doi.org/10.1108/01409171011083969

45. Young, op. cit.

46. Kumar, A., Mani, V., Jain, V., Gupta, H., & Venkatesh, V. G. (2023). Managing healthcare supply chain through artificial intelligence (AI): A study of critical success factors. *Computers & Industrial Engineering, 175*, 108815.

47. Dogru, A. K., & Keskin, B. B. (2020). AI in operations management: Applications, challenges and opportunities. *Journal of Data, Information and Management, 2*(2), 67–74.

48. Navathe, A. S., Troxel, A. B., Liao, J. M., Nan, N., Zhu, J., Zhong, W., & Emanuel, E. J. (2017). Cost of joint replacement using bundled payment models. *JAMA Internal Medicine, 177*(2), 214–222.

49. Gist Healthcare. (2022, March). Medical supply costs hit new highs amid supply chain disruptions. https://gisthealthcare.com/medical-supply-costs-hit-new-highs-amid-supply-chain-disruptions%EF%BF%BC/

50. Abdulsalam & Schneller, op. cit.

51. Stinson, Kenneth. (2019). Healthcare Group Purchasing Organizations: Who's really saving? An empirical investigation of hospital characteristics that influence supply expense for healthcare GPO members." [Dissertation, Georgia State University]. https://scholarworks.gsu.edu/bus_admin_diss/117

52. Coase, R. H. (1937). The nature of the firm. *Economica, 4*(16), 386–405. In Kronman, and Posner (eds). *The Economics of Contract Law*, Boston: Little Brown, 1979, pp. 31–32

53. Williamson, O. E. (1979). Transaction-cost economics: The governance of contractual relations. *Journal of Law and Economics, 22*(2), 233–261; Williamson, O. E. "Contract Analysis: The Transaction Cost Approach." In Burrows and Veljanovski (eds.). *The Economic Approach to Law*. London: Butterworths, 1981, pp. 39–60

54. Gaynor, M., Tuttle-Newhall, J., Parker, J., Patel, A., & Tang, C. (2020). Adoption of blockchain in health care. *Journal of Medical Internet Research*,

22(9), e17423. http://dx.doi.org/10.2196/17423. PMID: 32940618; PMCID: PMC7530694

55. Tsang, E. W. K. (2000). Transaction cost and resource-based explanations of joint ventures: A comparison and synthesis. *Organization Studies*, *21*(1), 215–242.

56. Abdulsalam, Y., Gopalakrishnan, M., Maltz, A., & Schneller, E. (2018). The impact of physician-hospital integration on hospital supply management. *Journal of Operations Management*, *57*, 11–22.

57. Ibid.

58. Nollet, J., Calvi, R., Audet, E., & Côté, M. (2008). When excessive cost savings measurement drowns the objectives. *Journal of Purchasing and Supply Management*, *14*(2), 125–135.

59. National Association of State Procurement Officials. Benchmarking cost savings and cost avoidance. Research Brief, September 2007. https://www.naspo.org/wp-content/uploads/2019/12/Benchmarking_Cost_Savings__and_Cost_Avoidance.pdf

60. Sheffi, Y. (2015). *The power of resilience: How the best companies manage the unexpected.* MIT Press.

61. Frederico, G. F., Kumar, V., & Garza-Reyes, J. A. (2021). Impact of the strategic sourcing process on the supply chain response to the COVID-19 effects. Business Process Management Journal, *27*(6), 1775–1803. https://doi.org/10.1108/BPMJ-01-2021-0050

62. Ibid.

63. Ibid.

64. Schneller, E. (2022). Best practices within the context of non-governmental Fully Integrated Supply Chain Organization (FISCO).

65. Polyviou, M., Ramos, G., & Schneller, E. (2022). Supply chain risk management: An enterprise view and a survey of methods. In Y. Khojasteh, H. Xu, & S. Zolfaghari (Eds.), *Supply chain risk mitigation. International series in operations research & management science* (Vol. 332). Springer. https://doi.org/10.1007/978-3-031-09183-4_2

66. Cardinal Health. 2016, Nov. 4). The biggest untapped resource at your hospital? Your supply chain. [Study fielded Oct. 19.]. https://www.cardinalhealth.com/en/essential-insights/the-biggest-untapped-resource-at-your-hospital--your-supply-chai.html

67. Cardinal Health. (2017). Survey finds hospital staff report better supply chain management leads to better quality of care and supports patient safety. https://newsroom.cardinalhealth.com/2017-02-15-Survey-Finds-Hospital-Staff-Report-Better-Supply-Chain-Management-Leads-to-Better-Quality-of-Care-and-Supports-Patient-Safety#assets_all

68. Christopher, M., & Peck, H. (2004). Building the resilient supply chain. *International Journal of Logistics Management*, *15*(2), 1–13.

69. Polyviou et al., op. cit.

4 Product Preference, Standardization, Value, and Clinical Integration— *You Can't Just Buy Anything*

4.1 Introduction

Standardization has long been a defining attribute for increased quality and cost containment across industries, especially where high reliability is sought. Variability, in both processes and outcomes, has characterized the health sector, where the autonomy of clinicians has frequently been put ahead of a systematic assessment of best practices.

Standardization of processes,[1] products,[2] data,[3] and communications[4] are critical for the existence of a high-performing healthcare system, one that moves healthcare delivery from a cottage industry to post-industrial care.[5] In the health sector, standardization is an important goal associated with the comparative effectiveness of therapeutic processes and products used in care delivery.

In general, product standardization entails developing and implementing acceptability standards based on the consensus of all stakeholders. Ultimately, it is the test of market suitability for a product. We have many examples of the usage of such acceptability standards, including the infamous "Good Housekeeping Seal of Approval,"[6] which designates a product is "assessed to perform as intended." The U.S. Food and Drug Administration (FDA) does this to some extent when determining whether a product is safe and effective for a specific indication. However, the FDA does not distinguish between equivalent products.

When sourcing the best products for patient care, hospitals, health systems, and clinicians must understand if products deliver the same, equivalent, or varying outcomes. Answering this question is key to managing the proliferation of similar products that may yield the same, equivalent, or varying medical outcomes. Unfortunately, a lack of evidence, especially regarding new technology, and a clinician's preference for a particular product (or manufacturer) can make it difficult to reach a consensus among the various players, including clinicians and procurement specialists. Too often, such preference has been tolerated, even when not justified.

Supply chain managers point to a variety of challenges resulting from a lack of standardization, including:

- Added complexity managing multiple products used for the same purpose;
- Need for additional training on product use;
- The potential for medical errors due to unfamiliarity with products;
- Limited ability to receive volume-based discounts in contracts;
- Reduced service levels from suppliers due to limited market share; and
- Additional costs for sourcing, ordering, and storing multiple products in the same category.[7]

Product standardization efforts for both new and existing products are intended to reduce these challenges and generate several positive outcomes for the healthcare system, including:

- Assurance that the most appropriate products are deployed in clinical practice;
- An optimal number of products sourced and kept in inventory based on both clinical and financial needs; and
- Increased leverage when negotiating contracts with suppliers.

With the move to more value-based healthcare systems worldwide, procurement leaders are increasingly tasked with sourcing products and services that meet clinical requirements while also considering the fiscal realities of healthcare delivery organizations, payors, and patients. Many of the strategies aimed at cost containment have existed for decades. At the same time, some approaches are being reworked and expanded to meet the demands of policymakers, purchasers, and consumers for better value for their healthcare dollars spent (as measured in factors including but not limited to quality and affordability).

Even before the passage of the Affordable Care Act (ACA), the American Recovery and Reinvestment Act of 2009 highlighted the importance of comparing the effectiveness of different therapeutic treatments. The legislation established the Patient-Centered Outcomes Research Institute (PCORI), which provides funding to support "the generation and synthesis of evidence that compares the benefits and harms of alternative methods to prevent, diagnose, treat, and monitor a clinical condition or improve the delivery of care."[8] PCORI's laudable goal has been to identify therapeutic options with the best health outcomes. From a supply chain perspective, the public-private partnership focused more on care processes than the products used in care delivery, even though some contribute significantly to the overall cost of care and reimbursement. As a result, the effort has generated little evidence for product evaluation and comparison.

Another challenge for medical devices is the relative lack of evidence generated from clinical trials prior to market approval compared to pharmaceutical products. With a drug, it is relatively easy to conduct randomized clinical trials in which subjects are assigned to groups with relatively similar patient populations, each given a different (and sometimes placebo) medicine to study what works best. With drug trials, several thousand people are ultimately involved in the research before the FDA or other regulators approve a product. It is far more difficult with medical devices, such as implantable devices, given the often-invasive nature of product use. As such, the FDA often allows medical devices to go through a less onerous approval process, whereby the manufacturer "*conducts comparative testing to predicate devices to demonstrate that a new device is substantially equivalent to the predicate.*"[9] In general, the number of patients involved in research prior to the approval of a medical device is far fewer than in pharmaceutical clinical trials. As such, the FDA and other regulators are increasingly interested in real-world evidence (RWE) as to how a product performs in routine clinical practice in order to identify any potential safety issues and to support future regulatory reviews for new approved uses and/or further iterations and innovations based on the existing product.[10] To support RWE generation, the FDA supported the creation of the National Evaluation System for health Technology (NEST) to "*more efficiently generate better evidence for medical device evaluation and regulatory decision-making.*"[11] More on NEST and the value of RWE later in this chapter.

This chapter also explores the role of value analysis committees (VACs), frequently referred to as value analysis teams (VATs), which seek to limit the proliferation of products in the same category, and their evolving relationship with clinicians as hospitals and healthcare systems move toward a more clinically integrated supply chain. We also review in detail a fundamental concept used widely in other industries, the total cost of ownership (TCO), which has only recently begun to be applied to healthcare sourcing decisions. And finally, we consider how, in the wake of the global pandemic, VATs are being asked to consider other factors when sourcing products, from supply chain resiliency to the environmental and health equity consequences of their sourcing decisions.

4.2 From Cost Analysis to Value Analysis

4.2.1 Defining Value Analysis

One of the most commonly practiced and effective procurement strategies employed by supply chain professionals is value analysis. Value analysis is an associated set of processes that can be traced back to practices first developed in response to shortages in raw materials and other components during World War II. The concept of Value Engineering (sometimes also called value analysis) was developed by General Electric engineers who were forced to look for substitutes when the part or material traditionally used was unavailable. They discovered that many of these substitute products resulted in lower total production costs, better quality, or both.[12] This is analogous to how clinical and supply chain leaders were forced to work together to find alternatives in the wake of critical shortages during the COVID-19 pandemic. In some cases, they were able to identify new products and new suppliers. Most importantly, they fostered new ways to collaborate to respond more quickly and simultaneously achieve their respective and common goals.

While value engineering is focused on finding alternative raw materials and components to support the production of a finished product, value analysis in healthcare procurement provides a systematic approach to evaluating and selecting products and services based on their ability to produce both clinically and fiscally acceptable results. Value analysis is foundational for the Cost, Quality, Outcomes Movement efforts described in Chapter 1. Without information on a product's contribution to patient care, the ability to select the best product to achieve optimal clinical and financial outcomes will be limited.

Value analysis (although not always referenced as such at the time) was first championed by healthcare supply chain consultants in the late 1970s and early 1980s to address rising hospital costs.[13] In just eight years after the passage of the law creating the Medicare and Medicaid system to cover healthcare costs for the elderly and the poor, national health expenditures had more than doubled. Hospital costs represented nearly 60% of total public outlays in 1972, and there was a growing recognition that a primary driver of rising hospital expenditures was advancements in medical technology and increased physician use of more sophisticated, higher-cost, and (presumed to be) more effective products.[14] Healthcare consultants at the time noted how changing reimbursement models, most notably the mid-1980s introduction of diagnostic-related groups (DRGs), a global episode of care payment to cover hospital stays (including most supplies), was a leading cost driver. These moves required supply chain professionals to adopt more robust cost containment practices like value analysis.

Before introducing value analysis, internal hospital committees evaluated products and services primarily from a cost-containment lens. The evolution of VATs represented an expansion of their work to include an interdisciplinary approach, especially regarding product use and performance.

Product selection and standardization are important FISCO functions, with mature organizations having well-established working groups that evaluate the impact of products on patient outcomes and link supplies to clinical pathways. Thus, a more extensive discussion of these two FISCO functions is warranted.

4.2.2 Product Selection and Standardization

The primary focus of early value analysis initiatives was product standardization (reducing the number of products or suppliers used for the same purpose) to negotiate better pricing with vendors in exchange for larger volume commitments. Despite these efforts, hospital expenditures and supplies have continued to climb.[15] The financing structure of the U.S. healthcare system under a fee-for-service model has made it difficult to control costs, as it creates incentives for hospitals and physicians (who influence the demand for care) to perform more services.[16,17]

Product standardization has remained a primary approach taken by most value analysis programs.[18] For many, the process is viewed as a "supply base reduction" exercise, whereby the number of active suppliers in the supply base is reduced to leverage better value from relationships. Product standardization has also begun to attract more clinician interest, given its ability to reduce unwarranted variation in clinical practice (including the products used) and, in turn, medical errors.[19,20]

Variation in supplies across a hospital or health system also adds complexity and workload for staff. The supply chain must manage more stock-keeping units (SKUs). At the same time, clinicians, especially nurses, must understand the differences between devices used for the same purpose and the different preferences of the physicians they support.[22] For this reason, nurses have been among the longest and most ardent supporters of value analysis.

The endurance of value analysis as a procurement standard of practice can be attributed to its relatively consistent ability to achieve savings without negatively impacting the quality of care. These savings have been achieved across multiple product types, from low-cost, high-volume products, such as sutures and gloves, to high-dollar implants that can account for a significant portion of the reimbursement paid for the procedures in which they are used. Side Bar 4.1 provides an overview of the factors that drive success in value analysis programs. Product categories most frequently considered by VATs include commodity medical supplies, reusable surgical supplies, high- and mid-cost preference devices, and drug-device items.[21]

New product introductions (NPI) are a primary function of VATs, given the continued and accelerated advancements in medical technology and the impact of acquiring new and more expensive devices on supply expense reduction efforts.[23] Most health systems have some level of centralized approach by which they consider a request (usually from a physician) to acquire a new product by first evaluating how it compares to the products already in use and the anticipated impacts on both costs and quality of care.

In addition to considering NPIs, VATs review the appropriateness of existing products. However, managing the multitude of reviews can be overwhelming, given the thousands of medical devices used in hospital settings and the thousands more approved by the FDA each year.[24] Policies are established to manage the extent and frequency of such reviews to balance time and resources.

Early value analysis pioneers encouraged greater involvement by physicians, given that doctors are responsible for 75–85% of the quality and cost decisions made in healthcare delivery.[25] Significant progress has been made in recent years in this area, judging by the increase in physicians participating not only on VATs[26] but also serving as supply chain medical directors.[27] Involvement by doctors, nurses, and other allied clinical professionals is also the foundation for the concept of a clinically integrated supply chain, which expands on many of the principles of value analysis and is discussed further in this chapter.

Side Bar 4.1

Value Analysis Success Factors

As with most things in healthcare, there is considerable variation in how individual health systems and hospitals structure and operate their VATs and initiatives, but there are a number of factors common to the most successful programs.

1. **Framework**
   a. Objective and evidence-based
   b. Systems-based, with attention paid to the upstream and downstream implications of the decisions made, for example,
      i. Will training be required on the new product?
      ii. Will the existing product need to be consumed and/ or disposed?
      iii. Are there implications for compliance with contracts for the existing product?
      iv. Are there guidelines for when the new product should or should not be used, for example, only in high-risk cases?

2. **People—Multidisciplinary:**
   a. Executive and clinical champions—The visible support of these champions validates the importance of the program while also helping ensure the adoption of the choices made by VATs.
   b. Key functional leaders/representatives from the following:
      i. Finance
      ii. Supply chain (including purchasing, contracting, inventory management)
      iii. Medical and Nursing staff
      iv. Respected clinical (physician and nursing) experts
      v. Service lines
      vi. Procedural areas, for example, OR/Cath Lab/Interventional Radiology
      vii. Infection Control
   c. Analytical support staff

3. **Process**
   a. Objectives of the program and specific initiatives are clearly outlined and communicated
   b. The process is transparent and communicated
   c. Decisions are communicated broadly
   d. The parties responsible for the implementation of decisions made are identified and supported
   e. The results of changes made are monitored both for compliance and realization of anticipated benefit

4.2.3 Evidence-driven Decision-making

Despite the progress, some physicians have remained reluctant to support product standardization for fear of losing clinical autonomy.[28,29] Medical quality experts have sought to overcome this resistance by highlighting how unwarranted variation in clinical practice leads to inappropriate care and significant waste in healthcare delivery, raising prices, reducing affordability, and too often causing patient harm and even death.[30] The solution has been to use clinical evidence to continually develop and revise best practice protocols as new information is acquired. Physicians, fearful of being relegated to following "cookbook medicine," are reminded that while they should standardize practice according to the latest clinical evidence, they can and should always be able to modify care processes when individual patient conditions warrant. Unfortunately, it is extremely difficult for even the most highly trained and educated physician to stay abreast of the latest evidence, given it is continually being updated, sometimes reversing what was considered to be best practice in the past.[31] In the absence of such information, physicians will often revert to what they know best, for example, a practice and product they first began using in medical school or upon which a preferred medical device manufacturer has trained them.

It is noteworthy that VATs are most challenged in the area of what has been termed "physician preference items (PPIs)," which most often include devices used in orthopedics, spine, and cardiology, and can have high variation in pricing despite equivalent outcomes.[32] When devices are purchased from various suppliers, hospitals and health systems have difficulty consolidating spending to achieve volume discounts and reduce clinical variation.

Given the high costs of PPIs, such as hip, knee, and spine implants, there are a variety of approaches to expense management. Some of the most common are listed in Side Bar 4.2.

A critical role for value analysis professionals is helping provide evidence to physicians and other clinicians to support their evaluation of the performance of various product options and how and when they should be used. For these reasons, value analysis professionals emphasize the importance of evidence in decision-making, as noted in the definition of value analysis espoused by the Association of Value Analysis Professionals (AHVAP):[33]

> *Healthcare value analysis contributes to optimal patient outcomes through an evidenced-based systematic approach to review healthcare products, equipment, technology, and services. Using recognized optimal practices to collaborate with organizational resources to evaluate appropriate utilization, clinical efficacy, and safety issues for optimal financial value.*

Side Bar 4.2

Modes of Reducing PPI Costs

- Standardizing devices in a hospital/IDN to facilitate better procurement terms;
- Setting cost savings targets for a given period of time and/or by clinical specialty (e.g., the spine unit is asked to meet specific cost savings in their procurement of PPI);
- Setting payment caps to items (e.g., spend up to a specific amount for specific devices);
- Reducing PPI inventory levels, including centralized distribution of PPI and closer collaboration with vendors/distributors on inventory management;
- Reducing approved PPI vendors, thereby reducing variations in PPIs in a hospital/IDN and monitoring of exceptions (i.e., requiring authorization to use devices not on approved lists or available through approved vendors);
- Developing closer working relationships with vendors/group purchasing organizations (GPOs) to drive costs down, including greater PPI price transparency and contract restrictions;
- Instituting greater accountability for item procurement and usage, including elaborate tracking of item utilization and costs generally or by specialty;
- Removing or reducing contact with PPI sales reps (for example, adopting a "repless" system where product sales reps are not allowed in operating rooms and/or have reduced interactions with physicians);
- Instituting systems in which cost savings from PPI procurement are shared with clinical unit/service lines that generate the savings; and
- Streamlining procurement processes, including training on Lean Six Sigma with greater supply chain personnel involvement in PPI procurement.

Adopted from Nyaga & Schneller.[20]

There are myriad sources for clinical evidence, from pre-market studies to peer-reviewed literature, with a growing business segment in healthcare comprised of companies that aggregate and evaluate the quality of such evidence, considering factors such as the methodology, potentially biased funding sources, and the size and diversity of the "n" to help ensure statistical significance and generalizability.

To support the work of the NEST and others to generate RWE, the FDA and its counterparts in the global regulatory community have introduced regulations requiring manufacturers to assign unique device identifiers (UDIs) to unambiguously identify their products through distribution and use.[34] As the director of the U.S. Centers for Devices and Radiological Health, Jeffrey Shuren, MD, JD, explained: "*By promoting the incorporation of UDIs into electronic health information, a vast quantity of untapped real-world data from clinical experience with devices housed in electronic health records (EHRs) and other electronic information sources may become available for use in understanding the benefit-risk profiles of medical devices.*"[35]

The generation of RWE depends upon the combined ability of healthcare supply chain, clinical, and technology leaders to ensure the data on products used in patient care can be accurately captured to support analysis of how the products contribute to quality care at an affordable price. Supply chain professionals are often in the best position to build the business case to support the necessary investments in people, process, and technology, as this data is needed for other activities, from meeting regulatory requirements around the use of EHRs to business functions such as charge capture and maintaining supply contract compliance. Aligning data on what products were used and in what quantities with other clinical and financial performance data, such as infection rates, length of stay, and so on, can help debunk beliefs that a higher price product always delivers better quality care or that a lower-cost product is always inferior. It is important to link specific products with performance and utilization data. For example, a product may have a lower per-unit price, but if you need to use more units to achieve the same results as a more expensive product, savings may be elusive, if not impossible, to achieve. Beyond price, supply chain professionals should consider a product's total cost of ownership (TCO), representing the entirety of costs incurred over the time the organization owns it. TCO is reviewed following a further discussion of the physician's role in value analysis.

4.3 The Physician's Role in Value Analysis

Reducing unwarranted variation in care processes to achieve more predictable and quality outcomes has become a key opportunity for supply chain and value analysis leaders to engage with physicians. Physicians are uniquely positioned in the supply chain between the administrative purchases and the patients, who are the ultimate beneficiaries of the purchased products. In this frame, the physician's role is akin to that of a restaurant chef who chooses the raw ingredients that go into the dishes, a professor who selects the textbooks for students to buy and study from, or an engineer who sources the most appropriate materials and equipment for a construction project. Physicians often act as "independent and detached experts with admitting privileges." Still, their expertise gives them greater influence over hospital management regarding patient care and, in turn, the ability to shape patient demand and drive revenue.[36] Hence, the physician acts as an informed agent and broker between the hospital and the patient, a role referred to in the academic literature as the surrogate buyer (or surrogate consumer in the marketing lexicon).

Surrogate buyers intervene on behalf of the ultimate consumer by researching and evaluating alternatives and entering into contracts for specific products or services. A need for a surrogate buyer arises when the consumer (in this case, the patient) has low shopping motivation or knowledge, combined with high perceived risk.

Exhibit 4.1 summarizes the more traditional triadic relationship among hospitals, independent physicians, and medical device manufacturers[37] under a fee-for-service model. It is worth adding that more value-based payment methodologies are shifting this dynamic, and with significant numbers of previously independent physicians becoming hospital employees.[38]

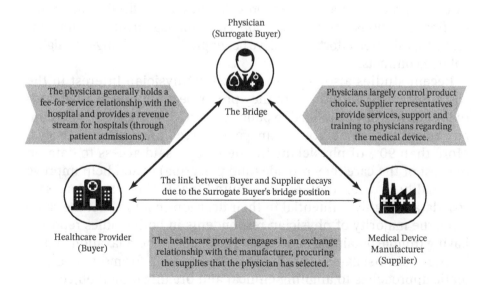

Exhibit 4.1: The professional service triad in healthcare purchasing.

Source: Abdulsalam, Y. J., & Schneller, E. S. (2021). Of barriers and bridges: Buyer–supplier relationships in health care. *Health Care Management Review, 46*(4), 358–366.

Under a fee for service model, with physicians acting as agents of the consumer but also with their own set of incentives and motives, reservations have been raised regarding their credibility and impartiality. Sometimes surrogate buyers have vested interests in selecting products that contribute to them personally. Arrangements between physicians and medical device manufacturers have also influenced physician judgment. This skepticism, further fueled by inappropriate decisions made by some physicians, led to legislative intervention outlining tighter boundaries and greater transparency of physician-manufacturer arrangements in the ACA, Section 6002, labeled the Sunshine Act.[39]

One of the objectives of value-based healthcare is to increase the alignment of incentives for hospitals and physicians, focusing on their respective abilities to deliver value to patients in the form of affordable quality care. Physicians can support this work by understanding where there is unwarranted variation and how to standardize based on what delivers the best quality outcomes with the most efficient use of resources. In such engagements, supply chain professionals assume the role of informed support teams that provide data on what products are being used, by which physicians, on which kinds of patients, and how that information relates to respective quality and cost outcomes such as procedural time, supply utilization, complication and infection rates, and length of stay. Armed with this data, physicians can identify the best pathways (including but not limited to supply usage) and create more alignment across the medical staff in adopting those protocols. In these cases, supply chain management provides the data. Still, clinicians make the final selections after which supply chain management can capitalize on standardization efforts to achieve better pricing in exchange for higher volume contracts.

Recent studies also point to a growing physician interest in the costs associated with the care they prescribe and provide. Such attitude changes may be related to policy changes that tie physician reimbursement to their ability to manage resource utilization effectively.[40] More than 90% of physicians in one study[41] said access to data on the cost of the care they provide (and prescribe) would help improve the quality of care. Another study found that 60% of physicians said cost data is highly influential in their decision-making.[42] At the same time, the majority of physician respondents in both studies reported having trouble obtaining or accessing such data. The relaxation of prohibitions against gainsharing[43] laid the foundation for more programmatic approaches to aligning clinical and organizational objectives, which have since been expanded through co-management[44] and other physician engagement initiatives.

4.4 Total Cost of Ownership

TCO is a process by which all the estimated expenses associated with purchasing, deploying, using, and retiring a product or piece of equipment are estimated. Although it has been practiced in other industries, it has only recently been used in healthcare organizations when sourcing the products or capital assets necessary to support healthcare operations.[45] Costs associated with products (particularly medical devices) include the time and resources required for sourcing, contracting, procuring, and receiving, as well as training, service, maintenance, and disposal. Capital assets have additional costs incurred for installation, connectivity to technology systems, ongoing operation, consumable supplies, and space requirements. TCO forces organizations to think beyond acquisition price to consider various activities and resources associated with the ownership of a particular product or piece of equipment and analyze what increases ownership costs and delivers the most value for money.[46] In more simple terms, it takes the focus off of price alone.

In healthcare, TCO is most frequently employed in decisions regarding capital assets, such as diagnostic imaging, biomedical equipment, and laboratory instrumentation, and higher-priced medical devices, such as ventilators.[47] TCO seeks to identify and quantify all the people-, process-, and tool-related expenses needed to operate and maintain equipment and instruments for various departments to help healthcare organizations make more informed business decisions on new purchases and dispositions based on both financial and non-financial factors. Frequently ignored are the human resources associated with product utilization. A TCO assessment for MRI scanners, from acquisition to decommissioning, included "installation costs; site modifications to comply with safety requirements; human resources including ancillary personnel; small equipment, supplies, contrast media; service contracts; IT; overhead; and upgrades." Human resources were the highest expense among them all.[48]

Disruption and failure risks should also be accounted for in an item's TCO. Disruption costs arise from inadequate product management processes and policies, poor reliability and performance, and compromised product efficiency, among others.[49] Such costs can make the purchase price of a good appear trivial. As organizations seek to standardize products that deliver value over time, the TCO process is an important adjunct to the value analysis processes discussed above. Side Bar 4.3 considers the TCO of ventilators used in intensive care units a capital asset critical to patient life. A ventilator's cost is heavily skewed toward maintenance and service support compared to the acquisition price.

Side Bar 4.3

Accounting for the Full Cost of Intensive Care Ventilators

Because intensive care ventilators entail ongoing maintenance and operational costs, the initial acquisition cost does not accurately reflect the TCO. Therefore, a purchase decision should be based on issues such as TCO, local service support, discount rates, nonprice-related benefits offered by the supplier, and standardization with existing equipment in the department or hospital (i.e., purchasing all ventilators from one supplier).

Hospitals should evaluate how they plan to use the ventilator; in particular, the decision to use disposable or reusable breathing circuits will affect the cost of operation. Hospitals can purchase service contracts or services on a time-and-materials basis from the supplier. Service may also be available from a third-party organization. The decision to purchase a service contract should be carefully considered. Purchasing a service contract ensures that preventive maintenance will be performed at regular intervals, thereby eliminating the possibility of unexpected maintenance costs. Also, many suppliers do not extend system performance and uptime guarantees beyond the length of the warranty unless the system is covered by a service contract. To maximize bargaining leverage, ECRI Institute recommends that hospitals negotiate pricing for service contracts before the system is purchased. Additional service contract discounts may be negotiable for multiple-year agreements or for service contracts that are bundled with contracts on other similar equipment in the department or hospital.

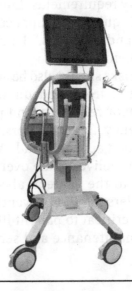

Notably, TCO is not just applicable to medical devices and capital assets. TCO is a concept that should be more frequently included in purchasing decisions, clinical or otherwise, where purchasing implications transcend price.

For example, when considering basic office equipment, Steelcase an office furniture company, suggests the following cost factors as necessary in measuring the TCO:[50]

- planning and design;
- selection process and purchasing activities;
- delivery and installation;
- orientation and training;
- movement of management and reconfiguration;
- refurbishing maintenance; and
- disposal.

Side Bar 4.4 depicts a methodical and disciplined view of the TCO that can be applied by supply chain managers to a variety of products associated with the healthcare delivery environment.

A focus on the total cost of ownership and its impact on the furniture configurations and the workplace does not exist in isolation. No company can be successful by focusing only on cost and the impact of this factor on the work environment.

As companies get a clearer picture of the true costs of ownership, businesses will also be focusing on issues such as:

- Financing alternatives: the new strategies being developed to more effectively leverage company investments in facilities and furnishings, creating an even more integrated approach to linking the workplace to business success;
- Organizational shape: the new structures, management styles, team patterns, and work culture and their collective impact in creating a new set of needs for the workplace; and
- Health and safety: the collection of issues that affect the safety, health, and comfort of the workplace and the impact of those issues on workplace design. A holistic integration of these and any other relevant workplace factors will ensure that a new approach to designing and furnishing the workplace will create a more effective place for people to work and companies to succeed.

4.5 The Vendor's Role in Value

Much debate persists about the role of medical device manufacturers and the potential conflicts of interest with regard to the value

Side Bar 4.4

Total Cost of Ownership

. . .it's possible that in identifying the total cost of ownership, a company may discover that a low-cost product may carry significant management costs. In this scenario, a company's most significant savings might be in streamlining management of the product in the workplace rather than trying to simply procure the product at a lower price. Or another strategy may involve selecting a different product that carries lower management costs. In this last option, a product whose purchase price is higher might actually offer a lower TCO.

A comprehensive understanding of the TCO is critical for leveraging the return on your company's investment in workplace furniture and furnishings.

Digital Equipment's Swedish operation in Stockholm redesigned their office for maximum flexibility. The redesign has produced a 50% reduction in space use, a 50% decline in energy consumption, a 60% decline in cleaning costs, and more highly motivated employees" (Personnel Management, Aug. 1993).

Exhibit 4.2 attempts to depict the allocation of the cost of ownership elements based on overall industry experiences. This is an illustration of how new views of lifecycle costs may affect the business impact of the workplace.

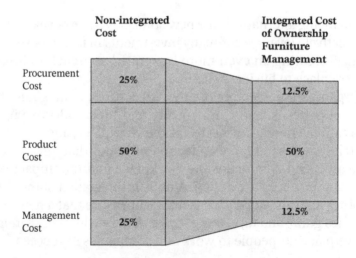

Exhibit 4.2: Cost saving of 25% from integrating cost of ownership.

Source: Schneller, E. S., & Smeltzer, L. R. (2006). Strategic management of the health care supply chain. Jossey-Bass.

they provide and the extent of their input and involvement in value analysis efforts and research. Supplier representatives, who are often part of the firm's sales force, are frequently deployed by their employers to work within hospitals to provide clinical support and education for their products, manage consigned inventory, and in the case of surgical items, provide support and coaching during the procedure. Many believe their presence can create multiple forms of risk, including "upselling" (switching the clinician to a more expensive product at the point of care)—all leading to an escalation in costs.[51] Policies often restrict such activities, with some hospitals refusing to pay for any products not already under contract, while others have banned supplier representatives from the operating theater or otherwise limited their access. Physicians, meanwhile, often value the product expertise and experience possessed by representatives and believe their presence is valuable.[52] To address this need, hospitals are increasingly utilizing technology, such as the use of web-based video services, to allow for physician-supplier engagement but in a more controlled manner.

Healthcare systems have recognized both the risks and values associated with supplier representatives.[53] There has been little research providing an understanding of how hospitals and surgeons define, recognize, and authorize appropriate supplier competencies and input.[54] To the extent that supplier representatives support both high-volume implant surgeons as well as those who do relatively few cases, it is possible that the role of suppliers may be overvalued in some cases and undervalued in others. While supplier representatives can bring critical knowledge to the operating theater, research has shown that their presence in coronary stent procedures has led to the implantation of a more significant number of stents than when such representatives are absent.[55]

A final issue related to supplier representatives is vendor credentialing, a process driven by government regulations[56] with additional requirements and standards established by The Joint Commission, the Association of PeriOperative Registered Nurses, the American College of Surgeons, and the Centers for Disease Control and Prevention. Credentialing covers the supplier organization, to help ensure it is financially sound, appropriately licensed, and not on any regulatory watchlists. Other aspects of credentialing consider the requirements of the representatives themselves, including their level of training and education, as well as whether they have had all necessary vaccinations and do not have a criminal or other compromising background.[57] While some healthcare systems may develop their own credentialing program, most outsource credentialing to commercial vendors.

4.6 The Clinically Integrated Supply Chain

As previously mentioned, many of the fundamentals of value analysis—from process to purpose—are inherent in what is referred to as the clinically integrated supply chain. The Association for Healthcare Resource & Materials Management defines it as "*an interdisciplinary partnership to deliver patient care with the highest value (high quality, best outcomes, and minimal waste at the lowest cost of care) that is achieved through assimilation and coordination of clinical and supply chain knowledge, data, and leadership toward care across the continuum that is safe, timely, evidence-based, efficient, equitable, and patient-focused.*"[58] Exhibit 4.3 provides a simple road map toward a clinically integrated supply chain.

Like value analysis, many of the earliest efforts around clinical integration, especially those supported by GPOs, focused on product standardization, both for cost savings and quality improvements stemming from a reduction in variation. Exhibit 4.3 provides a simple road map toward a clinically integrated supply chain.

More recently, clinical integration maturity models have considered the ability to capture data on products used in patient care to improve patient safety through better visibility of adverse events and to generate RWE on product performance. The result is not only lower costs but also better outcomes that, in turn, drive higher revenues under value-based

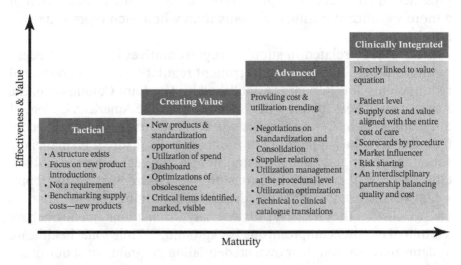

Exhibit 4.3: A maturity model for clinical integration.
Source: Stanford Health.

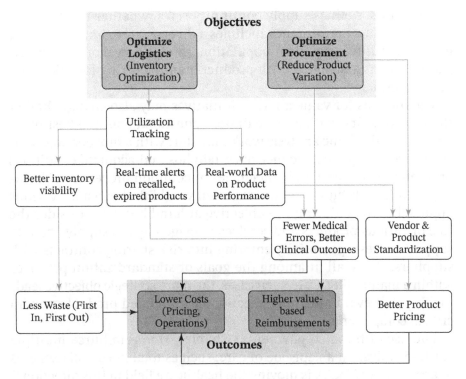

Exhibit 4.4: Clinically integrated supply chain value flow chart.

purchasing. Exhibit 4.4 depicts these multiple approaches and how they support both savings and quality.[59]

4.7 The Future of Value Analysis

From its inception, value analysis has been product-centered, often starting with a request to acquire and utilize a new product, with the quality and affordability of patient care guiding decision-making. As previously discussed, value analysis exists at various levels of maturity within healthcare systems. With the continued evolution toward a more value-based healthcare system (one that supports the creation of health, not just the provision of sick care), value analysis and supply chain professionals are aligning more with higher-level system objectives. This includes addressing major issues impacting both the healthcare system and society as a whole, such as reducing health disparities among socially and economically disadvantaged populations and reducing the environmental impact of healthcare operations. In the future, while cost and quality will remain the most important criteria for decision-making, value analysis professionals may also consider other factors, such as supply continuity risks, whether the evidence around product performance includes a diverse "n" to understand the efficacy for different patient populations, and the level of greenhouse gas emissions associated with product manufacturing logistics, use, and disposal.

The impetus for value analysis initiatives may also change. Rather than starting first with a more limited question about the best products to use, the value analysis work may start with a broader objective, such as reducing the incidence of certain hospital-acquired conditions or improving the cost and efficiencies of common procedures. This is depicted in Exhibit 4.5. Decisions then would first consider various approaches to achieving the objective at hand but also consider the role of various products and services managed by the supply chain to support success, potentially entering into risk sharing contracts with suppliers. These all fit among the goals of standardization practices within a mature FISCO. In such cases, the more strategic objective leads the way, but evaluation and selection of associated products remain critical components.

The use of bundled payments (Chapter 3) to reimburse multiple parties involved in an episode of care, such as total knee replacements or arthroplasty (TKA), is moving the healthcare field in this direction.[60] Together, participating organizations, which as an example can include the surgeon, the hospital, and a post-acute care facility, have a shared interest in not only the quality of care, but also the ability to control supply costs, some of which can represent a high percentage of the total reimbursement shared among the respective providers. As better data, including RWE, becomes more available, VATs can expand their focus beyond equivalent product alternatives to consider the contribution of

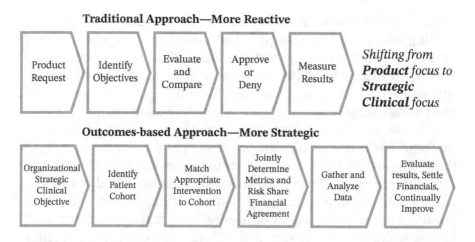

Exhibit 4.5: Value analysis—A more strategic approach.

products to the cost and quality of the total episode of care. Indeed, the lessons from TCO also apply. Along the way, value analysis and clinical-supply chain integration will assume increasingly important roles in achieving not just supply chain goals but also the strategic objectives of healthcare delivery organizations as well as the healthcare system as a whole.

Notes

1. Swensen, S. J., Meyer, G. S., Nelson, E. C., Hunt, G. C., Pryor, D. B., Weissberg, J. I., Kaplan, G. S., Daley, J., Yates, G. R., Chassin, M. R., James, B. C., & Berwick, D. M. (2010). Cottage industry to postindustrial care—The revolution in health care delivery. *New England Journal of Medicine, 362*(5), e12.
2. Montgomery, K., & Schneller, E. S. (2007). Hospitals' strategies for orchestrating selection of physician preference items. *The Milbank Quarterly, 85*(2), 307–335..
3. Wilson, N. A., & Drozda, J. (2013). Value of unique device identification in the digital health infrastructure. *JAMA, 309*(20), 2107–2108.
4. Vardaman, J. M., Cornell, P., Gondo, M. B., Amis, J. M., Townsend-Gervis, M., & Thetford, C. (2012). Beyond communication: The role of standardized protocols in a changing health care environment. *Health Care Management Review, 37*(1), 88–97.
5. Swensen, et. al., op cit.
6. Good Housekeeping. (2022) How the GH Limited Warranty Seal protects uou. Good Housekeeping website. Retrieved October 26, 2002, from https://www.goodhousekeeping.com/institute/about-the-institute/a22148/about-good-housekeeping-seal
7. Schneller, E. (2022). Best practices within the context of non-governmental Fully Integrated Supply Chain Organization (FISCO).
8. Chandra, A., Jena, A. B., & Skinner, J. S. (2011). The pragmatist's guide to comparative effectiveness research. *Journal of Economic Perspectives, 25*(2), 27–46.
9. U.S. Food and Drug Administration. Statement from FDA Commissioner Scott Gottlieb, M.D., on how modern predicates can promote innovation and advance safety and effectiveness of medical devices that use 510(k). Retrieved May 20, 2023, from https://www.fda.gov/news-events/press-announcements/statement-fda-commissioner-scott-gottlieb-md-how-modern-predicates-can-promote-innovation-and
10. U.S. Food and Drug Administration. (2021, March 16). Leveraging real world evidence in regulatory submissions of medical devices. U.S. FDA website. Retrieved October 29, 2022, from https://www.fda.gov/news-events/fda-voices/leveraging-real-world-evidence-regulatory-submissions-medical-devices
11. US Food and Drug Administration. National Evaluation System for Health Technology (NEST). U.S. FDA Website. Retrieved October 29, 2022, from

    https://www.fda.gov/about-fda/cdrh-reports/national-evaluation-system-health-technology-nest

12. Corporate Finance Institute (CFI Team). Value engineering: What is value engineering. https://corporatefinanceinstitute.com/resources/knowledge/strategy/value-engineering; https://www.mcgill.ca/ve/history

13. McFaul, W. J., & Lyons, D. M. (1983). Supply cost management: A new frontier. *Hospital Purchasing Management*, *8*(2), 10–12.

14. National Health Expenditures, 1929–1972. https://www.ssa.gov/policy/docs/ssb/v36n1/v36n1p3.pdf

15. Kurani, Nisha, Jared Ortaliza, Emma Wager, Lucas Fox, & Krutika Amin. (2022). How has U.S. spending on healthcare changed over time?" Peterson-KFF Health System Tracker (blog). Retrieved September 26, 2022, from https://www.healthsystemtracker.org/chart-collection/u-s-spending-healthcare-changed-time

16. https://www.cbo.gov/sites/default/files/cbofiles/ftpdocs/76xx/doc7665/91-cbo-001.pdf

17. Perl, J. R., Sheth, K. R., Shea, K. G., & Wall, J. (2021). Hospital value committees: The role of the surgeon in new technology adoption. *Surgical Innovation*, *28*(4), 401–402.

18. Survey and Report on Hospital Value Analysis. (2021). Greenlight Medical. https://insights.greenlightmedical.com/state-hospital-value-analysis.

19. Andel, C., Davidow, S. L., Hollander, M., & Moreno, D. A. (2012). The economics of healthcare quality and medical errors. *Journal of Health Care Finance*, *39*(1), 39–50..

20. Kumar, S., & Steinebach, M. (2008). Eliminating US hospital medical errors. *International Journal of Health Care Quality Assurance*, *21*(5), 444–471. https://doi.org/10.1108/09526860810890431

21. Lane E. Value Analysis Committees: What they are and why they exist. Advisory Board Company. May 2, 2021. https://www.advisory.com/topics/life-sciences/2021/05/value-analysis-committees

22. Creating value through strong partnerships in a clinically integrated supply. (2021). AHVAP Conference presentation.

23. Krantz, H., Strain, B., & Torewski, J. (2017). Medical device innovation and the value analysis process. *Surgery*, *162*(3), 471–476.

24. Darrow, J. J., Avorn, J., & Kesselheim, A. S. (2021). FDA regulation and approval of medical devices: 1976–2020. *JAMA*, *326*(5), 420–432.

25. Lumere presentation. (2019). AHVAP Conference.

26. Montgomery et al., op. cit.

27. Perl, op. cit.

28. Montgomery et. al., op. cit.

29. Nyaga, G., & Schneller E. (2018, October). Physician Preference Items Management: Challenges, opportunities and strategies. CAPS Research. https://www.capsresearch.org/media/2335/2018-10-01_physician_preference_items_management_challenges_opportunities_and_strategies.pdf

30. Lean Healthcare. (2022). 6 methodologies for improvement from Dr. Brent James. Retrieved June 16, 2022, from https://www.healthcatalyst.com/wp-content/uploads/2021/05/Lean-Healthcare-6-Methodologies-for-Improvement-from-Dr.-Brent-James.pdf

31. Laiteerapong, N., & Huang, E. S. (2015, 2015). The pace of change in medical practice and health policy: Collision or coexistence? *Journal of General Internal Medicine*, *30*(6), 848–852. http://dx.doi.org/10.1007/s11606-015-3182-0. Epub 2015 Jan 22. PMID: 25608743; PMCID: PMC4441682

32. Nyaga, & Schneller, op. cit.

33. Association of Healthcare Value Analysis Professionals. Creating exceptional value in healthcare. https://ahvap.memberclicks.net/overview (accessed April 19, 2023).

34. Federal Register. (2013, Sept. 24) Unique Device Identification System: A Rule by the Food and Drug Administration. https://www.federalregister.gov/documents/2013/09/24/2013-23059/unique-device-identification-system

35. Shuren, J., M. D., J. D. (2015, April 28) Statement before the Committee on Health, Education, Labor and Pensions. http://www.help.senate.gov/imo/media/doc/Shuren3.pdf

36. Nyaga, & Schneller, op. cit.

37. Abdulsalam, Y. J., & Schneller, E. S. (2021). Of barriers and bridges: Buyer–supplier relationships in health care. *Health Care Management Review*, *46*(4), 358–366.

38. Dydra, L. (2021). 70% of physicians are now employed by hospitals or corporations. *Becker's ASC Review*. https://www.beckersasc.com/asc-transactions-and-valuation-issues/70-of-physicians-are-now-employed-by-hospitals-or-corporations.html

39. The Patient Protection and Affordable Care Act. (2010).

40. Khullar, D., Bond, A. M., Qian, Y., O'Donnell, E., Gans, D. N., & Casalino, L. P. (2021). Physician practice leaders' perceptions of Medicare's Merit-Based Incentive Payment System (MIPS). *Journal of General Internal Medicine*, *36*(12), 3752–3758.

41. Falk S, Cherf J, Schulz J, & Huo A. (2019, Jan. 23). Cost and outcomes in value-based care. Physician Leadership Journal Website. Retrieved July 7, 2022, from https://www.physicianleaders.org/news/research-costs-outcomes-value-based-care

42. Deloitte Insights. Study: Volume to value-based care: Physicians willing to manage cost by lack data and tools. (2018, Oct. 11). Retrieved July 7, 2021, from https://www2.deloitte.com/insights/us/en/industry/health-care/volume-to-value-based-care.html

43. Hospital-Physician Gainsharing. (2006, March). Jones Day website. Retrieved October 29, 2022, from https://www.jonesday.com/files/Publication/66fdb136-0fa7-4b89-8ff6-003f06b27574/Presentation/PublicationAttachment/476ab65d-2da8-469b-8ca0-047cf8aa6dbd/March%20Back%20to%20Basics.pdf

44. Physician Co-management. Advisory Board website. Retrieved October 29, 2022, from https://www.idsociety.org/globalassets/idsa/

practice-management/compensation/cheat-sheet-series-hcita-
-physician-comanagement.pdf

45. Martinko, K. How understanding the total cost of ownership of your equipment or instrumentation can reduce costs, increase performance and improve workforce productivity. Thermo Fisher Scientific, Scientific Instruments Division, Madison, WI. Application note 01004. http://tools .thermofisher.com/content/sfs/brochures/D19489~.pdf

46. Ellram, L. M., & Siferd, S. P. (1993). Purchasing: The cornerstone of the total cost of ownership concept. *Journal of Business Logistics : JBL, 14*(1), 163.

47. ECRI Institute Europe. (2009/2010, Winter). Intensive care ventilators: Purchase considerations ICU, 9(4).

48. Jones, E. (2020). Total cost of ownership is a useful tool for life cycle management Abstract 4158 of MRI scanners and managing costs in an MRI department. SMRM & SMRT Virtual Conference & Exhibition, 0A08-14 August 2020 Abstract 4158.

49. Buczynski, M. (2002). Uncovering the total cost of ownership of storage management. Computer Technology Review, 45-446. https://www .thefreelibrary.com/Uncoveringthetotalcostofownershipof storagemanagement-a0110227170

50. Schneller, E. S., & Smeltzer, L. R., (2006). Strategic management of the health care supply chain. Jossey-Bass.

51. O'Connor, B., Pollner, F., & Fugh-Berman, A. (2016). Salespeople in the surgical suite: Relationships between surgeons and medical device representatives. *PLoS One, 11*(8).

52. Cleveland Clinic. (2021). Non-employee visitation and onboarding standard operating procedure. Supply Chain, Support Services and Protective Services.

53. Burns, L. R., Housman, M. G., Booth, R. E., & Koenig, A. (2009). Implant vendors and hospitals: Competing influences over product choice by orthopedic surgeons. *Health Care Management Review, 34*(1), 2–18.

54. Schneller, E. S., & Wilson, N. A. (2009). Professionalism in 21st century professional practice: Autonomy and accountability in orthopaedic surgery. *Clinical Orthopaedics and Related Research®, 467*(10), 2561–2569.

55. Sudarsky, D., Charania, J., Inman, A., D'Alfonso, S., & Lavi, S. (2013). The impact of industry representative's visits on utilization of coronary stents. *American Heart Journal, 166*(2), 258–265.

56. U.S. Department of Health and Human Services. (2013, May 8). Office of Inspector General. Effect of exclusion from participation in federal health care programs. https://oig.hhs.gov/exclusions/files/ sab-05092013.pdf

57. Smartsheet. (2021, Aug. 17). Get started with vendor credentialing in healthcare. https://www.smartsheet.com/hospital-vendor-credentialing

58. Association for Health Care Resource & Materials Management (AHRMM). (2018). Cost quality and outcomes. https://www.ahrmm.org/resource-repository-ahrmm/2018-ahrmm-cost-quality-and-outcomes-cqo-report-on-the-clinically-integrated-supply-chain-1.

59. Conway, K. (2021). The maturation of clinically integrated supply chain maturity models. *Health Purchasing News.* https://www.hpnonline.com/sourcing-logistics/article/21219040/the-maturation-of-clinically-integrated-supply-chain-maturity-models

60. Rana, A. J., & Bozic, K. J. (2015). Bundled payments in orthopaedics. *Clinical Orthopaedics and Related Research, 473*(2), 422–425.

5

Purchasing Strategies and Alliances— *Success Requires Good Partnerships*

5.1 Introduction

Supply management (sometimes loosely referred to as *procurement, sourcing,* or *purchasing*) is considered one of the three pillars of supply chain management, along with manufacturing, and logistics. The early- to mid-twentieth century brought about ample research and developments in manufacturing and logistics management, owing to innovative business models that incorporated mass production, assembly lines, automation, and other methodologies as well as military-inspired research initiatives that transformed the fields of operations management and operations research. It wasn't until later in the twentieth century that procurement received more recognition as a strategic differentiator toward organizational success. Peter Kraljic's 1983 publication in the *Harvard Business Review*, "Purchasing Must Become Supply Management," provided a paradigm shift for sourcing from a basement-level business function to a strategic one. Just as Ford Motors demonstrated how efficient manufacturing could lead to success, the 1970s and 1980s heralded many companies, such as Toyota and Walmart, that achieved competitive advantage via strategic sourcing. As seen in Chapter 3, sourcing carries many risk implications. Chapter 4 demonstrated that sourcing is also strongly associated with quality management, value, and clinical outcomes. This chapter dissects strategic sourcing by describing its core components in the health sector. Second, the sourcing environment is discussed to introduce the many essential intermediaries and models involved. Finally, the chapter provides insight into provider organizations' and suppliers' crucial relations.

Embedded within the purchasing role are the Fully Integrated Supply Chain Organization (FISCO) functions of product sourcing, product standardization, contracting, supplier relationship management (SRM), and supply chain risk management. When executed effectively, supply management ensures the organization can achieve its supply chain strategy and the broader mission for products and services. Large-scale empirical research on strategic sourcing indicates that this process can significantly impact a hospital or system's goals. Not all healthcare systems, however, capitalize on the opportunity related to cost reduction and risk management. In fact, for many years, healthcare supply management was viewed as immature and inefficient relative to other industries.[1]

Supply management in healthcare can quickly become complex. A typical hospital carries 30,000–40,000 active stock-keeping units (SKUs).[2] Product proliferation is vast, and the rate at which technologies, practices, and products evolve relative to other industries is high. To manage this complexity, healthcare systems outsource at least some sourcing activities to external parties or purchasing alliances. Purchasing alliances, commonly known as group purchasing organizations (GPOs), have become essential in the healthcare supply chain. They help hospitals lower costs, improve efficiency, and provide quality, safety, and services value. These third-party organizations deal with the affairs relating to healthcare sector purchases[3] and operate under a safe harbor from anti-trust, allowing for organizations, even if they are competing, to enter the market collaboratively.[4] The U.S. Congress has intended that GPOs could *"help reduce health care costs for the government and private sector alike by enabling a group of purchasers to obtain substantial volume discounts on the prices they are charged."*[5]

Purchasing alliances and consortia exist in other industries but are exceptionally prevalent and pivotal to the healthcare supply chain. The Healthcare Supply Chain Association (HCSA), the trade association that represents GPOs, defines a *GPO* as "*an entity that helps health care providers (such as hospitals, ambulatory care facilities, nursing homes, and home health agencies) realize saving and efficiency by aggregating purchasing volume and using that leverage to negotiate discounts with manufacturers, distributors, and other vendors.*"[6] The role and structure of GPOs continue to evolve with diverging business models and intense merger and acquisition activity among the large national GPOs. In addition, there has been a proliferation of regional GPOs associated with large integrated delivery systems and even specialty GPOs, such as Uro-GPO, servicing urology practices. Much research has been conducted to quantify the cost-savings or other benefits GPOs bring to hospitals with mixed and nuanced findings.[7] GPOs, like their counterpart for pharmaceuticals, pharmacy benefit managers (PBMs), are designed to avert a variety of market, strategy, and demand-related risks, as discussed in Chapter 3. Yet there continues to be a debate regarding the value proposition GPOs provide and whether they improve strategic supply management.[8]

The consideration of GPOs later in this chapter allows the reader to (a) understand the primary activities related to strategic supply management and how they pertain to the health sector, (b) recognize the outsourcing opportunities in this sector and major players involved, (c) understand the characteristics and history behind the different intermediaries and alliance types available to outsource to, (d) scrutinize the value that purchasing alliances contribute to hospital and system strategic supply management, and (e) project the trajectory of purchasing alliances and outsources as well as other emerging issues around this topic. Our consideration is the GPO as a principal purchasing partner. This aligns with our identification of Purchasing Partner Management (PPM) in Chapter 1 as a somewhat unique health supply chain concern. Those interested in a more in-depth assessment of GPO and PBM performance and their similarities and differences will want to consult Burn's critical review.[9]

5.2 Strategic Sourcing and Contracting

Many terms refer to supply management or parts of it: *purchasing, procurement, sourcing, contracting,* and so on. These terms are often used interchangeably in the popular press, but different labels refer to a subset of supply management activities. Let us disentangle some labels that refer to interrelated yet distinct activities. *Sourcing* is the act of identifying the organizational needs, followed by identifying sources that can fulfill those needs, whether internal or external, and leading to supplier selection. *Contracting* focuses on negotiating price and agreement terms with suppliers, tracking and amending existing agreements, and managing possible legal implications. *Procurement* is an umbrella term that covers sourcing and contracting activities. It constitutes all activities, from identifying the organizational needs to setting up the first purchase order with the selected supplier. *Purchasing* is a term used to describe the operational processes related to placing the necessary orders with suppliers, making payments, and ensuring timely and accurate delivery of supplies. More about purchasing is discussed in Chapter 6, as these processes naturally align with inventory management and replenishment processes discussed in that chapter. While sourcing and contracting generally include strategic and labor-intensive activities, automation is often sought for purchasing more repetitive processes.

The boundaries between these labels blur even further with activities touched by multiple business functions, such as managing requests for proposals (RFPs). Other processes and activities, such as supplier relationship management (SRM), are not confined to a single subcategory. Furthermore, different organizations may label and categorize their functional departments and activities differently depending on their history, industry norms, size, and so on.

To provide more coherence to the terms and activities related to supply management, a comprehensive model of supply management, derived from both academic research and consultants, is presented in Exhibit 5.1.[10] The sequential activities depicted in the model are applicable to sourcing activities carried out by a GPO or health system itself.[11] The activites include procurement activities, contracting, and SRM. Readers should be aware of the fact that entire textbooks are dedicated to detailing the procurement process, so we will suffice with a brief description of the major activities involved and how they manifest in the healthcare industry.[12]

5.2.1 Sourcing Activities

Category and Spend Analysis

A procurement strategy must be adapted to fit the nature of the supply strategy, which in the hospital industry can dramatically differ based on hospital characteristics and the population served. Products can generally be categorized based on multiple dimensions such as cost, durability, complexity and availability. To demonstrate, we consider three essential dimensions: (a) an item's reusability and durability, (b) cost, and (c) physician preference toward an item. Exhibit 5.2 illustrates the continuum

Exhibit 5.1: Procurement Activities

Supply management activity	Description
Sourcing	
Category and spend analysis	making informed decisions by knowing and managing supply and demand
Market analysis	knowing the supply market structure
Strategy development	researching and identifying strategic options
Supplier identification & analysis	knowing the product and supplier/manufacturer options
Supplier selection	the outcome decisions emanating from multiple processes, including value analysis decisions, for entering contracting
Contracting	
Cost/price analysis	the elements of the purchase price, as well as other costs of ownership
Fact-based negotiation	the process of seeking win-win outcomes in procuring a product or category
Compliance	reviewing and verifying adherence to the terms and conditions of a contract
Supplier relationship management	
Performance monitoring	Knowing how a supplier can bring value to both parties and growth in the relationship, including supplier capabilities, capacities
Buyer-supplier collaboration	collaborative strategies, including implementing continuous measurement to improve suppliers
Supplier development	Initiatives to improve supplier's performance

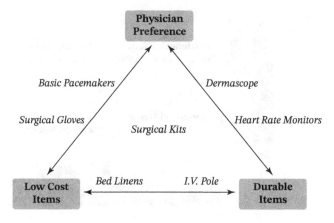

Exhibit 5.2: Categories of hospital supplies with examples.

of the categories with examples. For example, sterile surgical gloves are inexpensive, disposable goods, but are often subjected to physician preferences when considering the materials, brands, and sizes to buy. To add another layer of complexity, procurement analysts must also consider product bundles, such as surgical kits, that bundle commoditized products—such as sutures, durable scalpels, and implantable devices based on the procedure it was designed for and a particular surgeon's preferences. The complexity and divergent preferences in surgical kits have allowed distributors to carve out a market niche in customizing and selling surgical kits that cater to the needs of individual physicians. Exhibit 5.3 provides another more widely recognized framework to classify supplies on the item cost and risk (or complexity) dimensions, and it is discussed in finer detail further into the chapter.

Three levels of sophistication of spend analysis are identified: (a) spend summary, (b) category data, and (c) consolidated spend data.

- **Level 1: Spend summary**—Information on the dollar and quantity spent on specific items at individual sites. This influences buyers to develop sourcing strategies on perception rather than comprehensive fact-based summaries.
- **Level 2: Category data**—Categorical data typically classifies supplies into families of spending that offer the most significant leverage. Data on categories, such as paper and cotton goods, constitute categorical data. This level, while providing strategic direction, can also be deficient. The trouble is that a single supplier can provide multiple and different categories of goods. The consequence is that opportunities for leveraging spend, across the product groups of a supplier, may be lost. With the emergence of products that span pharmaceuticals and materials categories, such as drug-eluting stents, classification becomes even more difficult.

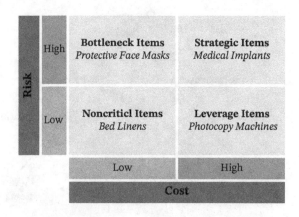

Exhibit 5.3: A framework for category management and analysis.

■ **Level 3: Consolidated spend data**—The aggregation of 100% of
the data into a single consolidated view of the spend. This level
of detail provides a clear view of spending with each supplier for
each commodity in the system at the hospital and buyer levels.

It is important to note that not all health systems have the information
systems necessary to conduct a spend analysis at Level 3. However,
even when spend analysis is at Level 1 or 2, it is still possible to use the
subsequent strategic sourcing steps on certain items. For instance, a system
might have a precise spend analysis of all hip replacements across the
four hospitals. This makes it possible to use strategic sourcing and drive
value on this particular category of items even though many other items
have poor spend visibility. Spend analysis and data aggregation may be the
foundation for supply chain improvements. Using business-to-business
(B2B) purchasing exchanges that not only automate purchasing, but also
normalize purchasing data, enables health systems to see a more comprehensive view of their purchasing to do more advanced spending and
opportunity analysis.

Category analysis requires classifying goods or services on the dimensions of risk and cost. These dimensions are portrayed in the 3x2. Kraljic
analysis (Exhibit 5.3), a standard tool in procurement, that supports a
simple yet valuable classification scheme.[13,14] In some variations to this
matrix, one axis is labeled product complexity instead of risk, and profit
impact or value is substituted for cost or spend.[15]

The products or services in each quadrant in Exhibit 5.3 require a
different sourcing strategy. Managing a low-risk, low-cost item differs
greatly from a high-cost, high-risk item. Also, the strategy will vary
depending on whether the product is a commodity, capital good, or physician preference item. Most physician preference items would likely
fit into the upper right-hand quadrant, and the subsequent purchasing
strategy would differ entirely from those in the lower left-hand quadrant.
The strategy would also differ if the hospital or health system had successfully standardized an item by gaining physician consensus to limit
the range of medical implant products. When using this framework to
develop the purchasing strategy, there are a number of common considerations for items in each quadrant:

■ **Noncritical items.** These goods require a focus on the reduction
of transaction costs. Disposable drinking cups are a good example
of such a product used throughout the hospital or system. For
these low-cost, high-volume, and noncritical items, progressive
hospitals and systems use purchasing cards, allowing vendors to
manage substantial aspects of their inventory. For highly competitive items with significant price pressure, further opportunities to

reduce price may be minimal. Outsourcing supply management and sourcing functions through purchasing partners such as GPOs and distributors can reduce transaction costs, especially for these items. Further price reductions may not justify the time that hospital and system employees would expend, hoping for minimal returns.

Intuition may tell many managers that low-cost, low-risk items do not justify their time and attention. However, some considerations may lead managers to engage the market to reduce costs for the system. Besides sourcing such items through GPOs or distributors, a reverse auction can be used. A reverse auction is an "*online, real-time dynamic auction between a buying organization and a group of pre-qualified suppliers who compete against each other to win the business to supply goods or services that have clearly defined specifications for design, quantity, quality, delivery, and related terms and conditions.*"[16] Ample supply chain research has examined reverse auctions to understand the risks and value they provide under various conditions and contexts.[17]

- **Leverage items.** A typical strategy in this quadrant is first standardizing products across divisions and then aggregating the purchase. In this manner, the entire system can have one contract for a product. Developing leverage in the marketplace for high-cost, low-complexity products is important. This applies to both clinical as well as administrative items. For example, a large health system used this approach for photocopy machines. It found that it was spending over $2.5 million per annum with four suppliers of photocopy machines. When it was standardized across hospitals so that the system used only one type of machine, it reduced the total cost by 20%. Short-term contracts may also be used to remain flexible as prices or costs change. At the same time, it is also important to actively analyze the supply base to identify new suppliers.
- **Bottleneck items.** Low-cost yet critical goods frequently lend themselves to long-term contracts. Common surgical instruments or simple implantable devices, such as a bare metal stent or a cochlear implant, fall into this category. In this instance, it is efficient to source via a purchasing alliance contract without much questioning price, given that product availability is generally more important. This strategy ensures the presence of supplies and reduces the need to develop new sources for goods, thus reducing transaction costs. The COVID-19 pandemic demonstrated how shortages in some low-cost items, such as PPE, can prevent clinicians from safely serving patients.

■ **Critical items.** This strategy requires a sophisticated supply effort on a long-term basis. This is a multifaceted situation because the market is complex, and the product's value is high. Health systems develop strategic partnerships with external entities to manage such goods while integrating clinicians for their judgment and buy-in. In progressive systems, value analysis teams are often formed to analyze categories of critical items and come to a consensus regarding the most suitable options for the hospital to buy. Effective teams bring together procurement analysts and clinicians who work to gain the thoughts, and eventually the buy-in, from fellow clinicians.[18]

Market Analysis

Market analysis determines the supply market structure, forces, and trends to determine how to best purchase items from the market. First, markets may be classified in complexity based on the number of suppliers in a given market structure, the presence of unique versus standardized/commoditized products, and new versus changing versus established technologies. It is essential to know the fundamental market structure—perfect competition, imperfect competition, oligopoly, or monopoly—to determine how much power the hospital or system ("the buyer") has in influencing pricing. For instance, in a near *monopoly*, where one supplier dominates the market for an item or category, the buyer has little power to influence pricing. Highly specialized capital equipment, such as a gamma camera, may represent this market structure. The buyer may be on a waiting list to receive the capital item. Conversely, in a *perfect* or *imperfect market structure*, many suppliers may exist, so it may be possible to have a greater influence on the market price, as is the case with items such as bedding, gauze, and gloves. Such markets are much easier to buy from as they have many suppliers, stable products, and mature technologies. An *oligopoly,* a market with very few suppliers, can exist with pharmaceuticals with patent-protected products. Although only a few competitors may exist initially in specific categories, patent expirations can introduce generic drugs, transforming the market into an imperfect competition market that drives prices downward. All-in-all, the buyer usually has little power in markets characterized by few suppliers, nonstandardized products, and new technology.

A major aspect of market analysis is to determine market trends. Possible trends include changes in price, cost, current and emerging technology, potential new entrants in the market, or possible company consolidation. However, it is difficult and costly to track all market trends. Many analytics tools have been developed to assist this task: driving insights from large amounts of decentralized data. Health systems rely on their clinicians/practitioners or external supply chain partners for intelligence. Publications, consultants, and purchasing partners, such as GPOs and companies that analyze evidence on efficacy, also provide important information for such decision-making. Sometimes advanced analytics techniques are applied (utilization, pricing, forecasts, etc.) to extract insights and predictions. Other times, market information is obtained by consulting colleagues and clinicians who are believed to have a good feel for the market. Even in the age of artificial intelligence (AI) and powerful computing, communication and interpersonal relationships among supply chain stakeholders remain an important source of intelligence, especially for fast-changing items with limited data to systematically analyze.

Strategy Development

After the product's cost and risk are analyzed, the market is studied to determine its complexity in terms of market structure, forces, and trends. These analyses then lead to the appropriate strategy for sourcing the product. No organization can be strategic with every supply item purchased and must consider what goals to pursue, including:

- A focus on negotiating better prices;
- Procuring the latest innovations; and
- Consideration of supplier reliability.

In addition to the preceding considerations, the organization needs to gauge its capabilities and recognize when to insource or outsource products and services. The alternatives here represent a broad spectrum of possibilities. For example, some progressive health systems utilize Consolidated Service Centers (CSCs) to manufacture and distribute specific categories of items.[19] Chapter 6 discusses CSCs in the inventory management and distribution context. The extent to which a hospital or system decides to outsource some of the sourcing activities to a GPO or distributor is also an important decision that carries many implications not only to the strategy, but also to present many risk implications. Other considerations may include *sole-sourcing* versus *multi-sourcing*, *near-sourcing* versus *global sourcing*, degree of automation via product data standardization and electronic data interchange.

An abundance of research and guidance continues to be published regarding strategy in supply management. The *Sage Handbook for Strategic Supply Management*,[20] a textbook co-authored by one of the authors of this book (Eugene Schneller), provides a rigorous and theoretical perspective of strategic supply management. Other outlets, such as the *Harvard Business Review*, provide more accessible articles that synthesize the more recent research in supply management strategy.[21]

Established trade journals also provide contemporary developments in the field, but are generally less theoretically rigorous.

Supplier Analysis

A critical step in the strategic sourcing process is identifying, qualifying, and selecting potential suppliers. Supplier analysis moves the focus from the product to the market and finally to the supplier. Before it is possible to identify suppliers, it is first necessary to clearly articulate the required specifications. In the case of services such as specialized temporary labor, this is the development of a statement of work (SOW), or the specification statement for products. Completing this step requires extensive deliberation by a cross-functional team to ensure that clinical and business perspectives are considered.

The supplier identification stage often starts during market analysis. While reviewing the market, more than likely, the major suppliers in an industry are identified. Supply management professionals use many sources to identify potential suppliers, such as internet sites, catalogs, industry associations, and even discussions with competitors. After identifying the potential pool of suppliers, it is necessary to determine the best supplier(s) and qualify them to determine if they can meet the health organization's needs.

Numerous dimensions must be considered when analyzing potential (and current) suppliers. Some transactional considerations are price, production capacity, size, location, and logistical capabilities. Beyond these dimensions, systems and hospitals consider strategic suppliers that can grow with the system and share mutual success. A supplier's capacity to innovate, research intensity, willingness to invest dedicated resources for the system, and commitment to sustainable practices are considerations for establishing long-term collaborative partnerships.[22] How a prospective supplier fits within the existing supply base of a system is also a consideration that has received more attention in the literature recently, which connects back to concepts of risk and resilience that isdiscussed in Chapter 3.[23] Increasingly, buyers are carefully considering a supplier's various manufacturing locations as well as the locations of the supplier's suppliers. This knowledge enables sourcing and contracting teams to manage supply disruptions caused by local or regional events effectively.

Supplier Selection

With all the aforementioned analyses in mind and having negotiated terms and conditions, hospitals and systems have enough information to select an adequate supplier.[24] Often, a balanced scorecard approach (Chapter 7) is used to apply weights to the various dimensions of the product, price, and supplier.[25] Risks should also be factored into the supplier selection decision. Even if the product's price and features excel in the market, hospitals may choose a less desired alternative if the manufacturer of the said product faces a high risk of bankruptcy, litigation, or supply shortage.

The supplier selection team may consider single-sourcing, dual-sourcing, or multi-sourcing after weighing the risks and benefits of each. The advantage of *single sourcing* (or sole sourcing) is receiving volume discounts and additional after-sale benefits and services from a more dedicated supplier. *Multiple sourcing*, or *multi-sourcing*, involves purchasing from multiple suppliers, where the major advantage is diversifying supplier risks (bankruptcy, shortages, etc.). Multi-sourcing provides increased product variety for end users, which can be important in complex product categories such as physician preference items.[26] Dual sourcing involves buying from two suppliers, sometimes with a 70–30 ratio split, to hedge supplier risks and maintain competitiveness in supplier offerings. Essentially, the secondary supplier acts as the backup if the primary supplier faces shortages, quality issues, or other contract compliance issues.

5.2.2 Contracting Activities

Cost and Price Analysis

Price and cost analysis is often considered part of supplier analysis. However, it is presented as a separate step because of its importance. *Cost analysis* implies the *total cost of ownership*, which is the sum of all the costs related to the acquisition, preparation (e.g., user training), use, and disposal of a service or product.[27] As discussed in Chapter 3, the analysis should include administrative and transaction costs associated with the supply. Price analysis is a product's historical pricing and comparing prices across brand names.

It is not uncommon to find that the purchase price represents only 50 or 60% of the total cost of ownership, with large swings in cost savings existing for products ranging from furniture to medical equipment. With highly sophisticated medical operating room equipment, maintenance and training can account for nearly 75% of the total cost of ownership. Although the total cost may be the most important analysis with capital purchases, it is imperative to realize that inventory and handling costs can also affect most types of goods and should be considered when making such purchases.

The total cost of ownership information can be obtained during the market analysis stage or the RFP stage of the process. However, conducting a simple price analysis is more common, requiring less data and research and providing a more straightforward comparison, even if sometimes misleading. When this occurs, the organization should not be surprised when it encounters the escalating costs associated with training and other incidents, which have previously been included in the price of other supplies.

Fact-based Negotiation

As a result of each of the previous steps in the process, the cross-functional team ideally should have extensive information about the product and its features, the market, price, and supplier services.

We reiterate that price is not the only item that needs to be negotiated. Other contract parameters may require greater attention than price, as they will affect aspects related to service and quality. Such items include the level of service support, delivery priority, clauses in the contract to modify future shipping quantities, quality assurances, training, and so on. These considerations should be combined in a typical contracting process for a comprehensive and fact-based negotiation brief. Fact-based negotiation, which can result in distributive or integrative approaches, is generally advocated in strategic sourcing, and differs from most traditional negotiations in four basic ways.[28]

1. Traditional negotiations are often based on personal perspectives, opinions, and biases. Fact-based negotiations, on the other hand, address facts derived from market analysis and supplier analysis.
2. In traditional negotiations, personal persuasion strategies are stressed and generally have adversarial overtones. In fact-based negotiations, emphasis is placed on providing objective, factual evidence derived from extensive research. Fact-based negotiation can take a collaborative approach. Chapter 4 discusses the involvement of multiple parties and comparative effectiveness in negotiating greater value.
3. In traditional negotiations, the negotiators' personalities are stressed. In contrast, facts and evidence are more important than the negotiator in fact-based negotiations.
4. As a result of these differences, traditional negotiation is more subjective, whereas objectivity dominates fact-based negotiations.

The sourcing team can clearly state its overall position with the negotiation brief, including the *Best Alternative to a Negotiated Agreement* (BATNA). This is the sourcing team's alternative if it cannot obtain a deal with the first party. The negotiation brief also outlines the *Least Acceptable Alternative* and the *Most Supportable Alternative,* along with the point at which the initial offer should be set.

Fact-based negotiation can either take an arms-length, competitive approach or a collaborative, problem-solving approach Exhibit 5.4.

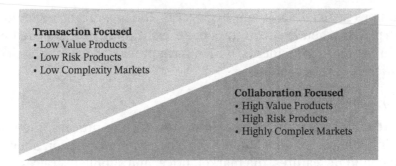

Exhibit 5.4: Contingencies for different relationship strategies.

The collaborative approach would generally be best for high-risk, high-cost products (the upper right quadrant of Exhibit 5.3), while the arm's length approach would be best for low-cost, low-risk products (the lower left quadrant of Exhibit 5.3).

Compliance

Another important activity in supply management is contract compliance. Beyond establishing a strategy and negotiating the appropriate relationships and contracts, the supply management team must ensure that the contracts and relationships remain in order. With potentially thousands of contracts in a health system's procurement portfolio, there is no shortage of contract turnover with new, expired, unfulfilled, breached, and so on. This activity is interdisciplinary, sharing responsibility between risk management, legal, procurement, and so on. The supply management team(s) needs to have visibility of the "pipeline" of contracts and resolve any potential issues before they cause disruptions to the flow of goods or services.

Soon-to-expire contracts can create an opportunity to renegotiate terms, seek a different supplier, or renew early to avoid service disruption. Many contracts, especially for commodity-type items, are often renewed automatically. Part of the supply management strategy is recognizing where to best allocate their efforts in re-negotiation and contract enforcement.

Identifying contract breaches and resolving disputes is also a crucial objective of this activity. Contract breaches may emanate from an incomplete job, undelivered goods, or incomplete or late payments. Health systems must also pay attention to anticipatory breaches, which occur when one party indicates they will not complete the commitment. Disputes arising from errors or minor issues frequently occur in business and can often be resolved via *negotiation*, especially when the parties value the long-term relationship. *Mediation* introduces a neutral third party to suggest solutions if the two parties cannot reach an agreement.

Neutral consultants, industry experts, or lawyers can serve as mediators. Mediation may escalate to *arbitration*, where a neutral third party provides a binding decision. Many law firms offer arbitration services. Finally, if the dispute is unresolvable, parties may seek *litigation* and take the issue to a court of law. Escalation of the dispute through these resolution alternatives increases time to resolution, cost, risk, uncertainty, and damage to the relationship. Dispute resolution that minimizes operational slowdown and losses (to both parties) is a good way to demonstrate commitment to the other party in moving toward long-term strategic relationships. There is even academic literature about restoring broken buyer-supplier relationships through effective apologies.[29]

5.2.3 Supplier Relationship Strategy

Supplier relationship strategy encompasses the nature and length of contracts, the number and mix of suppliers, and the mechanisms established to engage the supplier in various relationships. Managing supplier relationships intersects many supply management activities, from product analysis to contract compliance; importantly, as depicted in Exhibit 5.5,[30] how the procurement process can contribute to improving a full range of buyer and supplier engagement for continuous supply chain improvement.

A simple way to think about supplier relationship strategy is presented earlier in Exhibit 5.4, which distinguishes between a transaction and a collaborative focus. Strategies with a transaction focus generally have a short-term, arms-length arrangement, whereas strategies with a collaborative focus generally have a long-term, highly interactive focus. Another way to think of the transaction focus is by referring to it as cash-and-carry, in that the goal is to complete the transaction. Generally, there tend to be many suppliers for these products. However, because the organization may have low switching costs between suppliers, the amount of communication and the number of contracts maintained are frequently kept to a low level. This could be used for basic commodities such as alcohol swabs or tongue depressors, capital items such as bed frames, or administrative necessities such as paper forms. However, the collaborative approach is much more involved and requires the parties to develop

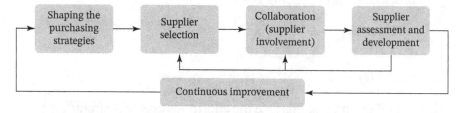

Exhibit 5.5: Supplier relationship management for continuous improvement.

The Sourcing Continuum						
Transactional		Relational			Investment	
Basic provider model	Approved-provider model	Preferred-provider model	Performance-based/managed services model	Vested business model	Shared-services model	Equity partnerships

Exhibit 5.6: The Sourcing Continuum.

and maintain a continuing relationship. This is especially important for, physician preference items and high-cost supplies. These include orthopedic implants, robotic surgical capital equipment, software, and temporary labor providers. Depending on the risks of the market and the number of suppliers, the organization will need to balance the number of relationships through depth and commitment.

Notably, relationships in the procurement arena are not simply dichotomous (transactional vs. collaborative) and thus can be segmented more precisely. The Sourcing Continuum (Exhibit 5.6) builds on Oliver Williamson's early work in transaction cost economics[31] and further parses the different levels of buyer-supplier commitments.[32]

Supplier Relationship Management continues to grow as an area of interest in the health sector.[33] A Gartner Inc. survey investigating hospital-manufacturer relationships revealed that over 90% of respondents reported a lack of trust between providers and suppliers.[34] Major relationship barriers include a lack of information sharing, a failure to recognize value beyond the lowest price, the differences between for-profit and not-for-profit organizations, and uncertainties in the business environment that encumber long-term commitments.[35] Clinicians also play an important role in tempering the relationships between hospitals and manufacturers, especially when they are engaged directly by the manufacturers. With supply chain management taking on a more strategic role in the healthcare environment, there is more awareness and understanding of the importance of effective supplier relationships. There are various levels of sophistication for SRM, and supply chain professionals in other industries find that most of the value comes from reducing risk, monitoring contract compliance and service levels, streamlining processes, and reducing costs.[36]

5.3 Strategic Outsourcing to Purchasing Alliances

Today, hospitals and systems face the enormous task of sourcing and contracting for products to accomplish their clinical and nonclinical goals.

Failure to meet the needs of internal customers can, as demonstrated in Chapter 3, exposes the hospital to substantial risk. In the complexity of the hospital and healthcare system, such assessment must be within the context of deciding the extent to which risk-related problems can be solved as the result of internal supply management or one of a variety of outsourcing options.

For over a century, hospitals and health systems have formed purchasing alliances to address the risks and complexity in procurement by outsourcing some part of the purchasing function to (a) purchase less (by consolidating volumes and engaging in aggressive negotiations), (b) buy better (by optimizing and increasing service), and (c) bring about better product use (through standardization of products and specifications). Over many years, these purchasing alliances have greatly evolved in structure and services. The term *GPO* is often used synonymously with *purchasing alliance* because it is the most commonly observed type of alliance. However, other forms of purchasing alliance structures have emerged, such as purchasing cooperatives and regional purchasing coalitions, offering complementary or sometimes competing value propositions over larger and national GPOs.

5.3.1 What Are Purchasing Alliances?

Outsourcing contracting activities in the health services sector has a long history in the United States. The first healthcare purchasing alliance was created in New York in 1910. The Hospital Bureau of New York first established a purchasing cooperative to centralize the hospitals' laundry services procurement. By the 1970s, the U.S. healthcare system had experienced extensive growth, resulting in more than 6,000 hospitals serving a nation with a growing population and a highly dispersed healthcare system. Small and rural hospitals seemed especially vulnerable to supplier pricing strategies in a marketplace characterized by inequities in knowledge, money, and managerial skills. With hundreds of thousands of supply-line items in multiple product categories, purchasing alliances were seen as an important strategic option to assist hospitals and healthcare systems achieve their purchasing goals. Today, 90% of hospitals engage with at least one purchasing alliance, and on average, 70% of hospital purchases are via contracts negotiated by purchasing alliances.[37] While purchasing alliances are most prevalent in the healthcare sector, they also exist in other sectors, such as food service, agriculture, education, and manufacturing.[38]

GPOs are purchasing alliances that negotiate contracts with suppliers on behalf of a group of hospitals or other healthcare providers (referred to as "members"). A GPO can leverage its large member base to negotiate better contract terms with suppliers. The purpose of purchasing alliances is to reduce the complexity of sourcing and contracting by leveraging centralization and economies of scale. This reduces the need for each member to conduct their due diligence regarding the market, suppliers, price and individual negotiations.

In exchange for their services, GPOs gain an administrative fee of approximately 3% from the vendors on all contracted purchases. While GPOs have other revenue streams (such as hospital membership fees), the administrative fee represents over 90% of the revenue, as observed by the largest GPOs in the United States.[39] More recent research shows that GPOs have since diversified their revenue streams, with administrative fees representing 67% of GPOs' revenue.[40] Emerging revenue streams include data benchmarking and e-procurement, each representing about 12% of the revenue. Exhibit 5.7 outlines the relationships between the various stakeholders concerninphysical goods and information flow.[41] Exhibit 5.8 presents a similar layout to Exhibit 5.7 but considers the cash flows between the same stakeholders.

Exhibit 5.9 summarizes the process of GPOs negotiating new contracts with suppliers that are then made available to the alliance members. Most negotiated contracts have three-year terms, with some longer contracts awarded for certain product categories where setup and training on such products or systems make it infeasible—or simply inconvenient—to switch every three years. Laboratory products, chemistry analyzers, and intravenous (IV) systems are examples of such

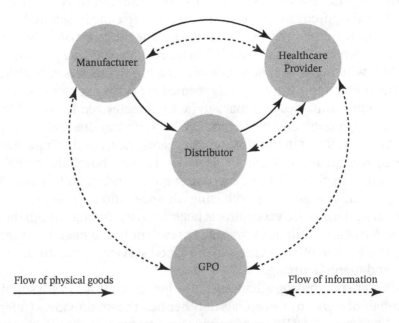

Exhibit 5.7: The flow of physical goods and information among procurement stakeholders.

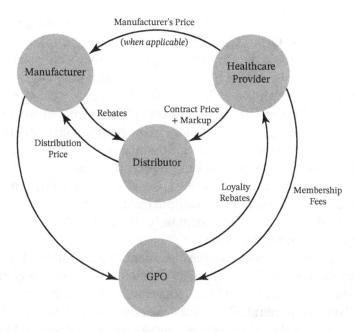

Exhibit 5.8: The flow of cash among procurement stakeholders.

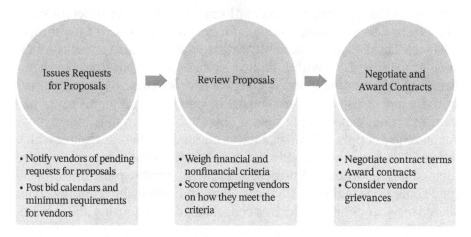

Exhibit 5.9: Process of negotiating contracts with manufacturers.

products. Many contracts also include *commitment provisions*, incentivizing hospitals to buy more from the same supplier. For example, greater product discounts are available if a hospital purchases 80% of its needs in this product category from that manufacturer.[42] GPOs also negotiate *bundled contracts*, which group related products for greater incentives and discounts for hospitals.

It is worth noting that in most arrangements, there is no guarantee for the suppliers that all the members of a GPO will buy into the negotiated contract. These GPOs are said to operate on a *voluntary membership* basis. Other GPOs operate on a *contractual membership* basis, where members commit to using the alliance's contracts to purchase a specified percentage of their needs. That percentage is referred to as the contract compliance level.[43] GPOs that enforce contract compliance levels with their members generally have a smaller membership base but gain leverage with suppliers by providing better estimates of the demand. Increasing contract compliance is an important target for both voluntary and contractual membership alliances, as it directly impacts their expenses and revenues. However, this is undermined by the hospitals' discretion to join multiple purchasing alliances to expand their purchasing options. Approximately 50% of hospitals are members of multiple and competing GPOs.[44,45]

There are several tiers of purchasing alliances: national level (the more traditional form of a GPO), regional level (often referred to as regional purchasing coalitions), and local level (sometimes referred to as purchasing cooperatives). In general, GPO classification is based on the alliance's member base and the geographic dispersion of the members. However, there is no clear delineation among the different GPO types, and some of the labels are often used interchangeably. Furthermore, each alliance, whether at the national, regional, or local levels, provides different value propositions, so it is not uncommon for hospitals to subscribe to multiple alliances. Local alliances generally cater to the customized needs of their smaller member base with high involvement and input from the members in the procurement process.[46] It is easier for clinical representatives from member hospitals to participate in value analysis teams to coordinate and better express their needs. This enables them to focus on more sophisticated supply categories, such as physician preference items, which larger GPOs have traditionally not been as successful in integrating into their contract portfolios. Furthermore, the geographic proximity of local (and sometimes regional) alliances allows for establishing supply chain shared service operations, such as consolidated warehousing and logistics centers.[47]

Many hospitals engage with multiple alliances at multiple tiers, and sometimes alliances of different tiers coordinate to reduce duplication and share best practices. Notably, regional alliances are frequently aligned with larger national purchasing groups, thus providing members access to a wide range of contracts. As there has been growth in the size of systems, some health systems have chosen to sponsor their own GPOs and even expanded these GPOs to other hospitals in their region. An example of a local regional GPO partnering with a national GPO is Captis, a GPO launched by Mayo Clinic in partnership with Vizient, a large national GPO.[48] Exhibit 5.10 presents the supply spend breakdown of hospitals that, in 2014, were subscribed to one of the five

Exhibit 5.10: Typical hospital supply spend.

Type of GPO/alliance	Supply spend (%)
National Alliance ("Group Purchasing Organization")	55
Regional Alliance ("Regional Purchasing Coalition")	10
Local Alliance ("purchasing cooperative," "shared service")	5
Self-negotiated Contracts	20
Off-contract purchases	10

Note: Data obtained from[50] 2014 data.
N = 899 hospitals surveyed.

largest GPOs in the country, which account for approximately 90% of all hospitals.[49]

5.3.2 Value of Purchasing Alliances

GPOs have received much scrutiny over the past two decades regarding the value they bring to hospitals relative to the potential risks, such as monopolization, anti-trust issues, and limiting supplier diversity.[51,52,53] This section examines both sides of the argument, guided by the latest available academic research.

The Healthcare Supply Chain Organization (HSCA), which represents GPOs in the United States, funded an empirical study in 2009 to identify the areas of greatest cost savings that GPOs provide their member hospitals.[54] To address the risk of bias, the data was collected by the independent third-party research firm Mathematica Research, Inc. The study estimated a $36 billion cost savings nationwide, with 50% of those cost savings in commodity-type items such as computers, food, janitorial services, office products, other clinical items, and so on. Medical-surgical items and pharmaceutical supplies represented the next two largest savings categories, accounting for 23% and 19% of the savings, respectively.

In addition to direct savings through the availability of better prices, the study also found that GPO membership reduces the number of full-time employees (FTEs) responsible for procurement activities at hospitals and healthcare systems. Surveyed hospitals estimated that the average number of procurement employees would need to be doubled to replace the GPO's role, from an average of 7.9 full-time equivalent employees (FTEs) to 17.1 FTEs.[55] A more recent study considering more localized purchasing alliances found similar results.[56]

One study considered the procurement activities for a hospital to establish a contract with a supplier and estimated the total cost of about $3,000 per contract.[57] The same metric was estimated when the hospital outsourced some activities to a GPO, finding an overall estimated cost avoidance of about $1,300 per contract. The GPO provided the most value by reducing the cost and time associated with RFP preparation and submission. Product evaluation, product/supplier selection, and contract compliance monitoring were the activities that generated the least cost savings from GPO involvement.

While there appear to be real cost savings brought forth by purchasing alliances, outsourcing some procurement activities for a portion of contracts to GPOs does not provide a hospital or system with a significant strategic advantage. Recent empirical research has demonstrated that membership in a national purchasing alliance did not significantly impact a hospital's supply expense ratio after controlling for other factors.[58] Nor did it have a significant impact on clinical performance

---

Side Bar 5.1

Safe Harbor for GPOs

The safe harbor for GPOs, which Congress enacted by statute and the Office of the Inspector General (OIG) interpreted at 42 C.F.R. Section 1001.952(j), potentially applies to the Proposed Arrangement. It excludes from the definition of *remuneration* certain fees paid by vendors to GPOs, which otherwise could constitute remuneration to induce, reward, or arrange for federal healthcare program business referrals. To qualify for protection under the GPO safe harbor, a GPO must have a written agreement with each individual or entity for which items or services are furnished. That agreement must either provide that participating vendors from which the individual or entity will purchase goods or services will pay a fee to the GPO of 3% or less of the purchase price of the goods or services provided by that vendor, or, in the event the fee paid to the GPO is not fixed at 3% or less of services, specify the amount (or if not known, the maximum amount) the GPO will be paid by each vendor (where such amount may be a fixed sum or a fixed percentage of the value of purchases made from the vendor by the members of the group under the contract between the vendor and the GPO). Where the entity that receives the goods or services from the vendor is a healthcare provider of services, the GPO must disclose in writing to the entity at least annually, and to the Secretary upon request, the amount received from each vendor with respect to purchases made by or on behalf of the entity.

outcomes or patient experience scores.[59] Researchers of one such study interpreted their findings as follows:[60]

> *Outsourcing the responsibilities regarding price negotiation and contract management may ultimately lower hospital capital expenditures and reduce operating margins, two financial metrics distinct from the supply expenses that we hypothesized that GPOs would directly affect.*[61]

Given that over 90% of hospitals in the United States subscribe to at least one purchasing alliance, it is then no surprise that membership participation alone is insufficient for sustaining a supply chain competitive advantage. Having a certain configuration of multiple purchasing alliances that matches the hospital or system's own procurement capabilities is a more apt strategy. For example, some hospitals report referring to GPO contracts as a benchmark or reference point to negotiate more customized and favorable contracts directly with manufacturers. Furthermore, researchers recognize that some GPO characteristics, such as members' geographic dispersion, play a role in the GPO's ability to improve members' supply expense performance.[62]

5.3.3 Criticisms toward Purchasing Alliances

Purchasing alliances have received criticism over the years for not being able to provide the promised cost-savings, and the U.S. Government Accountability Office has investigated the industry on multiple occasions. A major criticism the industry received is the inherent conflict of interest: the primary goal of GPOs is negotiating the lowest product prices for hospitals, but higher product prices translate to higher administrative fees for the GPOs, which continues to be their main source of revenue.[63] Others suggested that competition between the GPOs incentivizes them to keep prices low and points to the fact that as much as 70% of the collected administrative fees are eventually passed back to the members/owners of the GPOs.[64] The empirical evidence regarding the intentions, actions, and repercussions of GPOs remains sparse for both sides of this argument.

Another criticism received by GPOs is that they impede smaller and newer medical device manufacturers from reaching their customers, becoming a barrier to innovation. Established manufacturers hold similar criticisms regarding GPOs being gatekeepers that sometimes stifle medical innovations. This matter has been raised to the Senate, the Federal Trade Commission, and the Department of Justice. Consequently, there is increased awareness of these issues among all players involved, resulting in reduced sole-source contracting. Additionally, the large GPOs have begun working more closely with smaller and more focused purchasing coalitions to improve intermediation. As mentioned earlier in the chapter, smaller regional purchasing coalitions or other local alliance structures are better positioned to manage relationships with suppliers of more complex product lines for a more defined customer segment. As health systems assume responsibility for contracting activities for strategic items, they are experiencing improved relationships with strategic suppliers that provide advantages beyond those achieved via GPO intermediation.

5.3.4 Purchasing Alliances Are Not Silver Bullets

All-in-all, purchasing alliances represent a supply chain intermediary largely unique to the healthcare sector. Perhaps the most authoritative analysis of GPOs has been written by Lawton Burns.[65] Burns provides evidence that purchasing alliances can provide a service and bring cost savings to hospitals and carefully considers criticism regarding GPOs' true savings potential for the hospitals and other complexities they bring into this supply chain. Nonetheless, the fact remains that the vast majority of hospitals in the United States subscribe to at least one purchasing alliance. When surveyed, hospital executives (namely, vice presidents of materials management or supply chain) indicated that the role of the GPOs has increased in importance over the past decade, and they indicated overall satisfaction with their GPOs, finding the benchmarking and data analytics services that the GPOs provide to be of particular value.[66]

The decision to outsource a hospital's contracting activities to a purchasing alliance on its own is neither a necessary nor sufficient condition to realize cost savings. This decision needs to fit into a larger sourcing strategy that integrates a portfolio of sourcing and contracting alternatives and aligns with the healthcare system's overall clinical management strategy.

5.4 Supply Chain Diversity, Equity, and Inclusion

5.4.1 What Is Supplier Diversity?

Supplier diversity, providing contracting opportunities to suppliers representing minority or underprivileged groups, is a supply chain practice that took form in the United States primarily during the civil rights movement of the 1960s. In particular, General Motors was among the pioneers in implementing supplier diversity programs following one of the worst riots in American history, the 1967 Detroit race riot, which saw confrontations between the black community and the Detroit Police Department. The federal government later implemented laws encouraging government contractors to source from minority-owned businesses.[67] In the United States, issues of racial disparity have come to the forefront in recent years with the Black Lives Matter movement and the accentuated impact of the COVID-19 pandemic on lower-income minority populations, which carry higher rates of co-morbidities such as hypertension, obesity, and diabetes. Responsibilities for correcting these long-standing social issues fall on corporations as much as on government and individual actors. As referenced in Chapter 1, supply chain management holds a substantial role in any corporation's social responsibility efforts (in addition to the social responsibility toward its employees), perhaps most directly observed in socially responsible supplier selection practices and supplier diversity programs.[68]

Supplier diversity programs have matured, and all major organizations have dedicated supplier diversity teams within the procurement department. In addition to contracting opportunities, top programs also earmark funds to invest in supplier capabilities and mentoring. In 2021, a survey of over 100 large U.S.-based corporations (23% of which operate in the healthcare sector) found the median supply spend on diverse suppliers to be 8% of total spend, and over 80% of them indicated having a dedicated fund for supplier development activities.[69] As mentioned earlier in this chapter, GPOs have come under heavy criticism in the past for failing to adequately accommodate small and diverse manufacturers, culminating in Senate hearings and Federal Trade Commission rulings. GPOs have since invested significant efforts in developing supplier diversity programs and guiding member hospitals through developing their programs. The Healthcare Group Purchasing Industry Initiative (HGPII), a GPO membership organization, was formed in 2002 to provide a platform for GPOs to buffer themselves against criticisms and encourage a high level of social responsibility in procurement.[70] HGPII solicits information and reviews the performance of GPO adherence to ethical standards and best practices with an emphasis on GPO conflicts of interest, adherence to administrative fee threshold, fostering innovation, use of single, sole, dual, and multi-source contracts, and bundling of unrelated products and vendor diversity programs.[71]

5.4.2 Who Are Diverse Suppliers?

The definition of a *diverse supplier* continues to evolve, but generally, a certified diverse supplier is a business that meets at least one of three broad guidelines:

- 51% owned by one or more diverse people;
- Operates in an economically disadvantaged community ("HUB-Zone business"); and
- Small business (based on the number of employees or revenue).

These guidelines carry different interpretations across different entities. For example, "51% ownership by diverse people" includes Black-, Hispanic-, Native American-, women-, veteran-, minority-, LGBTQ-, and disability-owned suppliers are some of the qualifying categories. Such ownership groups are identified because they have experienced an unfair economic disadvantage in their business transactions, such as hindered access to capital and contract bidding. Some organizations also consider local suppliers in their programs, which benefits the local economy while diversifying the supply base,[72] shortening the supply chain, and hedging certain risks. Buyers looking to authenticate a supplier's claim for diversity can conduct a *diversity audit*, hire a firm to carry out this investigation or ask suppliers for certifications granted by the government or specialized agencies.

Organizations go about identifying diverse suppliers in several ways. Most commonly, diverse suppliers will bid for a contract and identify themselves as such. Other times, supplier diversity organizations help connect buyers with suppliers and provide the most value in identifying second-tier suppliers when needed. Large GPOs facilitate supplier diversity programs for their members by recommending diverse suppliers for new contracts and sharing best practices for integrating such programs into a health system's supply chain organization. In 2022, HGPII reported that all of their member organizations had promoted diverse ownership within the supply chain.[73]

5.4.3 Supplier Diversity Programs

Socially responsible supplier selection provides both indirect economic benefits to a corporation's community and directs financial benefits.[74] For example, organizations that dedicate a relatively higher portion of supply spending to diverse suppliers attribute 15–20% of their sales to their supplier diversity programs.[75] Other less tangible benefits to supplier diversity programs that organizations cite as motivators to increase program spending include:

- Providing sources for innovative products, services, or processes developed by diverse suppliers. Attractive diversity supplier programs also attract and retain niche, quality suppliers.
- Diversifying the procurement channels for the required goods and services. Dedicated diversity organizations or GPOs help health systems find solutions that may not be available in mainstream markets.
- Generating goodwill translates to increased market share. Sharing a supply network with diverse suppliers can provide positive network effects for both.

- Driving competition in prices and service levels. The buyer can negotiate favorable delivery terms and gain quality oversight when the diverse suppliers are local.

There is much social and institutional pressure to implement supplier diversity programs, leaving some corporations to rush into such efforts to appease shareholders or prop up a public image. This practice is akin to greenwashing, where companies cosmetically "implement" environmentally sustainable practices primarily for compliance and publicity. It is also not sustainable to accept lower product or service standards to qualify diverse suppliers in efforts to meet diversity thresholds. Instead, developing a diverse supplier's business capabilities can reap great long-term benefits for both parties. Examples include investing in their manufacturing capacity, recommending procurement standards and systems, or co-locating employees. It is important for hospitals and healthcare organizations contracting with smaller diverse suppliers to recognize that, unlike larger corporations, they cannot withstand dramatic shifts in the volume of purchases or withstand slow payment.

Supplier diversity programs must fold into a broader corporate social responsibility strategy with relevant and measurable key performance indicators. While diverse supplier spending is the most often cited measure of a program's size and success, leaders should seek more meaningful metrics. What is the cost saving from switching to diverse suppliers? How does the program' impact the local economy regarding jobs, health equity, or socio-economic status? Does the supplier diversity program correlate with market share, and does it resonate with diverse buyers? Finally, leaders must continue to ask what value propositions the diverse suppliers provide that mainstream suppliers do not (for the same price or service level). Plenty of examples exist, but some fit specific strategies better than others.

5.5 Chapter Summary

This chapter provides a general overview of procurement in the healthcare sector. Procurement begins with identifying the organizational needs expressed by the healthcare system's administrators and clinicians. FISCO functions of product sourcing, product selection, standardization, contracting, SRM, and risk management are key purchasing considerations.

One of the many ways to classify healthcare products is to consider three broad categories: (a) physician preference items, (b) commodities, and (c) capital goods. The sourcing team invests time to understand the type and nature of the required products or services, which for a medium-sized hospital, translates to somewhere around 30,000–40,000 stock keeping unit (SKUs). Understanding the required supply demands developing category and spend analyses, market analysis for product categories, and supplier analysis to identify appropriate candidates that can reliably provide the required materials. Progressive systems develop strategies to procure a complex collection of required supplies within the available time, budget, and other constraints. Tactical-level contracting activities complement these strategic-level activities. After proper research, the products and suppliers are selected, and contracts are negotiated. All activities above are cyclical and perpetual. There is a constant need to introduce new and innovative products as the science and technology of healthcare advances, which may be suggested by the suppliers or requested by hospital professionals. Similarly, on the contracting front, there is never a shortage of contract compliance issues that need to be monitored.

The inherently complex nature of healthcare and modern medicine brings a vast diversity of mission-critical supplies with a wide range of alternatives and potential suppliers. Most hospitals find value in outsourcing contracting activities to purchasing alliances, which have emerged as intermediaries in the procurement process. The primary role of purchasing alliances in the healthcare sector is negotiating contracts with manufacturers and supporting efforts to gain value for money. Member hospitals can then utilize these contracts, saving time and resources on research and negotiation. To that end, membership in a purchasing alliance does not provide a competitive advantage. Still, it merely allows healthcare systems to focus on developing a supply strategy appropriate to their context. Progressive systems develop a portfolio of procurement vehicles, utilizing GPOs, regional purchasing coalitions, and local alliances while directly engaging suppliers that they consider strategic partners.

Finally, it is crucial to remember the procurement function's social and ethical responsibility that transcends all alliances and strategies. This responsibility manifests through a supplier diversity program, which is vital to an organization's corporate social responsibility strategy.

Notes

1. Nachtmann, H., & E. Pohl, "The state of healthcare logistics: Cost and quality improvement opportunities" (Center for Innovation in Health Care Logistics, Arkansas, 2009).
2. Michael Darling, M., & Sandy Wise, S. (2010). Not your father's supply chain. Following best practices to manage inventory can help you save big.

Manage inventory can help you save big, Materials Management. *Health Care, 19*(4), 30–33.

3. Adobor, H., & McMullen, R. S. (2014). Strategic purchasing and supplier partnerships: The role of a third party organization. *Journal of Purchasing and Supply Management, 20*(4), 263–272.

4. Burns, L. R. (2022). *The Healthcare Value Chain: Demystifying the Role of GPOs and PBMs*. Springer International Publishing AG.

5. Conti, R. K. (2018, July 30; 2018, July 6). OIG Advisory Opinion No. 18–07. https://oig.hhs.gov/documents/advisory-opinions/750/AO-18-07.pdf

6. HSCA. (2011a). A primer on group purchasing organizations: Questions and answers. Washington, .https://www.google.com/search?q=hca+a+primer+on+group+purchasing&rlz=1C1GCEB_enUS918US918&oq=hca+a+primer+on+group+purchasing&aqs=chrome..69i57j33i160.6330j1j7&sourceid=chrome&ie=UTF-8

7. Burns, op. cit.

8. Ibid.

9. Ibid.

10. Smeltzer, L. R., Manship, J. A., & Rossetti, C. L. (2003). An analysis of the integration of strategic sourcing and negotiation planning. *Journal of Supply Chain Management, 39*(3), 16–25.

11. Ibid.

12. Harland, C. M. (2013). "Supply Chain Management Research Impact: An Evidence-Based Perspective."

13. Karljic, P. "Purchasing must become supply management," Harvard Business Review, 1983.https://hbr.org/1983/09/purchasing-must-become-supply-management

14. Ibid.

15. Polyviou, M., Ramos, G., & Schneller, E. (2022). Supply chain risk management: An enterprise view and a survey of methods. In Y. Khojasteh, H. Xu, & S. Zolfaghari (Eds.), *Supply chain risk mitigation chain risk mitigation* (pp. 27–58). Springer.

16. Stewart Beall, S., et al. (2003). The role of reverse auctions in strategic sourcing. *CAPS Research.*

17. Prashant, P. Abhishek Behl, & Padmanabha Aital, Systematic literature review on electronic reverse auction: Issues and research discussion, International Journal of Procurement Management 10, no. 3 (January 1, 2017): 290–310. https://doi.org/10.1504/IJPM.2017.083457; Pearcy, D., Giunipero, L., & Wilson, A. (2007). A Model of Relational Governance in Reverse Auctions. *Journal of Supply Chain Management, 43*(1), 4–15. https://doi.org/10.1111/j.1745-493X.2007.00023.x

18. Lang, K, & Eaton, B. "The value analysis team: A shared mental model," The Health Care Manager 28, no. 2 (June 2009): 165–71. https://doi.org/10.1097/HCM.0b013e3181a2cc61; Robert Yokl, "Value Analysis in the Age of Value-Based Competition," *The Journal of Healthcare Contracting*, July 2015. http://www.jhconline.com/value-analysis-in-the-age-of-value-based-competition.html

19. Abdulsalam, Y., et al. (2015). The emergence of consolidated service centers in health care. *Journal of Business Logistics, 36*(4), 321–334. https://doi.org/10.1111/jbl.12107

20. Harland, C. M. (2013). Supply chain management research impact: An evidence-based perspective. *Supply Chain Management, 18*(5), 483–496. https://doi.org/10.1108/SCM-03-2013-0108; Flynn, A. E., & Fraser Johnson, P. (2019). *Purchasing and Supply Management*, 15 (MC GRAW HILL INDIA); Keith, B., et al. (2016). *Strategic Sourcing in the New Economy: Harnessing the Potential of Sourcing Business Models for Modern Procurement* (1st ed. 2016 edition). Springer. Monczka, R. M., et al. (2020). *Purchasing & Supply Chain Management* (7th ed.). Cengage Learning. Harland, C., et al. (2013). *The SAGE handbook of strategic supply management*. SAGE Knowledge. https://doi.org/10.4135/9781446269886

21. Ramírez, R. McGinley, C., & Churchhouse, S. Why investing in procurement makes organizations more resilient, *Harvard Business Review*, Jne 17, 2020. https://hbr.org/2020/06/why-investing-in-procurement-makes-organizations-more-resilient

22. For example, Fawcett, S., Brockhaus, S., & Fawcett, A. (2015, Nov.). Sustainability as strategy: Caught in the luxury trap. *Supply Chain Management Review, 19*(6), 16. Lu, G., & Shang, G. (2017). Impact of supply base structural complexity on financial performance: Roles of visible and not-so-visible characteristics. *Journal of Operations Management, 53–56*(1), 23–44. https://doi.org/10.1016/j.jom.2017.10.001; Narasimhan, R., & Narayanan, S. (2013). Perspectives on supply network—Enabled innovations. *Journal of Supply Chain Management, 49*(4), 27–42. https://doi.org/10.1111/jscm.12026; Thomas, R., et al. (2020, Nov). Decomposing social sustainability: Signaling theory insights into supplier selection decisions. *Journal of Supply Chain Management*. https://doi.org/10.1111/jscm.12247; Wagner, S. (2012). Tapping supplier innovation. *Journal of Supply Chain Management, 48*(2), 37–52. https://doi.org/10.1111/j.1745-493X.2011.03258.x

23. Choi, T. Y., & Krause, D. R. (2006). The supply base and its complexity: Implications for transaction costs, risks, responsiveness, and innovation. *Journal of Operations Management, 24*(5), 637–652. https://doi.org/10.1016/j.jom.2005.07.002; Kim, S., Wagner, S., & Colicchia, C. The impact of supplier sustainability risk on shareholder value. *Journal of Supply Chain Management, 55*(1, 2019), 71–87. https://doi.org/10.1111/jscm.12188

24. Choi, T. Y., & Hartley, J. (1996). An exploration of supplier selection practices across the supply chain. *Journal of Operations Management, 14*(4), 333–343. https://doi.org/10.1016/S0272-6963(96)00091-5; Sarkis, J., & Talluri, S. (2002). A model for strategic supplier selection. *Journal of Supply Chain Management, 38*(4), 18–28. https://doi.org/10.1111/j.1745-493X.2002.tb00117.x

25. Hirakubo, N., & Kublin, M. (1998). The relative importance of supplier selection criteria: The case of electronic components procurement in Japan.

International Journal of Purchasing and Materials Management, 34(1), 19–24. https://doi.org/10.1111/j.1745-493X.1998.tb00044.x

26. Montgomery, K., & Schneller, E. S. (2007). Hospitals' strategies for orchestrating selection of physician preference items. *The Milbank Quarterly, 85*(2), 307–335.

27. Ellram, L. M. (1994). *Total cost modeling in purchasing.* Center for Advanced Purchasing Studies Studies. http://archive.org/details/totalcostmodelin0000ellr

28. Gan, I. (2017, Dec). Advancing a distributive-bargaining and integrative-negotiation integral dystem: A values-based negotiation model (VBM). *Social Sciences, 6*(4), 115. https://doi.org/10.3390/socsci6040115; Smeltzer, L. R., Manship, J. A., & Rossetti, C. L. (2003). An analysis of the integration of strategic sourcing and negotiation planning. *Journal of Supply Chain Management, 39*(3), 16–25. https://doi.org/10.1111/j.1745-493X.2003.tb00161.x

29. Mir, S., et al. (2021). Mending fences in a buyer–supplier relationship: The role of justice in relationship restoration. *Journal of Supply Chain Management.* https://doi.org/10.1111/jscm.12272

30. Park, J., Shin, K., Chang, T. W., & Park, J. (2010). *An integrative framework for supplier relationship management.* Industrial Management & Data Systems.

31. Williamson, O. E. (1981). The economics of organization: The transaction cost approach. *American Journal of Sociology, 87*(3), 548–577. https://doi.org/10.2307/2778934

32. Keith, B. et al., (2016, Dec.) *Strategic sourcing in the new economy;* Kate Vitasek, "Map your way to an effective sourcing strategy, Supply Chain Quarterly, https://www.supplychainquarterly.com/articles/1278-map-your-way-to-an-effective-sourcing-strategy

33. Abdulsalam, Y. J., & Schneller, E. S. (2020). Of barriers and bridges: Buyer-supplier relationships in health care. *Health Care Management Review, 1.* https://doi.org/10.1097/HMR.0000000000000278

34. Dominy, M. and O'Daffer, E. "Supply chain consultants and outsourcing providers for healthcare delivery organizations" (Stamford, CT: Gartner Research, July 5, 2011).

35. Abdulsalam & Schneller, op. cit.

36. SCMR Staff, "Current state: Supplier relationship management," Supply Chain Management Review, November 2018. https://www.scmr.com/article/current_state_supplier_relationship_management

37. Burns, L. R., & Briggs, A. (2018). Hospital purchasing alliances alliances: Ten years after. *Health Care Management Review..* https://doi.org/10.1097/HMR.0000000000000215

38. Curran, J. (2021, Aug.) Group Purchasing Organizations Industry Report Purchasing Organizations Industry Report. (IBIS World).

39. Government Accountability Office. (2010, Aug. 24). Group Purchasing Organizations. Services Provided to Customers and their Initiatives Regarding their Business Practices. Report to the Ranking Member Committee on Finance, U.S. Finance. chrome-extension://efaidnbmnnnibpcajpcglclefindmkaj/https://www.gao.gov/assets/gao-10-738.pdf

40. Curran, (2021, Aug.). Group Purchasing Organizations Industry Report OD5963. IBIS World. https://www.ibisworld.com/united-states/market-research-reports/group-purchasing-organizations-industry; also reported in Burns, L. R. (2022). *The Healthcare Value Chain: Demystifying the Role of GPOs and PBMs.* Springer International Publishing. Curran, J. ibid.

41. Jayaraman, R., Taha, K., Park, K. S., & Lee, J. (2014). Impacts and role of group purchasing organization in healthcare supply chain. In Y. Guan & H. Liao (Eds.), *IIE Annual Conference. Proceedings* (pp. 3842). Institute of Industrial and Systems Engineers (IISE).

42. Government Accountability Office, "Group Purchasing Organizations: Funding Structure Has Potential Implications for Medicare Costs," October 2014. chrome-extension://efaidnbmnnnibpcajpcglclefindmkaj/https://www.gao.gov/assets/gao-15-13.pdf

43. Curran , op. cit.

44. Burns & Briggs, op. cit.

45. Ibid.

46. Mark Thill, M. (2012, Aug.). Regional purchasing coalitions grow up, Journal of Healthcare Contracting.

47. Abdulsalam Y. A. et al., (2015). Op. cit.

48. Benton, D. (2020, May 17). Vizient partners with Captis healthcare network to launch supply chain innovation programme. Supply Chain Digital Magazine. https://supplychaindigital.com/technology/vizient-partners-captis-healthcare-network-launch-supply-chain-innovation-programme

49. Burns, & Briggs, op. cit.

50. Ibid.

51. Nollet, J., & Beaulieu, M. (2003). The development of group purchasing: An empirical study in the healthcare sector. *Journal of Purchasing and Supply Management, 9*(1), 3–10. https://doi.org/10.1016/S0969-7012(02)00034-5

52. Singleton, M. (2018, Summer). Group purchasing organizations: Gaming the system. *Journal of American Physicians and Surgeons, 23*(2).

53. Walker, D. M., et al. (2021). Examining the financial and quality performance effects of group purchasing organizations. *Health Care Management Review, 46*(4), 278–288. https://doi.org/10.1097/HMR.0000000000000267

54. Schneller, E. S. (2009). *The value of group purchasing—2009: Meeting the needs for strategic savings.* Health Care Setor Advances Inc.

55. Schneller, E. S. (2000). The value of group purchasing in the health care supply chain. Study 1 in Schneller, E. and Smeltzer L. The strategic management of the health ccare supply chain. Jossey Bass 2006.

56. Abdulsalam Y. A., et al., Op. Cit.

57. Schneller, E. S., The value of group purchasing, 2009 op. cit.

58. Nyaga, G. N., Young, J., & Zepeda, E. D. (2015). An analysis of the effects of intra- and iIterorganizational arrangements on hospital supply chain efficiency. *Journal of Business Logistics, 36*(4), 340–354. https://doi.org/10.1111/jbl.12109

59. Walker et al., op. cit.

60. Ibid.
61. Ibid., 10.
62. Ibid.
63. Singleton, op. cit.
64. Government Accountability Office, Group Purchasing Organizations: Funding structure has potential implications for Medicare costs.
65. Ibid., Burns.
66. Burns, L. R., & Briggs, A.D. (2020). op. cit.
67. Bateman, A., Barrington, A., & Date, K. (2020, Aug. 17)., "Why you need a supplier-diversity program," Harvard Business Review. https://hbr.org/2020/08/why-you-need-a-supplier-diversity-program
68. How CSC can supply chain meet the demand for health equity? Healthcare Purchasing News website. https://www.hpnonline.com/sourcing-logistics/article/21223123/how-can-supply-chain-meet-the-demand-for-health-equityPublished May 25, 2021. (accessed November 13, 2022).
69. The Hackett Group Inc., "Highlights from our 2021 Supplier Diversity Study," 2021.
70. Rahman, B., Schneller, E., & Wilson, N. (n.d.). In G. Racca & C. R. Yukins (Eds.), *Integrity and efficiency in Collaborative purchasing. Chapter 3 in Integrity and efficiency in sustainable public contracts: Balancing corruption concerns in public procurement internationally* (pp. 357–387). chrome-extension://efaidnbmnnnibpcajpcglclefindmkaj/ http://www.ius-publicum.com/repository/uploads/10_02_2015_11_07_RACCA_YUKINS_Integrity_and_Efficiency_in_Sustainable_Public_Contracts_Bruylant_2014.pdf
71. Healthcare Group Purchasing Industry Initiative. Healthgroup Purchasing Industry Initiative: Sixteenth Annual Report to the Public. January 2022, chrome-extension://efaidnbmnnnibpcajpcglclefindmkaj/https://hgpii.com/wp-content/uploads/2022/02/HGPII-16th-Annual-Report-Member-Final.pdf
72. Bringing supplier diversity home. (2021, July 26). Healthcare Purchasing News website. Retrieved November 13, 2022, from https://www.hpnonline.com/sourcing-logistics/article/21231053/bringing-supplier-diversity-home
73. Health Group Purchasing Initiative, op. cit. ibid., p. 3.
74. Thornton, L. M., et al. (2013). Does socially responsible supplier selection pay off for customer firms? A cross-cultural comparison. *Journal of Supply Chain Management, 49*(3), 66–89. https://doi.org/10.1111/jscm.12014
75. Amy, F. A., & Geoff Peters, G. (2019). *Supplier diversity: Moving beyond compliance drive meaningful value compliance drive meaningful value.* The Hackett Group.

6

Logistics Strategies and Alliances—*The Devil Is in the Details*

6.1 Introduction

Within every healthcare supply chain, *logistics* includes those operational activities that physically deliver the value created within the supply chain management system. These logistics activities are sometimes referred to as 'distribution services'. Whereas sourcing, purchasing, and risk management activities set up the framework and position the plans, it is logistics that actually drives the physical movement of products to the end user, the ultimate customer. Embedded within logistics are the Fully Integrated Supply Chain Organization (FISCO) functions of order processing, inventory management, receiving, and asset management.

This book provides a necessary level of detail in this area to enable a healthcare supply chain management practitioner to understand and master the field in general. Those interested in a very detailed examination of this specific topic will want to supplement this material with a specialized logistics operations textbook, such as Chopra and Meindl's book.[1]

The activities within the logistics system of a supply chain emanate from three core business processes: (a) inventory management, (b) order management, and (c) returns management. Each of these core processes includes numerous subprocesses, as shown in Exhibit 6.1.

To support the processes, the logistics system relies on a set of fixed and moveable assets to operationalize the process. These assets fall into two types: the first type is transportation assets that include vehicles and terminals. The second type includes warehouse assets, which are the physical warehousing facilities and the material handling equipment. Material handling equipment is a warehouse capital asset that is either stationary (such as racks, shelves, and conveyors) or an asset that is mobile (with a forklift being the most ubiquitous example).

For all of these processes and the related assets, there are two approaches for managing them: self-operated (insourced) and third-party operated (outsourced). Choosing between insourcing and outsourcing is the make-or-buy decision applied to logistics services. In most cases, either of these approaches will work effectively. However, depending on the circumstances, one of these approaches will prove more suitable. The choice depends on a combination of corporate readiness and market conditions. Furthermore, there is a continuum of insourcing and outsourcing, and many hybrid models involve insourcing and outsourcing different combinations of logistics functions.

This chapter explores the preceding three processes in-depth, the associated assets used to manage them, and the decisions regarding insourcing and/or outsourcing. Also explained is how all of these processes link to each other. It is due to this integration that changes to one process can affect others. By carefully managing the resources applied to specific activities, the effective supply chain manager can optimize the

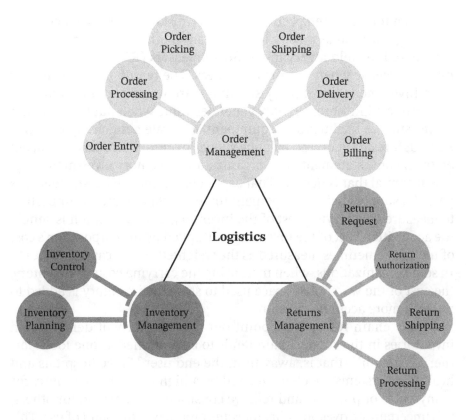

Exhibit 6.1: The major processes and subprocesses of the logistics function.

performance of a supply chain to generate significant value. To achieve this high level of performance and value creation, supply chain managers will design and apply certain strategies. A number of more powerful strategies are identified at the end of this chapter.

6.2 Inventory Management Process

Management, in general, is defined as the planning and controlling of any business endeavor. Consequently, inventory management is about the planning and control of a logistics system's inventories. Why should a business be concerned about inventory management? It is the core supply chain process that ensures that when a customer wants a certain product, it will be available for them to order and subsequently receive. While there cannot be 100% certainty of inventory availability at any time due to unforeseen circumstances, when inventory management is done well, the likelihood of not satisfying the demand from a customer is very low. When it's not done well, the likelihood of a disappointed customer will be high.

From a financial perspective, inventory resides on the balance sheet of an organization as an asset. Compared to other assets, inventory is considered to yield a very low return on assets (ROA), an important financial metric when valuing a business. The reason is that inventory is an investment that simply sits in a warehouse and does not generate value while at rest. It only generates value when put to use. Other assets, such as facilities and equipment, generate a much higher ROA. Although residing on the balance sheet, inventory also has an impact on the income statement of an organization. Inventory investments represent capital that is tied up. That capital has a financial cost. Hence, as part of a supply chain management financial statement, it is important to measure the carrying cost of the inventory. The calculation is simply the acquisition cost of the inventory multiplied by the corporation's cost of money, sometimes measured as the weighted cost of capital (WACC). In some organizations, when measuring the carrying costs of inventory, the cost of the warehouse space used to store the inventory is added to reflect a more accurate measure.

Supply chain researchers point out that volatility of demand and inventories in the supply chain tends to be amplified as one looks farther 'upstream'—that is, away from the end user.[2] Since hospitals and healthcare systems are characterized by a high level of uncertainty for many kinds of products and relative consistency in demand for others, this uncertainty drives volatility for some products at the point of use. This bimodal characteristic of product demand in the sector makes managing the internal supply chain difficult for hospitals. For products and processes in healthcare that are characterized by frequently changing circumstances, predicting demand further up the supply chain becomes even more difficult. For example, when drug-eluting stents were introduced to the market, there was still uncertainty about both their intended use by surgeons and their demand. This made it difficult for suppliers to forecast demand. Anticipation of demand is made even more difficult as surgeons develop new, off-label applications for products. When these stents first came onto the market, some hospitals reported difficulty in securing sufficient quantities of the product, while competing hospitals with long-standing relationships with the manufacturer enjoyed the ease of access.

The amplification of demand volatility is described as the "bullwhip effect" or "volatility amplification."[3] The primary cause of this arises from poor communications throughout the supply chain. Demand signals at the point of use are misinterpreted at each succeeding upstream level. Demand information is then distorted as it passes through the supply chain. Relatively minor perturbations at the point of use become amplified through misinterpretation at the next level. See Exhibit 6.2.

This phenomenon often leads hospitals to use distributors to buffer themselves (by holding inventory) against the erratic demands at the

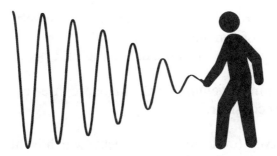

Exhibit 6.2: The bullwhip effect.

hospital or other end-user level. At the same time, clinical end users, faced with process-driven increases in the activity to support their work (or what is described as clockspeed amplification),[4] rely on their supply chain professionals and distributors to develop communication systems that provide accurate product demand information upstream to suppliers. This collaboration and effective communication is critical for information sharing that enables high-performance inventory management to ensure a smooth working environment. Today, with better communications and collaboration throughout the supply chain, such information misinterpretation is less likely but still occurs.

Within the inventory management process, there are two separate undertakings with different objectives and processes: inventory planning and inventory control. These are described below.

6.2.1 Inventory Planning

Inventory planning addresses how much inventory of a specific product should be held at each location of an enterprise's operation. To ensure that there is neither too much nor too little product, inventory planners apply forecasts of product demand along with estimates of expected delivery lead times for each product. This requires access to databases on product usage, vendor contract commitments, and awareness of special events that might cause demand to vary significantly. Hence, while it is a scientific process, it is also an inherently inaccurate one due to a range of unknown factors, some of which can arise unexpectedly.

The essence of inventory planning is to determine the amount of inventory required for each specific product at any one point in time. This is based on the characteristics of the flow of that product. These characteristics are tied to the following:

- Arrangements and capabilities of product suppliers in meeting demand requests;

- Behaviors of the users' demand for the specific product (e.g., reliability of demand forecasts); and
- Amount of inventory on hand at a specific point in time.

When planning inventory levels, there are three core variables that planners must consider:

- Stock levels (cycle and safety stocks) which is the actual amount of inventory on hand;
- Economic order quantity (EOQ), discussed in some detail later, is a calculation setting the amount of the replenishment order; and
- Inventory turns, which are the number of times that the inventory amount is completely used during a given time period.

The next sections describe each of these variables in detail.

◆ Cycle Stock and Safety Stock

Inventory planners take this information into account to calculate two types of inventories that are combined to form the total inventory needs.

a. **Cycle stock**—the amount of inventory needed to satisfy average product demand while a replenishment order from the supplier is in process.

b. **Safety stock**—the amount of inventory needed to cover two types of fluctuations in demand:
   - Delays in delivery time from supplier to warehouse (i.e., average time vs. actual time); and
   - Fluctuations in end-user demand (i.e., average user demand while awaiting a supplier replenishment vs. actual demand during that time).

In a calculation to determine required inventory safety stock, there are five variables that must be determined based on current and historical events. These are:

- Forecasted demand for the product for a particular time period;
- Variance in the historical demand forecasts;
- Lead time from the time that the order is issued to the vendor until the time that the product is delivered to the warehouse;
- Variance in the historical lead times for the vendor for the specific product; and
- Desired level of service, measured as line fill rate, is the percentage of times that the order for that product is completely filled as requested.

Embedded in the calculation of safety stock is this final variable that specifies the desired level of service for the customer. Since 100% in-stock performance is an almost impossible, if not very expensive, target to achieve, planners and supply chain managers must establish an acceptable level of in-stock performance. A 98% service standard (or fill rate) would imply that 2% of the time, the required amount of product would not be available for customers when they want it. For many products, a 98% fill rate would be quite suitable. However, for certain highly critical products in a healthcare system, 98% is not sufficient, and higher levels, such as 99% or 99.5%, are more appropriate.

Businesses often view inventory as a very low-performing asset. It is an investment in a stock that provides no margin or profit. Consequently, organizations do their best to minimize inventory held. However, when insufficient inventory is held, service quality deteriorates.

Without going into the technical details, a mathematical formula is applied to the five aforementioned variables to calculate the amount of inventory safety stock required. The input and output variables are summarized in Exhibit 6.3. For an in-depth explanation of the formulas and their application, see Chopra and Meindl.[5]

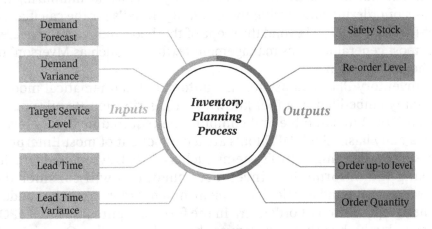

Exhibit 6.3: The inventory control process inputs and outputs.

◆ *Economic Order Quantity (EOQ)*

The sum of the cycle stock and the safety stock equals the amount of inventory required at any one time. However, as you decrease the inventory level through regular usage, you reach a point where the inventory on hand is below this sum. If not replenished, the inventory on-hand may not be sufficient to satisfy the demand. Consequently, at a

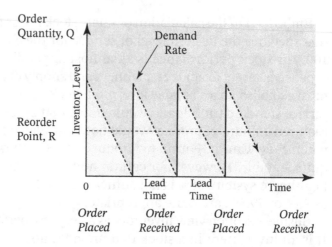

Exhibit 6.4: The "sawtooth" inventory replenishment diagram.

certain point, the inventory needs to be replenished. This point is known as the *Reorder Point* (ROP). This dynamic is illustrated in Exhibit 6.4. This sawtooth pattern is universal and applies to all inventory planning situations. Inventory planners must calculate the ROP. It is based on yet another inventory planning concept, the *Economic Order Quantity* (EOQ). It is defined as the optimal amount of inventory to reorder at any point in time to meet the required inventory level while minimizing the costs of ordering and storing the inventory. Details for the calculation of ROP and EOQ go beyond the scope of this book and are fully covered in most general logistics management textbooks, such as Myerson[6] or Chopra and Meindl.[7]

Inventory Planners use formal, automated mathematical models usually embedded in a tool known as a Distribution Requirements Plan (DRP) to assemble and compute the required inventory levels on a daily basis. Such DRP tools are a component of most Enterprise Resource Planning (ERP) systems such as SAP, Lawson, and Oracle. Using this information, inventory schedulers will consider the inventory on hand to calculate replenishment orders from the vendor. These replenishment orders are in the form of a purchase order (PO) issued by the healthcare system to the product vendor. Once issued, it becomes a contractual relationship driving delivery dates, quality, and payment terms.

◆ Inventory Turns

When measuring the performance of an inventory planning process, the number one metric used is the calculation of the inventory turns for each product. This measurement is an indication of the performance of the inventory held. For a supplier, when the number of turns is high, say 20 turns for explanatory purposes, it means that for every unit of inventory held, it generates 20 times the sales value of that product per period, typically measured on an annual basis. Conversely, if the number of turns is low, say two turns, that unit of inventory only generates two times the sales value for that same period. Clearly, the objective is to have all inventory turn at a high amount. However, that is unlikely since some products are simply not as popular as others. These are known as slow-moving items. Unfortunately, not every product is popular, and in every healthcare system, there will be slow-moving products.

To manage this situation, inventory managers often classify each product as an A, B, or C product. There are different ways to assign products to ABC classifications, but most typically, A products are the top 20% of the highest-selling products (often 80% of the total sales), while C products are at the bottom, generating 5% of the sales. B products are the balance, representing about 15% of the sales. Based on a product's ABC classification, inventory managers will make different decisions on stock location, inventory levels, and distribution strategies. These strategies lead to improved operating performance and product sales.

Often in cases where products are very slow turning, it may not be economically prudent for a healthcare organization to actually stock the items in their warehouse. In these cases, each time that the product is ordered by a unit in the hospital, that order will be forwarded to an outside supplier for subsequent delivery to the hospital. In such cases, the delivery times are extended; however, since these items have such a low level of demand, the delay is usually acceptable. In cases where the item may be critical for patient care, such items would be upgraded to a stocked item.

6.2.2 Inventory Control

Whereas *inventory planning* determines how much inventory is needed, *inventory control* ascertains whether the amount of inventory that should be in every location is actually in that location. This is crucial when ordering products from an internal stocking location, such as a warehouse. It assures the reliability of the warehousing process and, ultimately, the fulfillment process. The inventory control process includes knowing exactly where that inventory is in a specific location within a warehouse (e.g., a rack slot or shelf/bin denoted by a location-unique ID). This guarantees that whenever an order is placed for a product in a particular quantity, the warehouse or storage location can easily and accurately fill the request.

The control process begins when inventory is received at the warehouse. All items that reside in the storage location (warehouse) are subject to the inventory control process until those items are picked for an order. Embedded in the inventory control process are the following warehouse activities:

- Product receiving:
  - Warehouse dock staging of incoming product to enable easy putaway;
  - Product quality control (Is the received product exactly as described on the PO?);
  - Data entry of receipt information; and
  - Purchase Order (PO) reconciliation.
- Product putaway:
  - Location assignment; and
  - Product transfer from dock to storage location.

All of these activities require care not to damage the product as well as accuracy in counting and in putting away items in specific storage locations. Often corporate auditors are engaged to carefully review the activities and ensure the integrity of the process.

To make sure that the inventory level and locations are accurate at any one point in time, a supply chain management organization employs inventory control specialists whose primary role is to provide that certainty. Aside from requiring an ongoing practice of hygienic warehousing methods (e.g., reliable and accurate product movement within the warehouse), control specialists employ either *physical counts* or *cycle counts* for reconciling and adjusting inventory records. Either of these methods is appropriate. However, the physical count process is quite time-consuming and often requires the warehouse to suspend its normal operation while the count is in process. The best practice among most companies is the cycle count method.

The *physical count* method entails a complete wall-to-wall enumeration of every item, location by location, in the storage location. The actual physical count of the items is compared to the virtual amount recorded in the organization's inventory management system. In a large warehouse, this is a very lengthy and tedious process where nothing can be overlooked. Upon completion, the system record is updated with the actual physical count. Typically, corporate auditors oversee the process to ensure that the process and the outcome are consistent with corporate accounting standards. Any discrepancies result in a financial adjustment to the balance sheet as a write-off or write-on. Since such undertakings involve a substantial investment of time and a disruption to the business, physical counts are often limited to once per year.

In a *cycle count* program, products are counted periodically during the year according to two conditions: regular periodic counting and incident-related counting. The cycle count process has several advantages over the physical count process. It is far less time-consuming, it does not disrupt the business, and it is an ongoing process that most often identifies and corrects inventory discrepancies before they cause a fulfillment process failure. Almost all corporate auditors endorse the cycle count process as an acceptable alternative for inventory control purposes.

With regular periodically counted products, the frequency of counting a particular stock-keeping unit (SKU) depends on the velocity of its movement. Fast-moving items (referred to as A items in an ABC classification, typically representing the top 80% of total transaction value) might be counted monthly. Slow-moving items (C items representing 5% of total transaction value) might be counted only once per year. This process significantly reduces the amount of time spent reconciling inventory but yields an acceptable level of reliability.

With incident-related counting, which is done in addition to regular periodic counting, any item involved in an order that was not fulfilled due to an inventory discrepancy is flagged as an incident for immediate counting. This helps to quickly eliminate any further disruptions to the fulfillment process.

In addition to the counting processes for inventory control, accompanying any warehouse/storage function is adherence to good warehousing practices. To achieve this standard, all operating practices and processes require regular review and, if necessary, modification to ensure that all product flows/movements are transparent and recorded in the inventory database. This maintains information on product identity, quantity, and physical location before and after any product movement.

6.2.3 Best Practices in Inventory Management

This section identifies a series of best practices for inventory management processes. These practices are utilized by leading healthcare supply chain organizations to support their high-performance operations and are fundamental to the achievement of a FISCO.

Collaboration. The key to successful inventory management is the ability to know and predict changes in product flows, both upstream (supply side) and downstream (demand side). The best and only way to do this is through collaboration with partners throughout the supply chain. While some organizations fear that such collaboration outside their own businesses would compromise 'competitive' information, the benefits achieved far outweigh the risks. Collaboration may be done on a formal or informal basis. Whichever way it is done, it is key that the information obtained on changes to the above supply chain flows is accurate and shared with the appropriate people on a timely basis.

Information transparency and visibility. The principles of transparency and visibility are closely tied to collaboration. High-performance supply chains recognize that business decisions are best made when complete information on the operation of the extended supply chain is available to a broad number of business partners. Without information transparency, collaboration becomes limited, and difficult to generate value. For example, if a supplier withholds information about an upcoming planned shutdown, the customers will want to build inventory prior to the shutdown. If this plan was widely shared, then the customers could adjust their inventory levels at the appropriate time.

Despite the benefits of transparency, many organizations are opposed to sharing information in such detail, believing that their organization will be compromised if others (including some competitors) have access to some of their supply chain information. They view this information as proprietary. While it is a valid point that some information may be proprietary, quite often, most of it is not. However, sharing such non-proprietary information might, in fact, include contractual information from suppliers that is covered under a confidentiality clause in a supplier contract. This requires careful attention within collaboration and transparency practices.

The message is: carefully consider the information you place behind a firewall, assessing whether it is truly confidential or whether that information is better shared throughout the supply chain, enabling partners to make better inventory management business decisions.

Real-time information. Businesses operate at lightning speeds and 24 hours per day. Decision-makers cannot rely on batch-created reports and databases that were updated 12 or 24 hours previously. With today's cloud-based information enterprise resource planning (ERP) systems, all information is processed immediately and updated to databases within microseconds. This is real-time information processing. Despite the logic of such immediacy, there are still some legacy systems that operate on a batch mode with information updated on a daily basis. Think of the importance of banking transactions in real-time versus batch mode as an example. Today, best practice organizations have upgraded all or most of the information systems to ensure that the information databases reflect the actual position at the exact time that the information is requested. Consequently, a failure in inventory positioning can no longer be possible due to outdated information. However, the adage that "information from a computer is only as good as what goes in" still applies. Users must always remain wary of the information generated and apply a reasonable test to all information reports.

Measurement of forecast accuracy. Inventory management relies on forecasts of customer demand and supplier lead-time reliability. The accuracy (or inaccuracy) of these forecasts has a very significant impact on the usefulness of the inventory management plans that result. Interestingly, many organizations fail to track forecast accuracy and, more importantly, to learn from the mistakes of past forecasts. Best practice organizations incorporate demand and supply forecast accuracy into their planning processes and key performance indicators. Further, they modify their forecast parameters and practices as they learn from both the successes and failures of the past.

ERP processes. Today, most organizations have implemented broad-based ERPs. These powerful tools incorporate global best practices that control and direct all financial, human resources, and operations in a fully integrated manner. Managing a large healthcare organization without the support of such tools in today's highly complex environment is almost impossible. While most refer to these as computer systems, they are, in fact, a set of tools for establishing and operating fundamental business processes, such as financial reporting, purchasing, payroll, and people management. The major providers of these systems are Oracle, SAP, Infor, MediTech, and Workday.

Vendor Managed Inventory (VMI) and Vendor Owned Inventory (VOI). Some healthcare provider organizations have found that when the supplier participates in the management of inventory, the process improves and the outcomes are quite beneficial. Two types of programs are used with this arrangement, VMI and VOI. Such programs require careful design and control, but often result in considerable advantages. These advantages include reduced inventory investment, better control systems, and lower inventory write-offs from expired products. VOI programs are similar to consigned inventory. In this case, the supplier owns the inventory that is stored on the provider's premises. When inventory is used by the provider, an invoice for the cost of that product is generated. Simultaneously, the vendor's inventory planning process recognizes the withdrawal and adjusts its replenishment program accordingly. With VMI, the inventory investment is made by the provider. However, the supplier has total control over the planning and control of the inventory that resides on the provider's premises.[8] When following this approach, providers must ensure that they carefully examine the terms and conditions of the program established by the suppliers. Note that although the burden of inventory investment and management shifts from the provider to the supplier, such transfers are not without cost to the provider. There is never a "free lunch." Suppliers simply recoup the costs of such programs through product sales margins. However, inventory managed or owned by the suppliers is often a more efficient program. Hence, the total cost of ownership is usually lower.

EDI (Electronic Data Interchange). In its early incarnation, when hospital computer systems were not broadly aligned to the outside world, EDI was a separate process often managed by external partners to facilitate the transmission of business-related messages between market partners. These messages between providers and suppliers include a purchase order for a product's replenishment; confirmation of the order (including price) from the supplier, advanced ship notices indicating what is being shipped and when, and if any items are on backorder; and invoices for the products. All of these messages are time-sensitive, enabling a hospital manager or a supplier to act immediately on the new information. Timely and swift actions like these result in hospitals providing better quality service at lower costs. Today the vast majority of hospitals and suppliers use a business-to-business exchange to handle their EDI transactions in a one-to-many manner. These exchanges are linked directly to the hospital's ERP system.

Automation and machine learning tools. With the development of artificial intelligence (AI) tools, hospital supply chain managers can benefit from advanced tools that enable decisions to be made automatically and with greater precision than conventional manual methods. AI mimics the decision-making processes of industry experts. While not a perfect replacement for human intervention, these tools can improve the reliability of decision-making and lower costs. For many standard clerical activities, a branch of such automation methods, called robotic process automation (RPA), is particularly useful for automating many of the mundane inventory management processes.

Global risk management. Supply chains today are global. Events happening halfway around the world can disrupt access to inventory throughout a hospital system. To illustrate this, note the impact that Hurricane Maria had on the medical supplies manufacturing capacity of Puerto Rico. As it turned out, a very significant share of the global manufacturing capacity for saline solutions and intravenous (IV) bags was produced there. When the hurricane hit in 2017, manufacturing plants were taken offline. Subsequently, healthcare systems faced severe shortages of this critical product. As well, events happening close to home can equally disrupt inventory access. The COVID-19 pandemic created an inordinate and unexpected demand for personal protection equipment (PPE) products and critical care supplies. Consequently, leading supply chain managers tap into the expertise of global risk managers. Knowing immediately when and where such events happen and how they will impact the supply chain is crucial for inventory managers. Leading practice organizations have links to global threat awareness systems and have well-developed business continuity plans at their ready. Healthcare organizations can choose to have their own monitoring program or can subscribe to services from outside vendors.

Performance management system. No organization or operation will function at a high level unless it knows and responds to performance-level changes. Best practice healthcare organizations have well-developed and broadly communicated performance management systems tracking the key metrics of the organization. Such systems comprise a set of metrics that measure the most important aspects of the organization. Many organizations will categorize their metrics along four dimensions known as a "balanced scorecard": financial, process, quality, and people.

In addition, as metrics are created, best practice suggests that they should adhere to the principles of SMART (specific, measurable, achievable, relevant, and time-based). In addition to the metrics embedded in the performance management system, an effective system requires realistic targets. These targets should be achievable but also sufficiently challenging to maintain the market competitiveness of the organization.

6.3 Order Management Process

The order management process is at the heart of the logistics process. It connects the supply system to the end customer. It delivers the tangible value of the supply chain. The process typically begins with an expression of need by the customer, which is transmitted as an electronic requisition to the ERP system, which generates an order, sent internally, for example, to a warehouse management system (WMS), or externally to a supplier usually sent over a business-to-business (B2B) exchange. A number of steps, many of which are also electronic, follow until the product is physically delivered to the customer. In the healthcare world, much of this process is automated for lower cost, higher volume products, which are delivered to storage locations, such as nursing floors, where they are consumed as needed. For higher dollar items, some hospitals use automated replenishing cabinets that document when products are taken and by whom. However, in some situations, certain products are ordered on an as-needed basis under a blanket or standing order. Exhibit 6.5 displays the order management subprocesses that will be presented in this section.

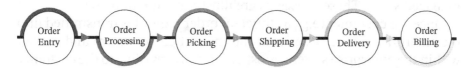

Exhibit 6.5: The order management subprocesses.

6.3.1 Order Entry

An order is simply a request from one person or one computer system to another for the fulfillment of a need. To act on this need, the order management process begins with the entry of an order into an order management system. It may be done manually or through a variety of technological systems. In the manual mode, end users of the product transmit their need through some form of expressed communication, either physical (e.g., written, oral, fax, etc.) or, increasingly, electronic requisitions. In either case, an order for a specific amount of a specific product to be delivered to a specific location at a specific time is transmitted to the materials management information or ERP system, which can send the order directly to the supplier or through a B2B exchange.

In the 1970s, as automated ordering began to grow, the healthcare industry agreed on a standard format to support electronic data interchange (EDI) transactions. Many types of order communications protocols were mapped to create an industry standard for communications of purchase orders, order confirmations, order status messages, and many more. The basic structures of these message formats are still in use today, most notably the purchase order request (referred to as an 850 EDI message), the purchase order confirmation (an 855 EDI message), advanced ship notices (856 EDI messages), and invoices (810 EDI message). Since that time, the process for automated ordering has evolved to benefit from solutions provided by data exchange organizations and other technology.

Manual order entry modes (such as phone calls, fax, and emails) are less structured, with customer service agents and others making one-off corrections to orders but not often making changes to prevent similar errors in the future. Automated transactions require data synchronization between buying and selling organizations to support fewer exceptions and more touchless orders.

6.3.2 Internal Order Processing

Hospitals and healthcare systems, especially those with consolidated service centers (CSCs), will also support internal order processes. The following describes processes that are similar in nature to what happens between health systems and suppliers, but this time, with their internally managed stock. These processes are illustrated in Exhibit 6.6.

Once the customer (e.g., a clinician) order request is transmitted into the enterprise system, a series of internal subprocesses are undertaken within the enterprise system. Most of these are invisible to the customer and to the staff fulfilling the order. But they are critical to ensure that an order can proceed. To understand the order management system, it is important to be aware of these background subprocesses.

1. **Order policy compliance**
   Embedded within all order management processes is a set of criteria that specify the characteristics of an acceptable order. These criteria are established not only to ensure a smooth flow of orders from the shipper, but also to ensure that only qualified customers place an order and that they order an appropriate quantity of the

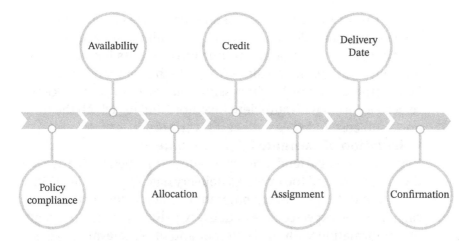

Exhibit 6.6: Order processing workflow.

product. For example, in the healthcare setting, the order system will usually only permit a clinical department to order products that are typically used in that department. For example, the system would typically have product category restrictions for example not permitting a nurse in a cardiac ward to order an orthopedic implant. As well, the order policy would control the quantity ordered to ensure that an order for an unreasonable amount of product (usually made in error) is not processed.

2. **Inventory availability verification**
   In order for an order to be processed, there must be sufficient inventory available to fulfill the order. The order processing step will determine whether and where inventory is available to process the order. In this step, it is needed to ascertain if there are multiple inventory stock locations that can be accessed, and which is the optimal one from a cost and service standpoint.

3. **Inventory allocation to the order**
   After determining that there is sufficient inventory to fulfill an order, the system goes through a process to formally allocate and reserve the inventory for that order. This is to ensure that another order does not capture that same inventory, leading to a possible situation where there is insufficient product to ship.

4. **Customer credit verification**
   An order is a contract to purchase a product. If the customer is unable to pay for the product, then the order cannot proceed. Even in healthcare settings within a hospital, while there is no formal payment, there are budget allocations in place. If a department does not have sufficient budget to order a quantity of products, then the order would be flagged and possibly suspended until the budget issues are resolved.

5. **Assignment of the order to a specific storage location**
   Inventory for an order may be located in multiple storage locations/warehouses. As part of an optimization process for smooth and efficient fulfillment, a location from which to ship the order must be identified. The order processing routine within the ERP will select a location with sufficient inventory and for which the transportation cost and speed are best for the order.

6. **Calculation of estimated delivery date**
   Key to customer-friendly order fulfillment is the transparency of the order flow and the expected delivery date for the order. Within a modern order processing program is a step whereby the system calculates the expected date of delivery to the customer and shares that information with the customer and other relevant parties.

7. **Confirmation of the order acceptance issued to the customer**
   Once all of the previous steps are completed, which in an automated system amounts to a couple of seconds at most, the plans for the balance of the order fulfillment process are communicated to the customer. At this point, these plans will constitute:
   - Acknowledgment of receipt of the order;
   - Confirmation that sufficient inventory is allocated to the order;
   - Estimation of the time/date when the order will be delivered to the customer; and
   - This confirmation is transmitted electronically to the customer.

8. **Transmission of the order instructions to the warehouse/storage location**
   The final step in the order processing stage is the transmission of the order information to the warehouse or storage location. Once again, this is an automated step within order management whereby an electronic message is transmitted to the system that manages the warehouse or storage location. In complex facilities, the warehouse information system may be a specialized WMS. In simpler facilities, it is a part of the order management system.

   When describing an order, we refer to both the quantity of lines and the quantity of items. Each order will have one or more lines, each line specifying a particular product or SKU. Particularly in healthcare, the line item will state the lot number and/or serial numbers of the product. Often these numbers will not be assigned to the order until the order line is picked, or in the case of implants, not until after the product is used in patient care.

   Within each line, the order will specify the number of units of the product that is ordered. It is important for the order line to clearly specify the unit of measure assigned to that particular line. Since the very same product could be sold as individual items, boxes, cartons, cases, or pallet loads, when the unit quantity is stated, the amount of product could vary considerably. In order management systems, the unit of measurement specification is taken very seriously since a mistake here could lead to an order of magnitude or more difference in the amount of product shipped. Increasingly, hospitals and healthcare systems are using global data standards managed by standards bodies such as GS1, Health Industry Business Communications Council (HIBCC), and International Council for Commonality in Blood Banking Automation (ICCBBA) and assigned to products by their manufacturers, and sometimes mandated by regulators as part of unique device identification (UDI) regulation.

6.3.3 Order Picking

Essentially, an order is only a virtual message. At this point, it exists only on paper or in a database. Needed is a connection between the virtual order with physical products stores in the warehouse. That is the order picking stage. When the order is received at the warehouse, it enters a queue with other orders in a specialized system module called a WMS. An advanced WMS has an optimization routine whereby orders are queued in a sequence to minimize the labor requirements while maximizing the speed of picking the order.

Further, to optimize the order picking process in a warehouse when an order has multiple lines, any individual line in an order may be picked along with items for other orders in a similar section of the warehouse and then consolidated with the other lines of the order, which may have been picked in a separate process. In large warehouses with thousands of orders being picked daily, this consolidation process is not simple, but it is manageable and can lead to considerable operational efficiencies.

6.3.4 Order Shipping

While the order items have been picked, they may be in various parts of the warehouse. They need to be assembled in one place and packaged for shipping. Once the consolidated order is brought from the picking area to the shipping area, the packaging process begins. A transportation method is chosen based on the size, weight, destination, and urgency of the order. Typically, automated warehouse management and transportation management systems are used to determine the shipping method.

The most complex step of this part of the process is the consolidation process, especially given that order lines are picked in different parts of the warehouse and at different times. Given the large number of orders that are processed every day and the immense size of these warehouses, such consolidation can get complex. Special consolidation systems, conveyor belts, and robotics are used for this purpose. Such systems send the picked order components to a specific location in the warehouse at a particular time. At that point, a mostly manual process takes over where the component order parts are located and physically placed together. For the first time, the order has materialized in an assembled state.

Packaging of the order will depend on the weight and cube of the assembled products. Once again, automated WMS have embedded modules to recommend the type and size of packaging. For example, a physically large order with a weight over 100 pounds would likely be palletized and then shrunk-wrapped for protection. A smaller-sized order of 10 pounds would be packed into a corrugated carton and stuffed with soft material to protect the contents from excessive movement.

6.3.5 Order Delivery

An order fully picked is of no value unless it is shipped to the customer or user of the products. This section describes how products get from the stock location (warehouse) to the user. Since orders could be sent from the warehouse to anywhere, the distance could be short or could be long. This will impact the type of transportation carrier chosen for delivery. Also, the speed by which the order needs to be delivered will impact the transportation mode and carrier chosen. The decision made will depend on economic, customer service, and availability concerns. As with packaging, the embedded transportation management system considers these factors and selects the optimal carrier for the order.

While transportation arrangements can be relatively straightforward (a request creating a transportation order for vehicle pickup and delivery), operational problems can interfere with the timely action of these arrangements, particularly for orders that depend on external parties or factors. In particular, global transportation equipment supply disruptions, labor issues, and natural disasters can lead to a lack of capacity and delays. Supply chain managers must carefully consider and account for the possibility of delays, whether international, national, or local transport moves are planned.

6.3.6 Order Billing

Since receiving payment for goods and services provided is important for businesses, this subsection describes how the orders are billed. Once an order has been shipped, a message is sent to the customer billing module of an ERP system to generate an invoice for the customer. For orders within a health system, this invoice is an internal accounting process. Inventory that was held on the balance sheet is expensed to the department receiving the product.

For shipments issued by external parties, the invoice to the health system will be based on the terms and conditions contracted between the shipper and the customer. It will reflect and specify pricing arrangements, discounts, and payment terms for the order. The invoice is typically issued and sent separately from the order, increasingly by electronic means.

6.3.7 Best Practices in Order Management

As with inventory management best practices, leading organizations have developed best practices for order management processes. Many of these practices are similar to those for inventory management. For example, performance management systems and information transparency provide similar levels of organizational effectiveness.

Consolidated warehousing. Many of the processes previously described reference the use of consolidated warehouses, especially by organizations operating many healthcare delivery facilities. A. large integrated healthcare organization may have hundreds of stock-keeping locations spread across its network of facilities. Some of these may be as small as a storage cabinet in a clinical area, but others may be standalone large or small warehouse facilities in a metropolitan area. Consolidation of these many facilities to one or two centralized facilities often delivers great value both from an economical and quality point of view. Economies of scale matter. Leading healthcare systems have established consolidated warehouse facilities to store efficiently and effectively, pick, pack, and ship products to user sites within the hospital.

Smaller healthcare organizations can also benefit from this type of solution. The economies of scale enable the system to invest in material handling equipment that reduces cost, speeds up order processing, and increases the accuracy of the order delivery. Note that while similar, it is important to differentiate consolidated warehousing from CSCs. The latter is a broader entity that includes consolidated warehousing along with consolidated sourcing, purchasing, and contracting services. CSCs are discussed in more detail later. CSCs are particularly applicable for large health systems with a critical number of facilities in regional areas or when multiple healthcare organizations partner together to be serviced by a single joint supply chain management organization (as discussed in Chapter 4). In some cases, a CSC owned by a health system will offer its services to other disparate organizations within the same region.[9]

Supply chain mapping, a practice initiated by sourcing and contracting teams, provides critical information about the location of shipping points by SKU. When utilizing global sourcing strategies, supply chain managers must maintain an acute awareness of global disruptions due to environmental, political, or other factors. Order managers must ensure that orders are placed with suppliers who will have the capability to process the orders successfully. While waiting for the supplier to report its capability for fulfillment is one tactic, a more proactive approach is to know of these disruptions prior to order placement and to redirect order requests to those suppliers with the ability to fulfill the order.

6.4 Returns Management Process

While the two previous logistics processes focused on the movement of product from the supplier to the patient, there is another logistics process that focuses on the sometimes necessary movement of product from the user (patient) to the supplier. This is the returns management process. While many medical products are not returnable due to hygiene reasons, circumstances sometimes arise, necessitating the return of products. Reasons for return may vary but are essentially driven by either an order placed by mistake (wrong item ordered or incorrect quantity ordered) or due to a recall of a medical product. The latter is critical, while the former is a nuisance. The circumstances ensuing from a product recall are discussed in Chapter 3. This section focuses on orders placed by mistake, although the processes for returning recalled goods are similar.

The returns process comprises four subprocesses—the request, the authorization, shipping, and the returns processing. Each is discussed in the following sections.

6.4.1 Return Request

When a healthcare system's logistics operation determines that it has excessive unexpired product due to an error in ordering (likely due to inaccurate demand forecast), it will submit a request to the vendor for authorization to return the product. Until the authorization has been granted, the product is placed in quarantine while awaiting the response.

If the product is being returned due to a recall from the manufacturer, the return request is actually initiated by the supplier, usually the manufacturer. The healthcare organization is required to return or dispose of the product in strict accordance with the terms stipulated in the return request notification.

6.4.2 Return Authorization

Manufacturers and distributors receiving the return request will assess the request based on a number of factors, including the product's condition:

- Product condition (days available before expiry and untampered packaging);
- Reason for the return request; and
- Terms in the sales contract.

Based on the manufacturer's discretion, they will issue to the hospital a returns authorization code, which must be clearly marked on the shipping label and documentation accompanying the returned product.

6.4.3 Return Shipping

The product owner (typically the hospital) is usually responsible for shipping the product back to the manufacturer. For recalled products, the manufacturers will typically pay the shipping charges. In some cases, the manufacturers will simply tell the healthcare organization to destroy the product instead of returning it. Upon proof of destruction, in these cases, the manufacturers will credit the healthcare organization.

6.4.4 Return Processing

When the manufacturers receive the returned product, they will inspect it for conformance to the conditions of the return program, including verifying lot numbers and packaging integrity. Invoice credits will be applied to the customer. While most of the products returned will be in sellable condition, to avoid any concerns with tainted products being released back into the marketplace, the manufacturers will often destroy the returned products.

6.4.5 Best Practices in Returns Management

Managing the returns of healthcare products can get overwhelming and messy very quickly. Products arrive unexpectedly in nonstandard packaging, often with incomplete documentation. Building processes and facilities to deal with this is usually beyond the scope and interest of most supply chain organizations. However, due to the value of healthcare products, such returns are necessary. To manage this, healthcare organizations often turn to specialized returns processing organizations with capabilities for managing unexpected receipts from users and programs to process individual items randomly received in varying conditions. These specialized processors are able to keep costs low and maximize the percentage of salvageable products that can be put back into stock. Since the integrity of the returned product is particularly critical for healthcare products, salvageability is an important consideration.

6.5 Make versus Buy Decisions for Logistics Services

The processes and practices described in the previous sections of this chapter lay out the fundamentals of effective and efficient logistics services to support healthcare systems. Success in execution depends on a well-designed supply chain management organization with well-trained and experienced staff. Such organizations require investments in people, facilities, and systems. Getting to best-in-class capabilities in this field takes considerable time, resources, and effort. Many health-care systems have made the strategic decision that this is not the type or size of investment that suits their organization. This is a strategic decision. Fortunately, they have an option. All of these services can be outsourced to an external service provider. This is the "make or buy decision" applied to logistics management processes.

This section describes and discusses the choices that healthcare orga-nizations have available to source logistics functions from outside pro-viders. The outside provider (or partner)—usually a national or regional distributor—establishes a fiduciary responsibility through contractual terms to service the healthcare organization in a manner as if it was their own business. The outside provider typically brings expertise and spe-cialized assets that are not available inside the healthcare organization. A successful outcome of this relationship is when value is created that otherwise could not be gained either practically or at a cost less than what the provider charges for the services.

As an added aspect of complexity for a healthcare organization, when deciding to outsource, a commonly adopted hybrid solution is for some products to be outsourced, and others insourced. Some organizations have found it efficient and effective to outsource their commodity-type products (i.e., those that are relatively low value and for which there is not significant differentiation among various manufacturers). These organizations, however, will insource their strategic (clinically preferred) products which are highly differentiated and often high-value items. Refer to the decision model in Chapter 2 for these designs.

When considering the external provision of services, there are four types of deals available. Exhibit 6.7 displays these four types and the structures often used in each type. For further insights into this endeavor,

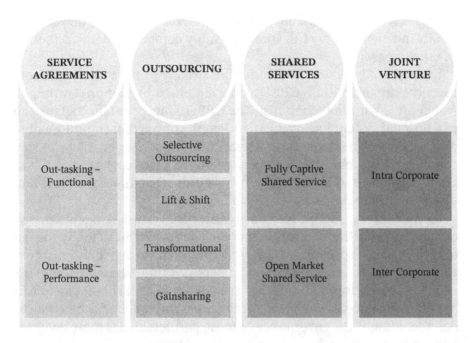

Exhibit 6.7: Types of service provision deals.

which is a well-developed field of its own, we refer you to Willcocks and Lacity,[10] Vitasek et al.,[11] and a 2022 Deloitte report on outsourcing practices.[12]

Fortunately for healthcare organizations, there are many service providers and options from which to choose. This section considers three types of organizational relationships that healthcare organizations can utilize to outsource some or all of their supply chain management needs. Just as purchasing partner management was identified as important for engaging group purchasing organizations (GPOs), purchasing partner management capability is a key consideration in the development of partnerships for distribution.

6.5.1 Collaborative Partnerships

Collaborative partnerships, by definition, are ventures between two or more organizations with a common interest to achieve a set of outcomes. A common example of such a partnership is a shared services organization, where multiple healthcare organizations (sometimes from disparate parent organizations) collaborate to fund and operate a joint supply chain services organization. These organizations are businesses with the intent to provide valuable services at a market price. In some cases, the shareholders of the business are the beneficiaries of the services. In other cases, the shareholders are arm's length organizations. The users of a shared services organization may be corporately related, or they may be totally independent organizations, possibly competing with each other in other areas.

Such shared services are sometimes referred to as common pool resource organizations (CPRO), a term coined by Elinor Ostrom,[13] a Nobel-prize-winning economist. The CPRO concept entails that instead of a hospital system having an arm's length contractual commitment to products through a large commercial entity, regional players (who may compete with each other for many goods and services) can collaboratively participate in a jointly governed venture that directly sources and distributes these products.

As businesses, shared service organizations must strive to operate efficiently, providing services that are needed and contractually subject to performance expectations. Consequently, such partnerships must continually adapt to meet the changing needs of their shareholders. This is not as straightforward as it may seem since not all shareholders will have the same needs when the partnership is formed, nor as time moves on. Accordingly, the governance of these partnerships is more complex and more important than in a conventional business.

Partnerships for shared services organizations can take many forms, ranging from informal communications (e.g., weekly conference calls) among unrelated organizations focused on solving a specific problem to formal joint venture organizations with common assets, contractual commitments, and governance structures (e.g., CSCs). Exhibit 6.8 displays the continuum of shared services solutions. Some are structured, while others are quite informal and may only be temporary solutions to a joint problem. During the COVID-19 pandemic, many healthcare organizations formed collaboratives in some form or another to jointly deal with the supply problems created by the excessive demand for personal protective equipment (PPE) and other supplies.

The Continuum of Shared Services Solutions

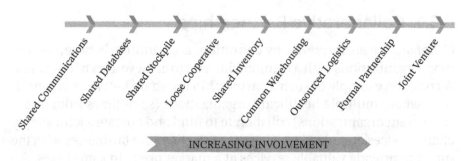

Exhibit 6.8: The continuum of shared services solutions.

Source: Adapted from Center for Outsourcing Research and Education.

In the healthcare setting, such collaborative partnerships often take the form of CSCs. These operations consolidate the logistics and sometimes procurement operations of multiple healthcare systems. Value is achieved through five distinct capabilities:

- Reduced *cost* through economies of scale;
- Reduced *risk* in supply through a broader set of customers/users;
- Increased *capability* through concentrated centers of expertise;
- Increased *opportunity* through experience and exposure to multiple operational settings; and
- Increased *predictability* through larger, more sophisticated operations.

The value gained through such capabilities is very difficult to replicate in standalone operations. Healthcare systems that commit to such CSCs have created significant competitive advantages.

Some healthcare collaborative partnerships are established among multiple healthcare systems to provide a common service operated by a single entity. While the focus of this book is on supply chain management services, such partnerships can function in many other healthcare system disciplines, some clinical and some administrative. Examples of others include laboratory services, facility management, biomedical engineering, laundry, food services, and diagnostic imaging services.

In very large complex healthcare systems extending over multiple regions, where each region traditionally has its own independent corporate structure, a shared service among the corporate regions can generate value through scale and reduction of redundant operations. Conversely, multiple healthcare systems in a particular region that may normally compete with each other in clinical services might find value in a shared service for a more administrative function such as supply chain management. In the U.S. healthcare system, both corporate shared services organizations and regional competitive shared services organizations thrive.

Among the forms of shared services organizations, there are two principal types of partnerships. One is voluntary, where each corporate entity may choose to participate or not. Alternatively, there is the mandated type whereby all entities are required to participate by virtue of a corporate policy. For each, the motivation for participating differs. However, for either type, unless the shared services entity generates more value as a whole than the sum of the individual members can do on their own, the shared service is of limited value and usually not sustainable.

In terms of the structure of the relationship, the shared services organization parallels the third-party outsourced relationship described in the following section. Central to its existence are service-level agreements entered between the shared services organization and each of its member shareholders. These agreements outline the details of the services performed, the performance expectations, the transfer price of the services, and obligations if the service levels are not met or payment for services is not forthcoming. In essence, these agreements become the basis of the contractual relationship between the parties. To complete the contract, a master agreement is crafted to specify terms and conditions for:

- Term of the services agreement;
- Liability limitations;
- Indemnification for damages;
- Termination provisions; and
- Dispute resolution.

In establishing the organization, as previously indicated, structuring an effective governance process is critical. Governance details the framework by which decisions are made in four areas:[14]

- Setting expectations for performance;
- Granting power to act;
- Verifying that performance is achieved; and
- Ensuring that risks are adequately monitored and managed.

The outcome of good governance results from meeting the five objectives inherent in all governance systems. These objectives, whether or not the relationship is arm's length or internal, are designed to:

- Achieve desired business objectives;
- Enable and ensure fulfillment of accountability;
- Provide the ability to rapidly identify and resolve issues;
- Maintain alignment of buyer/provider objectives; and
- Rapidly adapt to change.

In selecting executive committees/directors for the system, representatives are typically chosen from the shareholders, in other words, the sponsor organizations. However, it is not unusual to bring in some external directors who can bring an unbiased, objective viewpoint and with capabilities and skills not represented among representatives of the shareholders.

There are many good examples of collaborative supply chain management partnerships among healthcare systems. Among the leading partnerships, many have generated above-average value for their members and continue to drive value and innovation in health-care supply chain management. These collaboratives tend to be either multi-system operations or a multi-state integrated delivery network.

Some of the more notable collaborative healthcare system partner-ships across North America are listed in Exhibit 6.9. These partnerships provide a range of valuable services delivered efficiently and effectively. Some of these services include:

- Supply chain management services:
  - central sterile/instrument reprocessing,
  - supply distribution,
  - receiving,
  - recall management,
  - crash carts,
  - inventory management,
  - mailroom,
- Consolidated Service Center operations, and
- Logistics management

Exhibit 6.9: Notable healthcare supply chain management partnerships in North America.

United States	Canada
LeeSar[a] in Sarasota, FL	BC Support Services[b] in Vancouver, BC
ROi[c] in St Louis, MO	Plexxus[d] in Toronto, ON
Banner Health[e] in Phoenix, AZ	
Intermountain Health[f] in Salt Lake City, UT	
Common Spirit[g] in Phoenix, AZ	

[a] https://www.leesar.com.
[b] http://www.bccss.org.
[c] https://roiscs.com.
[d] https://www.plexxus.ca.
[e] https://www.bannerhealth.com.
[f] https://intermountainhealthcare.org/supply-chain-organization.
[g] https://www.commonspirit.org.

Several of these partnerships were discussed in depth in an article describing three collaboratives, labeled alpha, beta, gamma.[15] Exhibit 6.10 highlights some of the value metrics and performance for these three collaboratives.

6.5.2 Distributors

A major logistics solution used extensively within the healthcare industry is the distribution of products through specialized companies called

Exhibit 6.10: Impact on supply chain performance of three healthcare collaboratives.

	Alpha	Beta	Gamma
A. Percentage reduction in total number of med/surg. *suppliers*	Reduced by 10%	Reduced by 20%	Reduced by 10%
B. Percentage reduction in total number of med/surg. *direct*	Reduced by 90%	Reduced by 10%	Reduced by 50–75%
C. Expected *reduction* in FTEs at the hospital	5+ FTEs	15 FTEs	3 FTEs
D. Expected *additional* FTEs needed at CSC to service the hospital	2 FTEs	8 FTEs	1 FTE

Note: Abdulsalam, Y., Gopalakrishnan, M., Maltz, A., & Schneller, E. (2015). The emergence of consolidated service centers in health care. *Journal of Business Logistics, 36*(4), 321–334, 327.

distributors or wholesalers. There are many distributors in the market that provide a wide range of logistics services but essentially aggregate the demand from multiple providers and their customers, then efficiently deliver those products to their customers.

In the United States, at the time of publication, the major medical distributors include Cardinal Health, Owens & Minor, Medline, McKesson, and Concordance. In addition to these major distributors, there are many smaller, local, and regional distributors. They all provide similar services on a geographically specific basis, although some, due to their scale, are able to generate higher value for their customers.

Just as the distributor is actually being paid by two masters (manufacturers and healthcare delivery organizations), the distributor also has two sets of servants. First, distributors do their best to provide valuable services to both their buying and selling masters and generally have established a comfort level with the subsequent tensions. Perhaps this is because the distributor is also actually serving two very fragmented customer sets (supply chain managers and clinicians). While this may seem to create a market advantage, distributors continue to operate on fairly low margins. This occurs due to (a) intense rivalry among distributors and (b) distributors not clearly distinguishing themselves from a new set of either added or needed value products.

While manufacturers have been advised by business experts to treat distributors like partners in revenue creation,[16] the same has not been strongly advocated for healthcare providers that have abdicated some of their business control to distributors. To improve distribution and inventory, healthcare executives need to ask critical questions about value, control, and power. Accordingly, it is imperative to determine the extent of control the executive team wants over the expenses and services represented in these processes. In addition, the depth of desired knowledge must be determined. And third, the power within the supply chain must be assessed. The information provided from these strategic discussions can help form a more strategic approach to the supply chain.

Despite these limitations, many healthcare providers have a very strong, dedicated, loyal, and often dependent relationship with their distributors. For smaller providers, the distributor is often the only means for them to acquire a broad range of products, and they consequently rely on the distributor for almost all product purchases. For larger providers, their internal supply chain management organization is larger and has the capability to directly source products from manufacturers. These providers will typically use the distributor for commodity-type purchases and then source strategic products (e.g., high-value, high-complexity products) directly.

Due to the large purchasing power of a distributor and their inventories of products in warehouses across the country (and around the world), distributors have developed the capability to efficiently handle many small quantity orders and deliver them quickly to the provider facilities. As a result, they have developed just-in-time (JIT) inventory systems for their provider customers. Although over-reliance on JIT has been called into question in the wake of the recent global pandemic, JIT has enabled hospitals and healthcare systems to acquire products quickly and avoid holding inventories. Many providers have taken advantage of this solution, although more are seeking access to their own backup stockpiles. While JIT strategies have been under attack, a more appropriate view of JIT is to recognize it for what it is and to manage its use responsibly. In a well-written HBR article by Sodhi and Choi, they argue that JIT systems should be better designed to handle uncertainties.[17]

While distributors provide healthcare providers a wide array of valuable services, these services are not without a cost. Since distributors purchase products from manufacturers and then resell and deliver these products to the healthcare providers, in addition to the value (and margin) they create from physical distribution, they also generate margins for themselves from the buy/sell function. Typically, these buy/sell margins are significantly greater than the physical distribution function margins. Because these margins can be substantial, some healthcare providers with large purchasing power have chosen to repatriate their sourcing through distributors by doing it themselves. Internal sourcing staff will purchase products directly from manufacturers, usually under

GPO or local contracts. These purchases often require large order quantities necessitating warehousing in provider-owned or leased facilities. For high-value strategic items, this approach is quite effective. However, unless providers have capacity for large inventories, for low-cost commodity items, the distributors often offer better arrangements. Each provider organization, through its supply chain management organization, makes these decisions as part of its strategic sourcing and organizational design policies and practices. They apply a make versus buy decision.

6.5.3 Third-party Logistics Providers

A popular solution for healthcare providers is to outsource a significant proportion of their logistics operation to an arm's length provider organization such as a third-party logistics provider. Aside from the economic scale that such arrangements bring, a subtler rationale may exist. Healthcare institutions, given their culture, operate at a well-defined pace, consistent with the precision and high-quality demands that delivering great medical care requires. Supply chain operations, on the other hand, operate in a fast-paced environment affected by factors as varied and unpredictable as global conflicts and local road traffic conditions. Consequently, the "clockspeed" of these operations differ and will demand different intra-organizational cultural conditions. As is discussed in the introduction, Charles Fine[18] of MIT has argued that organizational design needs to consider alignment with the clockspeed and capabilities of the specific function in a rapidly evolving world. Accordingly, some have found that outsourcing the fast-paced functions of a healthcare organization's supply chain to third-party companies that regularly operate in that environment will provide improved performance.[19,20]

Many of the large global supply chain logistics companies, such as DHL, FedEx, and UPS, offer these services through subsidiaries. Notably, unlike traditional healthcare distributors, third-party logistics providers (3PL) do not own the inventory, nor do they generate margins from the sale of the goods. Their only margin is attributable to the value they create in the physical handling of the goods and the information that they process. Their breadth of experience and narrowly focused high degree of expertise brings value to healthcare organizations that the healthcare organization could not (easily) create on its own.

Outsourcing a service function such as logistics can generate numerous tangible benefits for the healthcare provider. The leading value-creation sources emerge from:

- Facilitating corporate focus on core functions;
- Sourcing innovative solutions;

- Accessing readily available "in-house" expertise;
- Implementing technology immediately, without the investment;
- Accessing specialized asset base;
- Sharing risks;
- Sharing gains; and
- Clarifying accountability: Single point of contact.

With any change in the source of value comes changes to accountability and responsibility. Organizations pursuing this strategy need to understand this and adapt to it (see Exhibit 6.11). While the accountability for the outsourced service shifts from the internal group to the external group through a contracted relationship, the responsibility for the service never transfers. The hospital or healthcare system retains responsibility and must structure its organization accordingly.

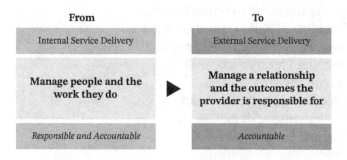

From	To
Internal Service Delivery	External Service Delivery
Manage people and the work they do	**Manage a relationship and the outcomes the provider is responsible for**
Responsible and Accountable	*Accountable*

Exhibit 6.11: Accountability and responsibility changes.

There are several ways to structure a 3PL relationship. All provide value. The choice depends on the breadth and depth of outsourcing that the healthcare system desires. Typical structures include:

- Full service (infrastructure and labor provision);
- Infrastructure only (healthcare system provides labor);
- Warehouse space together with material handling equipment;
- Information systems and business processes; and
- Labor only (healthcare system provides the infrastructure).

When deciding to consider this strategy for logistics services, there are a set of well-established practices that leading organizations follow. Many of these are drawn from the IT outsourcing field. The steps (Side Bar 6.1) reflect the best practice in outsourcing management, and hence, apply equally to establishing a successful 3PL provider relationship.

Side Bar 6.1

Steps for Establishing a Successful 3PL Organization

- Develop the strategy for outsourcing:
- Establish expectations and goals
- Identify core competencies and expertise
- Identify the scope of services to be outsourced
- Develop the model to be used
- Build the business case
- Establish performance specifications
- Target qualified providers
- Design the service delivery program
- Identify the services
- Construct service level agreements
- Draft preliminary contract terms
- Establish dispute resolution process
- Issue RFP and select a provider
- Negotiate terms and conditions
- Set pricing structure
- Execute a services contract
- Implement services
- Manage the provider
- Govern the relationship
- Measure performance
- Continuously improve
- Manage risks.

6.5.4 GPOs in Healthcare

GPOs, discussed extensively in Chapter 5, are widely used by healthcare organizations to manage all or a part of their product sourcing needs. While sourcing is not a logistics activity, it is included here for completeness since GPOs are, in fact, outsourcing organizations for procurement activities. Their focus is on sourcing and contracting. As such, these require the same oversight and corporate development practices as an outsourced third-party logistics provider. The very same principles outlined in the previous sections apply equally.

6.5.5 Best Practices in Outsourcing

As with the other aspects of logistics processes within supply chain management, there are some important best practices in outsourcing that cause highly successful organizations to perform as well as they do. Many of these are similar to those in insourced logistics processes, but some are unique to outsourcing. Noteworthy are the following best practices:

Executive support. Foremost to the success of any outsourcing initiative is the explicit endorsement of an outsourcing arrangement by the senior executives (and particularly the CEO) of the organization. Since outsourcing has a direct impact on corporate assets (both physical and human), such initiatives are clearly strategic. An endorsement sends a strong message throughout the organization that the initiative is important and a strategic imperative.

Business-case driven. Any major undertaking in a business must have a strong business case to support it. The business case demonstrates to everyone in the organization (and externally) that the initiative has merit and indicates where and how the value is created. Powerful business cases indicate the financial, operational, customer, human resources, and risk impacts of the initiative.

Effective governance. Due to the multi-party relationships in an outsourcing arrangement, the parties must be carefully monitored and controlled. The process by which a business does this is called governance. Governance is the system of rules, practices, and processes by which an organization is directed and controlled. All significant decisions regarding the outsourcing arrangement, including investments, changes to service conditions, and pricing should be passed through a governance council. The council should be comprised of representatives of the parties involved (the clients and the providers). Typically, clients would have voting rights while the providers would not.

Service-level agreements. To define the work being done and the expectation of associated service quality, formal service-level agreements are prepared to specify the nature of the work and the performance levels expected. Note that best practice organizations specify the service in terms of the performance level rather than through a functional specification that details exactly how the operation should run. In addition, these agreements indicate actions to take when service levels fall below a specified threshold.

Transparency. Throughout all supply chain management practices, including logistics, transparency into the workings of the supply chain is critical. Anyone making a business decision affecting a supply chain action needs the ability to view all necessary aspects of the supply chain's status, including inventory positions, supplier arrangements, and demand forecasts. While some of this information may be proprietary, there are ways to share the information in a manner that does not disclose proprietary or other competitively sensitive information. Too often, guidelines are excessively strict, and the sharing of valuable information is unnecessarily restricted. There are usually ways to structure the disclosure and share the information to those who need it without compromising anyone's competitive position.

Physician engagement. Unlike other industries, healthcare has an important extra component to its supply chain—the physician. Although the patient is usually considered the customer, the physician (and other clinical staff) act as agents for the customer dictating the use of particular medical products in the form of protocols. These protocols form the basis of medical practice. As such, these agents (physicians) have a critical role in the decision-making for supply chain management. That being said, physicians do not want to be directly involved in the day-to-day operations of the supply chain. Consequently, healthcare supply chain management involves a delicate balancing act of ensuring that physician needs are met without requiring them to get deeply involved. When logistics is outsourced to a third party, this balancing act is even more delicate and difficult, but must be incorporated into the business processes.

Change management processes. In all large, complex business endeavors, a formal change management process is incorporated into the introduction of new or modified business processes. For outsourced logistics processes where the operators are one step removed from the core business, a formal change management process with the inclusion of a broad representation of the parties is needed even more. Best practice organizations formally incorporate this as part of the contractual arrangements. Operators then place special emphasis and resources on its application.

Dispute Resolution. An outsourcing arrangement is a contractual arrangement between two or more parties. When any party in the outsourcing deal has a significant disagreement with another party, a formal dispute is formed. Within a good contract is a set of processes and remedies for resolution. Often through internal escalation of the matter, the issues can be resolved between the parties. In cases of very complex disputes, the use of arbitration may be warranted.

Communications. The farther away from the center of a business, the more important frequent and thorough communications become. When outsourced, the operations are more opaque to the suppliers and customers. Hence, even greater attention is needed for effective communication. Any changes in the supply chain management practice, unusual occurrences, disruptions, or changes in staffing need to be communicated. Sometimes this may seem like excess communications, but due to the extra organizational distance between the outsourced activity and the core customers/users of the supply chain, the excess is appropriate.

6.6 Successful Logistics Strategies

Successful logistics managers apply a set of well-established strategies when designing a logistics system and when operating it day-to-day. These strategies differ from "best practices" that apply to performing a specific function. Most strategies for a high-performance link to the concept of making trade-offs and deciding which option for the operation is best. A classic example of this is trading off holding more inventory in exchange for lower transportation costs. Discussed in the following are the most common strategies employed to improve operating performance.

Trade-offs in integrated logistics. There are many ways to operate a supply chain's logistics system. Assets can be deployed in multiple ways and in multiple locations. Inventory levels can be raised to offset transportation delays and uncertainties. Service levels (speed and quality) can be set higher or lower to meet customer and financial needs. As a result, there is a multitude of combinations and permutations to design and operate a logistics system.

When deciding which path to follow, decision criteria are required. Cost is not the only criterion. Decision-makers must also consider service quality impacts, regulatory, environmental, and social impacts, as well as risk mitigation. A low-cost solution could have long-term negative impacts on service quality and patient outcomes. The optimization process requires thoughtful consideration.

Deciding how to configure the logistics system with so many variables to consider takes a sizeable effort. Each one of the variables (e.g., inventory levels, transportation modes, packaging modes, warehouse facilities, etc.) has many dimensions to consider. More importantly, the configuration of one of the variables impacts the requirements (and costs) of others. In other words, this is a highly dynamic system where each variable impacts the others. For example, if slower transportation services are procured between two locations, need is increased investment in inventory to achieve the same level of service.

The overarching challenge for configuring a logistics system is understanding the outcomes of the myriad combinations of investments and service levels. To achieve a high-performing supply chain, managers focus on these trade-offs and design logistics systems that optimize the system. Using specialized computer-aided tools and algorithms, managers consider hundreds of design scenarios to establish the optimal solution. Then, on a regular basis, they review these solutions in light of a changing environment. The work of a logistics manager is never done.

Decision postponement. One of the secrets of supply chain management, and logistics management in particular, is that inventory acquisition, which hides many sins of the supply chain, can be deferred. And when deferred, significant benefits can accrue. Typically, supply chains have carried too much inventory—and inventory is viewed as a necessary evil. By deferring decisions to issue purchase orders until better information about future demand is available, inventory levels can be reduced, and in some cases, future write-offs avoided. By incorporating decision postponement strategies into the logistics process, purchase spend, inventory levels, write-offs, and order transactions can be lowered, resulting in a higher performing supply chain. All of this must also be viewed in light of the experience of the global pandemic. Hospitals and healthcare systems must balance resilience and economics.

Postponement can also apply to other parts of the logistics processes. In transportation, by holding shipments until a consolidated load is larger, shipping costs, as well as increasingly important carbon emissions, can be lowered. In order picking, by establishing minimum order policies, small uneconomic orders can be eliminated, resulting in larger, more efficient order picking and shipping. Postponement does not mean procrastination. By knowing the capability of the supply chain to react to an order and associated need, precise timelines can be set and trusted. Consequently, supply chain managers can initiate actions after more information about needs and supply chain operations becomes available. In highly competitive situations or where product availability is limited, such deferred decision-making capability can add significant value to supply chain performance.

Network optimization. The number and specific geographic locations of the warehouses and transportation routes used to distribute products has a very significant impact on the cost and service quality of product distribution. Generally, having more warehouses spread proportionally throughout a market area will speed up the delivery of orders to customers. However, the size and complexity of logistics infrastructure can be costlier to operate and requires a significantly higher investment in inventory. Hence, the objective in designing an optimal network is fourfold:

- minimize the number of warehouses;
- locate them in the ideal location from a transportation, real estate, and labor market standpoint;
- minimize the amount of inventory required; and
- ensure that the required customer service levels are met.

Given the vastness of the country, the number of combinations and permutations from these variables is immense. Calculating the optimal design based on these variables becomes a monumental task. Fortunately, highly effective computerized algorithms are available to create an optimal design. By inputting the customer demand, the cost of inventory, the transportation network options, labor costs, and the required customer service levels, potential network designs can be created. Typically, the results of such computer-generated design work will require minor tweaking to adjust for reality. But more often than not, these algorithms can suggest network designs that may otherwise not have been considered competitive.

Allocation when supply is limited. Increasingly, medical product suppliers face product shortages due to manufacturing disruptions or unexpected demand. Such disruptions occur due to a number of reasons, including:

- regulatory restrictions,
- equipment failure,
- raw material shortages,
- staffing shortages, and
- unexpected demand.

These shortages ripple through the supply chain impacting healthcare organizations' inventories and, consequently, patient care. As seen during the COVID-19 pandemic, such shortages have a wide and profound impact on the delivery of patient care as well as on the safety of medical professionals and staff. Dealing with these shortages requires careful consideration and logistics system adjustments. When inventory stocks are not limited, orders can proceed without restrictions. Any customer requiring product replenishment can order and receive regular amounts of products.

When a disruption occurs, and less product is available for shipping to customers, the manufacturers' logistics staff, in conjunction with marketing and sales staff, spring into action. Difficult decisions must be made to determine exactly how much product each customer will receive. Manufacturers and distributors will consider several factors, some of them arbitrary, in this decision:

- Contractual commitments,
- Historical shipment volumes, and
- Medical priorities.

Based on these factors, each customer will be assigned a maximum order quantity as well as an order frequency. In all cases, suppliers try to be fair, but in such situations, this can be very difficult due to competing priorities. Experience has taught us that manufacturers that perform the best in such situations take a long-term view and focus on long-term relationships with customers. Consequently, the impact on the customers could be severe.

For the customers (the healthcare organizations), the strain of reduced shipment volume is particularly difficult. In extreme situations, life or death decisions must be made to determine which patients (or staff, such as in the case of personal protective equipment) will receive the product. In such cases, medical ethicists are engaged in developing prioritization schemes for the allocation of products. In addition, supply chain staff need to actively involve clinical staff in these decisions as they are critical, if not the ultimate, decision-makers regarding the choice of products used in patient care.

6.7 Chapter Summary

Embedded within the logistics activities that are discussed in this chapter are the important FISCO functions of order processing, inventory management, receiving, and asset management. While other supply processes create the arrangements for product supply, these operational logistics functions that physically deliver the goods are critical to generating value from the supply chain management system.

The sections in this chapter explained how inventory levels are determined and managed, how suppliers respond to product order requests from providers, and how the product gets from the point of production to the point of consumption. Highlighted in each section were the best practices employed to generate a high-performance supply chain management solution. Also explained was how high-performing organizations decided which functions to perform themselves and which ones to outsource to an outside party, such as a logistics provider or a distributor. Healthcare organizations can use these guidelines to determine which approach to follow.

Notes

1. Chopra, S., & Meindl, P. (2021). *Supply chain management strategy, planning & operation* (7th ed.). Pearson.
2. Schneller, E. S., & Smeltzer, L. R. (2006). *Strategic management of the health care supply chain*. Jossey Bass.
3. Ibid.
4. Fine, C. (2000). Clockspeed-based strategies for supply chain design. *Production and Operations Management*.
5. Chopra & Meindl, op. cit.

6. Myerson, P. A. (2015). Supply chain and logistics management made easy: Methods and applications for planning, operations, integration, control and improvement, and network design. Pearson Education.
7. Chopra & Meindl, op. cit.
8. Hossain, M. I., & Parvez, M. S. (2020). Investigating the effect of extended vendor managed inventory in the supply chain of health care sector to enhance information exchange. *International Journal of Information and Management Sciences*, *31*(2), 171–189. http://163.13.238.245/IJIMS/files/recruit/774_548737df.pdf
9. Abdulsalam, Y., Gopalakrishnan, M., Maltz, A., & Schneller, E. (2015). The emergence of consolidated service centers in health care. *Journal of Business Logistics*, *36*(4), 321–334.
10. Willcocks, L., & Lacity, M. (2015). *Nine keys to world-class business process outsourcing*. Bloomsbury Information.
11. Vitasek, K., Manrodt, K., & Kling, J. (2012). *Vested: How P&G, McDonald's, and Microsoft are redefining winning in business relationships*. Palgrave Macmillan.
12. https://www2.deloitte.com/us/en/pages/operations/articles/global-outsourcing-survey.html
13. Ostrom, E. (1990). *Governing the commons: The evolution of institutions for collective action*. Cambridge University Press. ISBN: ISBN 0-521-40599-8
14. Center for Outsourcing Research and Education. (2015). Governance and relationship management, governance fundamentals. http://proc.conisar.org/2015/pdf/3662.pdf
15. Abdulsalam, op. cit.
16. Anderson, J. C., & Narus, J. A. (1984). A model of the distributor's perspective of distributor-manufacturer working relationships. *Journal of Marketing*, *48*(4), 62–74.
17. Sodhi, M., & Choi, T. (2022, Oct. 20). Don't abandon your just-in-time supply chain, revamp it. *Harvard Business Review*. https://hbr.org/2022/10/dont-abandon-your-just-in-time-supply-chain-revamp-it
18. Fine, C. (2000). *Clockspeed-based strategies for supply chain design, production & operations management*. MIT Press.
19. Skipworth, H., Delbufalo, E., & Mena, C. (2020). Logistics and procurement outsourcing in the healthcare sector: A comparative analysis. *European Management Journal*, *38*(3).
20. Beaulieu, M., Roy, J., & Landry, S. (2018, Dec). Logistics outsourcing in the healthcare sector: Lessons from a Canadian experience. *Canadian Journal of Administrative Sciences*, 635–648.

7

Performance Measurements and Maturity Models—*You Only Get What You Measure*

7.1 Introduction

Hospitals and healthcare systems are continually challenged to improve their performance. Performance, as a construct, can be abstract and subjective without defining how it is measured. The concept of organizational maturity provides a framework to measure the quality of an organization and its functions.[1] Maturity models provide "*a sequence of levels (or stages) that together form an anticipated, desired, or logical path from an initial stage to maturity*."[2] Such models allow organizations to make assessments and engage in management development to adapt to the variety of challenges in their environments and clockspeeds that characterize the environment. Recognizing which metrics to seek for specific aspects of performance is an essential skill for healthcare managers. Tracking performance indicators effectively and consistently provides a foundation for understanding an organization's level of maturity in its various business processes and subsequently, the development of a strategy.

This chapter defines and discusses performance measurements at three levels: (a) metrics, (b) metric sets, and (c) performance measurement systems. In doing so, we highlight some key performance indicators (KPIs) that a supply chain manager would benefit from tracking and provide context for why, when, and how often these KPIs should be reviewed. In unison, supply chain metrics steer strategic decision-making and integrate into a more prominent host of clinical, managerial, regulatory, and other KPIs. As such, metrics and metric sets integrate into performance measurement systems, forming a framework for monitoring hospital supply chain performance. Organizations develop their performance measurement systems or adopt previously developed performance measurement frameworks. Numerous performance measurement systems assess and guide organizational maturity.[3,4] Several performance measurement systems are presented introduced in this chapter, but a deeper dive is taken into the Fully Integrated Supply Chain Organization (FISCO) model, which is highly grounded in metrics for the various FISCO functions. This framework, already discussed in multiple chapters and contexts, enables healthcare managers to assess their current supply chain maturity and work toward its development.

To begin, we start with a discussion of the nature of metrics related to performance and how families of metrics group together to form metric sets that can be integrated into performance measurement systems.

7.2 Metrics and Measurements

Measuring performance is a core component of evidence-based management. Many performance metrics exist that consider different aspects of a healthcare provider organization. Measurements are taken at all levels of an institution: individuals, products, processes, departments, institutions, and so on. In other words, a mature organization meticulously measures the performance of all internal stakeholders, products, processes, and groups. Performance measurements serve many purposes. Commonly employed metrics allow for:

- Comparing different entities or a single entity across time;
- Identifying weaknesses or improvement opportunities;
- Evaluating for compensation, promotion, or termination decisions;
- Forecasting future outcomes;
- Estimating throughput and operational flow; and
- Reporting to owners, regulatory entities, or other stakeholders.

A metric is a single quantitative measurement or statistic representing an event or trend. Event metrics capture a single point in time, such as an organization's current cash balance or inventory on hand. Trend metrics capture changes over a period of time, such as an organization's annual revenue. Metrics commonly represent continuous measurements, categorical variables (including binary variables), or rank-order values. Multiple metrics can also be combined into new, more meaningful metrics, such as percentages (e.g., supply expense per total expense) or ratios (e.g., supply expense per patient). There are obviously thousands of potential metrics that can be tracked—some of greater importance than others.

KPIs are a subset of metrics that get differentiated from the rest for providing broader indications of an organization's current state and precisely measuring its performance against its set objectives. In short, metrics serve three primary functions:

- Communication;
- Control; and
- Improvement.

Good metrics and KPIs are necessary for truly understanding an organization's current state. Robert Handfield, a leading supply chain scholar, reminds us that *"it is always better to focus on a critical few, and select them wisely."*[5] Too often, managers base decisions on misaligned or mismeasured metrics, resulting in suboptimal outcomes without clear indications as to the source of the problems. As decisions will be informed by a metric, identifying and considering stakeholders is critical in the development of a "good metric." Stakeholder input should guide the components of the metric, support plans for how the data will be captured, confirm the need for accuracy, and help to shape the level of metric granularity. The design of a flagship hospital supply chain management KPI, "supply expense per patient," a KPI of relevance to both supply chain and finance executives, and potentially to clinicians, reveals the complexity of metric and KPI design. The following are questions one might ask in determination of what should be included in the design of the KPI:

- How are overhead supplies (e.g., thermostats) or other nonmedical supplies (e.g., linens) considered?
- What difference does calculating the metric based on patient admissions versus patient discharges versus patient days make?
- How can this measure be normalized for comparison across hospitals of different sizes and patient complexities?
- Will this metric provide guidance to clinicians as we engage them to work to reduce costs?

■ Are we capturing the data in a sufficiently granular level to fine-tune costs for different kinds of admissions or episodes of care?

No metric or KPI is perfect, and managers must always consider all such nuances and consider multiple metrics for decision-making.

In scrutinizing the fitness of metrics for measuring objectives, managers need to consider a metric's validity and reliability. A measurement's reliability refers to the consistency of a measure over time and if using different measurement tools or sources.[6] A high-reliability measure generates the same result when measured (under the same conditions) by different people or at different times. For example, if multiple nurses measure a stable patient's blood pressure using the same instrument and arrive at the same result, we can conclude that the measurement is reliable. On the other hand, if, for example, accounting records of inventory (based on orders and sales) significantly mismatch the physical counts of the inventory (due to loss, spoilage, theft, etc.), then we say that the accounting record is unreliable. Achieving high reliability in measurement becomes increasingly challenging when measuring abstract and complicated constructs such as employee performance, buyer-supplier trust, and customer satisfaction. Different methods of measuring these examples can paint different impressions about the situation.

Validity is concerned with whether the measurement truly reflects what it is intended to measure. This requires judgment and understanding of the measure's underlying intention. Validity issues are sometimes overlooked in analyzing metrics, even among experienced managers. If, for example, the goal of a metric "supply cost per procedure" is to support the work of a value analysis team in its deliberations over equivalent products, merely including the cost for the products, without consideration of the costs associated with the longer time needed in the operating room by one of the contending products, may not be a valid measure of costs for a episode of care.

Issues of reliability and validity become even more nuanced when assessing subjective or abstract constructs. What does a metric that measures supply department employee morale look like? Attempts to take such measures include surveying employees and aggregating results in specific ways. Much is to learned from the psychometrics discipline which blends statistics and psychology to develop and refine measurement scales to reduce reliability and validity risks in assessing employees. Applications in the healthcare supply chain setting may include measuring customer/clinician satisfaction, supplier relationships, the performance of negotiators engaged in strategic sourcing, patient attitude toward supplies, physician performance in supply standardization, service quality, and so on. Decision-makers need to form judgments based on a collection of interrelated metrics to maximize overall reliability and validity.

7.3 Metric Sets in Health Sector Supply Chain Management

Chief Supply Chain Officers and Materials Management Directors rely on many metrics to track routine operations and long-term performance. The specific metrics observed depend on the question they are asking or the issue they are trying to diagnose. With the potential hundreds or thousands of metrics that organizations can track, a methodical system of organizing these metrics is warranted. Supply chain metrics can be further into categories or *metric sets*. The following lists some of the standard metric sets used by managers, with examples of standard metrics in each set:

Financial metrics track expenses related to supplies. Labor expenses related to supply chain activities are also tracked under this category. Financial metrics provide a broader overview of the supply chain's health and performance, providing a basis for observing long-term performance and steering strategic decisions. Such metrics are generally reported in monetary values and adjusted for patient volume. For example, the *supply expense per CMI-adjusted patient discharges* estimates the supply expenditure per patient while accounting for the overall complexity of the patient pool using the case mix index as an adjustment factor. Other standard metrics include *supply accounts payable, spend under management, and supply chain labor expense per CMI-adjusted discharge*.

Risk metrics observe patient safety issues such as recalls and expiry management. Other internal or regulatory compliance issues are measured and tracked in this category. Some quality management metrics may also be grouped in this category. Like operational metrics, executives and directors need to keep a keen eye on these metrics to identify and react to disruptions and patient safety concerns quickly. The *percentage of expired inventory* and the *total number of product recalls* in a period are closely tracked metrics in this category.

Operational metrics track the workflow of orders, inventory, and logistics. Productivity, cycle time, and quality metrics are commonly included. Employee statistics and performance measures related to supply chain activities are also part of this category. Operational and risk metrics require frequent updating and monitoring since these metrics bring attention to any disruptions or risks that inevitably arise across a health system's supply chain environment. Examples of operational metrics include *distributor fill rate* (tracking the percentage of packages successfully shipped on the first attempt), *backorder rate* (percentage of backorders for a distributor), *perfect order rate* (the rate at which purchase orders go through the various steps of the purchasing process without errors), and *supply chain FTEs per $1M supply expense*. Inventory metrics, such as *inventory turnover* and *days of supply*, are also essential metrics considered in this category.[7]

Procurement metrics report on the organization's supply base and contract management.[8] These metrics consider supplier concentration, tracking the status of strategic suppliers, supplier performance, and supplier turnover. Other metrics are also needed to track the status and contract terms of thousands of procurement agreements with suppliers. Some procurement metrics provide a long-term overview of operations to assist strategic decision-making. Such metrics include ones that report on the composition of supplier base and product category metrics. Other procurement metrics with a more operational scope help track and manage tactical issues such as delinquent suppliers, new sourcing opportunities, or contract compliance issues.

Sustainability metrics track the amount of waste (in pounds) per patient, medical device reprocessing, and other recycling activities. As environmental and social issues receive increased attention, so must the metrics that track progress and issues on these fronts. There is less of a consensus across organizations as to which metrics to track and how often. The scope and breadth of these metrics depend on the organization's maturity and commitment to these causes. Typical metrics include *waste pounds per adjusted patient day, percentage of reprocessed medical supplies*, and *percentage of environmentally-preferable products purchased* (vendors indicate which products are environmentally preferable, based on U.S. Environmental Protection Agency (EPA) standards.

   The Association for Health Care Resource & Materials Management (AHRMM) provides a comprehensive guide to essential KPIs, with information about how they are defined and measured.[9] Its metrics and metric sets are tailored to the healthcare supply chain industry, thus making it a good reference for healthcare supply chain professionals. While not healthcare system-focused, CAPS Research also provides insight into how metrics allow for benchmarking for procurement across various sectors. Healthcare supply professionals can learn a great deal about implementing metrics for organizational excellence through scrutiny of the CAPS/Research.[10]

7.4 Toward a Performance Measurement System

With many metrics properly measured and considered, a more holistic impression of the organization takes shape, allowing decision-makers to assess where they stand and move toward higher performance. To bring coherence to the hundreds of important metrics, they must be synthesized into a framework or model to answer the question: "how are we doing overall?"[11] Thus far, this chapter has discussed *individual metrics* and *metric sets* (financial, operational, risk, etc.). The performance measurement system is the third and highest level of metric aggregation, which aligns metrics across functions and levels of management (strategic, tactical, and operational).

Consultants and academics have designed many performance measurement systems which differ in their customization and focus (organizational level vs. functional level). A few common performance measurement systems are introduced in this section, followed by a deeper dive into the FISCO model as a performance measurement system to assess the maturity of a healthcare supply chain organization.

7.4.1 The Balanced Scorecard Approach to Metrics

Organizations often develop a customized performance measurement model via a balanced scorecard approach. First introduced by Robert Kaplan and David Norton in 1992, the *balanced scorecard* pulls together multiple metric sets and places weights on each set, allowing one to aggregate them into a single composite score or "grade" for overall performance.[12] The balanced scorecard was further popularized following its adoption by large, successful companies such as Apple and Advanced Micro Devices (AMDs) in the 1990s.[13] Given its versatility and range of applications, it remains a dominant performance measurement system. Kaplan and Norton have continued to develop their scorecard throughout the past three decades, elaborating on its use for measuring intangible assets like human capital, information capital,[14] and strategic alliances.[15]

7.4.2 Metrics for Financial Performance

A financially driven performance measurement system is the *strategic profit model*, also known as the Dupont Profit Model,[16] which lays out how improvements on operational metrics link to financial metrics that top management is often most interested in. Although not a maturity model in the classical sense, this model can be helpful for operations managers to communicate to executives the impact that their supply chain initiatives will have on the organization's financial performance.

7.4.3 The SCOR Model

The *supply chain operations reference (SCOR) model* is a standardized and functionally-focused model that measures supply chain performance guided by over 200 metrics and standards (Exhibit 7.1). It has become a widely adopted model for organizations across industries to assess their supply chain maturity and identify improvement opportunities. Like the strategic profit model, the SCOR model is industry-agnostic and has been adopted by many organizations across many industries. Achieving this critical mass of adoption enables ongoing updates, discussions, and developments on the model with diverse perspectives.[17] Research carried out by the Health Sector Supply Chain Research Consortium provides essential insights into the applicability of the SCOR model for the healthcare sector.[18]

Exhibit 7.1: The supply chain operating reference model.

SCOR Process and components	SCOR Primary attributes
Plan	Agility
SourceMake	Asset management efficiency
Deliver	Costs
Return	Reliability
Enable	Responsiveness

7.5 FISCO Framework as a Maturity Model for the Healthcare Supply Chain

As noted earlier, many organizational maturity models cater to healthcare supply chains, each carrying slightly different philosophies and frameworks. Nonetheless, the ultimate objectives of all such maturity models are highly overlapping: improving value (cost reduction, higher productivity, and optimized production levels), improving quality, improving risk management, and improving innovation.

The model presented throughout this book, the FISCO model, is rooted in supply chain integration as an enabler of innovation, value, quality, and resilience. Definitions of supply chain integration can be inclusive and fluid, as demonstrated by multiple literature reviews that have gathered and synthesized dozens of academic research publications surrounding this topic.[19,20] For our purposes, *supply chain integration* can be defined as the degree to which an organization strategically brings together internal functions and external supply chain members to manage the intra- and inter-organizational processes. Robust supply chain integration is necessary to achieve effective and efficient flows of products, services, information, money, and decisions to provide maximum value to the customer.

We proposed the FISCO model to depict a robust effort to gain control over related organizational processes and meet critical operational and strategic goals. The idea of a FISCO model was first developed at Arizona State University's Department of Supply Chain Management (in the W.P. Carey College of Business) to scrutinize healthcare systems that had successfully implemented a shared service organization. The concept was further refined in studying and advising healthcare systems implementing a wide range of supply chain management and integration functions to bring high-quality healthcare services, within the U.S. Department of Defense, to warfighters and their dependents.

A FISCO model evolves from decisions enabling control and alignment of internal, external, and outsourced functions. The hallmark of a FISCO model is the reduction of complexity. The most progressive healthcare systems are genuinely integrated delivery systems where supply chain management significantly contributes to the enterprise's success. Current industry trends are integrating clinical requirements, patient outcomes, and supply chain performance. The FISCO characterization is based on our knowledge of integrated health systems and their consolidated service centers and learnings from various nonhealth sector organizations. The intended outcome from striving toward a FISCO ideal includes:

- Cost—reduction of expenses through
    - Leverage,
    - Standardization,
    - Innovation, and
    - Quality management;
- Risk—management of risks;
- Predictability—the creation of defined support services budgets;
- Capacity—increased capacity for healthcare system growth; and
- Opportunity—identified opportunities for systemic improvement.

Akin to the classical "people, process, technology" framework that has been around since the 1960s as a tool to balance operations and improve efficiency, the dimensions of the FISCO framework, as introduced in Chapter 1, Exhibit 1.1, and reproduced in Exhibit 7.2, are organized into three categories: (1) the supply chain processes, (2) technology tools, and (3) organizational support and governance. Each area consists of a

Exhibit 7.2: The FISCO framework.

SCM processes	Technology tools	Organization support
Product sourcing	System integration architecture	Organization structure
Product selection and standardization	Key performance indicators and Metrics	System training
Contracting		Governance of the supply chain
Supplier relationship management	Item master management	
Accounts payable (AP)	Electronic health record integration preparedness	
Order processing		
Inventory management		
Receiving		
Asset management		
Supply chain risk management		

number of the essential dimensions required to achieve integration at the highest levels. The dimensions are listed in Exhibit 7.2.

Initially, for each dimension, one must identify the universal and health industry best practices and then consider the organization's capabilities relative to the best practices. Finally, decision-makers should prioritize specific dimensions based on their needs and resources and develop plans to bridge gaps between capability and best practice. The following sections briefly describe each of the dimensions. Appendix 1 provides further details on each dimension with a maturity scale based on Gartner's five-point scale for logistics maturity: (1) react, (2) anticipate, (3) integrate, (4) collaborate, and (5) orchestrate.[21]

Managers value assessing their own organization's performance against industry best practices. Exhibit 7.3 provides insight into the maturity of these organizations across the FISCO functions. We note that the prevalence of the number of organizations that achieve industry best practices remains to be established.[22]

7.5.1 Supply Chain Management Processes

Product sourcing is the supply chain process involved in identifying, investigating, and deciding to acquire products to fulfill a clinical or business need. In the healthcare field, the sourcing process is led by experienced managers with industry and product knowledge of the specific branches of medicine such as cardiac, orthopedics, neuro, and oncology. Considerations related to this process are discussed in Chapter 4.

Exhibit 7.3: Current Industry Best Practices (IBP).

FISCO Functions	Level 1 react	Level 2 anticipate	Level 3 integrate	Level 4 collaborate	Level 5 orchestrate
(1) Product Sourcing				IBP	
(2) Product selection and standardization				IBP▪▲	
(3) Contracting and purchasing					IBP
(4) Supplier relationship management/vendor Performance management					IBP▲
(5) Accounts payable					IBP
(6) Order processing				IBP▪▲	
(7) Inventory management				IBP▪▲	
(8) Receiving				IBP▪▲	
(9) Asset management					IBP
(10) Supply chain risk management				IBP	

SCM Business processes

(continued)

Exhibit 7.3: (continued).

	FISCO Functions	Level 1 react	Level 2 anticipate	Level 3 integrate	Level 4 collaborate	Level 5 orchestrate
Technology tools	(11) System integration/architecture				IBP	
	(12) Key performance Indicator (KPI)/metrics				IBP	
	(13) Item master management strategy			IBP ▪▲		
	(14) Electronic health record integration preparedness				IBP	
Organization support	(15) Organization structure					IBP
	(16) System training			IBP ▪▲		
	(17) Governance of the supply chain					IBP

Product selection and standardization processes are carefully orchestrated supply chain processes that ensure that the best and most appropriate products are chosen for use in the healthcare system. Much of this process is discussed in Chapters 4 and 5. Exhibit 7.4 provides, as an example,

Exhibit 7.4: Example FISCO Maturity Scale: Product selection and standardization.

Maturity level	Examples
1 React	Little attention to product standardization, leading to an extensive product base for the clinical services provided
	Formulary of frequently ordered items that lack accompanying standardization
2 Anticipate	Limited or sporadic product standardization programs
	Standardization of work and evaluation of vendor products, product selection decisions, and contracting processes as applicable
	Compliance metrics gathered and reported
3 Integrate	Promotion of product standardization programs, although broad-based clinical engagement may not be achieved
	Standardization of working groups; market research; evaluation of vendors/sources, vendor products, product decisions, and contracting processes as applicable; risk management review
	Compliance metrics gathered and reported
4 Collaborate	Formalized product standardization programs with clinical staff appreciating the value of standardization but not fully engaged
	Standardization of working groups and standardized clinical pathways (including equipment, supplies, and quantity to be used, not just clinical procedure)
	Standardization determined by the working group and based on the clinical pathway and market research; evaluation of vendors/sources, vendor products, product decisions, and contracting processes as applicable; risk management review
	Compliance metrics gathered and reported
5 Orchestrate	Similar to Level 4 but adding:
	Standardization of programs that are part of the culture—all clinical and administrative staff are fully aware, appreciate, and are committed to the process
	Standardization of working groups and standardized clinical pathways
	Patient outcomes are also monitored, and compliance or deviation from the clinical pathway is determined; re-evaluation of the clinical pathway is for potential modification

the maturity scale for the product selection and standardization process. Maturity scales are available for each FISCO dimension and in Appendix 1 of this book.

Contracting. The contracting process establishes formal arrangements for acquiring products and services at predetermined terms and prices. The purchasing process describes the steps involved in conveying a demand for a product to the supplier of the goods. It may be electronically or manually communicated, and it may be through a central purchasing department or by individual users.

Supplier Relationship Management (SRM) is the business process involved in bilateral communications between suppliers and buyers to ensure that each side understands its role and best meets its obligations. Scorecards are often prepared to track the performance of the relationship and each party's contribution to the relationship. A more detailed discussion is contained in Chapter 5.

Accounts Payable is the business process of paying a supplier for the delivery of its products following the agreed-on commercial terms. Before a payment is made, a three-way match (physically or virtually) of purchase, receiving, and invoice is required. This process and the upcoming three are discussed in Chapter 6.

Order Processing. Moving requisitions to purchase orders and transmitting those orders to the suppliers is paramount. Failure to complete this process efficiently can result in duplicate supply requests, stockpiling supplies with requestors due to a lack of faith in the process, and insufficient suppliers to support the organization's needs. Some key leading practices must be implemented to support a highly functioning, modern supply chain.

Inventory management and distribution encompass the process of moving sourced and purchased products from the supplier to the intended recipient within the healthcare organization. This movement of a product also encompasses the management of fixed inventories. Management in this context is further defined as the planning of inventory levels to ensure that the products stocked are appropriate for the type of location and customer.

Receiving is an essential function in inventory management. When done correctly, it systematically enables high efficiencies for all downstream processes. If done incorrectly, the negative impacts can be far-reaching, resulting in lost products, overstocks, and mistakes when fulfilling orders. Leveraging automation and clear procedures will drive efficiencies into your organization, resulting in cleaner data and knowledge of what items are in the warehouses.

Asset management is the process of identifying requirements for the nonexpendable moveable property, procuring it, assigning accountability and responsibility for it, maintaining it throughout its lifecycle, and planning for its replacement.

Supply chain risk management is a cross-functional process to identify, assess, mitigate, and monitor relevant risks (e.g., natural disasters, accidents, sabotage, or production problems) that can disrupt an organization's supply chain operations. Refer to Chapter 3 for an in-depth discussion of risk and resilience.

7.5.2 Technology Tools

System integration and architecture is a FISCO dimension that evaluates the supply chain information technology systems to determine their level of integration. Enterprises with disparate systems are inefficient, while those with tightly coupled or highly integrated systems are more efficient. Chapter 8 covers the information technology issues related to healthcare supply chains.

Use of KPI/metrics. This dimension evaluates the enterprise's use of metrics and performance measurement systems to determine the health of the supply chain. As discussed earlier in this chapter, using reliable and valid metrics allows an enterprise to anticipate and resolve issues before they occur.

Item master management. Developing a modern item data strategy that drives the integrity of supplies and implant data is critical yet often overlooked in many organizations. Many hospitals traditionally address the individual "pieces" of master file maintenance (purchasing, standardization, agreements) but do not align the individual functions with interacting collaboratively. High-functioning organizations maintain current product data integrity through integration across various systems enabled by a master data maintenance group and a robust governance model. As enterprise systems grow in size and complexity, industry leaders embrace the importance of data as the lifeblood of their organizations to provide valuable insights across a clinically integrated supply chain.

Electronic health record (EHR) integration preparedness. With the rapid expansion and use of the EHR across the healthcare continuum, supply chain data, or more specifically, the item master, is evolving to become a strategic asset. As the single source of truth for item information, this data is being leveraged to support clinical documentation and patient billing, including supply and implant capture at the point of use. With this increased use of the data, a new set of challenges arise that the supply chain team is faced with solving. Accuracy, breadth, and consistency, to name a few, are all critically important, and the EHR is leading to an exponential growth of the item master and associated maintenance.

7.5.3 Organization Support

Organizational structure. The organizational structure defines the design of the organizational relationships and the roles of the leaders of each of the entities. It also portrays and defines the relationships among the multiple entities within the enterprise. Chapter 8 examines organizational structures and implications.

System training. The process for training users of the information systems and the supply chain business processes how to fully use the systems to gain the maximum value from their use. The training should help the users understand how to use the systems and why the system and related business processes are essential for fulfilling the mission.

Supply chain governance. The structures and rules for governing supply chain business processes and systems. Key to governance is specifying the levels of authority for decisions and complex situations where multiple organization entities are involved in the decision-making processes.

7.5.4 Finding the Right Strategic Fit

While it is possible to characterize hospitals and systems along a continuum or developmental stages (whether via the FISCO framework or any other maturity models), a number of the supply chain management characteristics present in very mature organizations are also present in organizations that might be judged as being rather nonprogressive. At the same time, very progressive organizations frequently are characterized by some practices that one would not associate with organizational "best practices." Some health systems are uneven in the extent to which system hospitals and departments progressively engage their supply environment. Furthermore, as corporate best practices diffuse across system hospitals, practices may vary due to technical, cultural, or political elements, triggering different adoption patterns.[23] Incorporating an academic health center, with a strong focus on demonstrating the value and performance of multiple equivalent products, may hamper the broader system of single sourcing. Such discrepancies may constitute a challenge for the system-level supply chain executive.

Those wishing to develop a supply strategy for hospitals and systems will find it helpful to think of the stages as "ideal types," and the more mature stages being aspirational. Systems may have the vast majority of hospitals at a single stage with a good number of higher achievers and laggards. Thus it is important to think about the contradictions observed within hospitals and systems and the observation that not all hospitals continue to aspire to move to the next stage of maturity. Healthcare organizations engage in purchasing within the parameters of the legal actions that characterize their systems. Progressive organizations seek strategic fit in aligning their goals with the opportunities they encounter in their marketplace. Contingencies that "*are both environmental and organizational*" must be considered in seeking such a strategic fit.[24] Firms face a conflict in seeking "*a fit between its strategy and its environmental situation vs. a fit between its strategy and its unique competencies.*"[25] Strategic fit is essential in the health sector, where organizational cultures are powerful, and clinician engagement is central to producing successful outcomes. When purchasing partners do not allow the organization to achieve its goals or purchase within the framework of its culture, the purchasing organization may attempt to change its existing purchasing partner's strategy or seek alternative partners.

For example, Chapter 5 explored the idea of strategic fit for hospital involvement in purchasing alliances, such as group purchasing organizations (GPOs). In that context, strategic fit was discussed regarding the demand for products and the supply chain's responsiveness to providing needed goods to hospitals and systems. As hospital and system supply chain maturity is discussed in this chapter, a more macro and dynamic view of strategic fit is implied—one that can consider the broad spectrum of issues associated not just with purchasing partners (such as GPOs or distributors)—but with managing the variety of internal stakeholders, customers, processes, and design of the organization itself.

7.6 Chapter Summary

Up to this chapter in the book, many major supply chain roles and functions have been discussed, including strategy development, risk management, value analysis, procurement, and logistics. Important across all these functions is the ability to assess their performance adequately and reliably. Various industry associations and similar organizations make many resources and frameworks available for supply chain managers to measure the performance of supply chain core functions holistically. This chapter formalizes some fundamental characteristics of good metrics and their uses. Different metric sets are intended to describe various facets of the healthcare supply chain. Important to remember is that measurement, in itself, is not the objective of employing a robust system of metrics and KPIs.

Performance measurement systems are often operationalized as balanced scorecards that combine and weigh numerous metrics to give decision-makers a better sense of the supply chain's overall status and health. Balanced scorecards, when carried out effectively, are a value-enhancing tool to link measurement to strategy and elevate the role of measures from an operational checklist to a comprehensive system for strategy implementation.[26]

On a broader scale, maturity models provide a framework to measure the various supply chain functions and processes strategically, allowing for identifying shortcomings relative to best practices and industry peers. The FISCO framework is one maturity model that focuses on the health of the supply chain concerning cost-effective performance and how well it enables clinical performance. Different hospital and organizational structures (discussed in the next chapter) naturally call for different expectations and measurements to gauge their success. Hence, we emphasize that no specific framework or metric is "ideal" to compare. Organizations must seek strategic fit between their respective organizational structure and strategy to guide their performance benchmarks and metrics. This chapter has provided insights and tools for achieving excellence in the management of supplies and their relationship to an organization's vision and strategy.

Notes

1. Wendler, R. (2012). The maturity of maturity model research: A systematic mapping study. *Information and Software Technology, 54*(12), 1317–1339.
2. Pöppelbuß, J., & Röglinger, M. (2011). What makes a useful maturity model? A framework of general design principles for maturity models and its demonstration in business process management.
3. DeSarbo, W. S., Anthony Di Benedetto, C., Song, M., & Sinha, I. (2005). Revisiting the miles and snow strategic framework: Uncovering interrelationships between strategic types, capabilities, environmental uncertainty, and firm performance. *Strategic Management Journal, 26*(1), 47–74.
4. Zajac, E. J., Kraatz, M. S., & Bresser, R. K. F. (2000). Modeling the dynamics of strategic fit: A normative approach to strategic change. *Strategic Management Journal, 21*(4), 429–453.
5. Handfield, R. (2015, April 1). Supply chain metrics: Make sure they are aligned with your strategy! Supply Chain Resource Cooperative. North Carolina State University. https://scm.ncsu.edu/scm-articles/article/supply-chain-metrics-make-sure-they-are-aligned-with-your-strategy
6. Jhangiani, R. S., Chiang, I.-C. A., Cuttler, C., & Leighton, D. C. (2019). *Research methods in psychology: 4th edition*. Independently published.
7. Strategic Marketplace Initiative. (2007). Perfect order: A new healthcare supply chain metric. Implementation Process & Automation Roadmap. https://www.smisupplychain.com/wp-content/uploads/2022/09/perfect_order_metric.pdf
8. CAPS Research. (2021). *Procurement metrics index*. CAPS Research.
9. AHRMM. (2020). *AHRMM keys*. American Hospital Association. https://www.ahrmm.org/keys
10. CAPS. Research. Library access at: https://www.capsresearch.org/library

11. Melnyk, S. A., Stewart, D. M., & Swink, M. (2004). Metrics and performance measurement in operations management: Dealing with the metrics maze. *Journal of Operations Management, 22*(3), 209–218.

12. Kaplan, R. S., & Norton, D. P. (2005). The balanced scorecard: measures that drive performance. *Harvard Business Review, 83*(7), 172.

13. Kaplan, R. S., & Norton, D. P. (1993). Putting the balanced scorecard to work. *Harvard Business Review.* `https://hbr.org/1993/09/putting-the-balanced-scorecard-to-work`

14. Kaplan, R. S., & Norton, D. P. (2004). Measuring the strategic readiness of intangible assets. *Harvard Business Review, 82*(2), 52–63.

15. Kaplan, R. S., Norton D. P., and Rugelsjoen, B. "Managing alliances with the balanced scorecard." Harvard Business Review, January 1, 2010. `https://hbr.org/2010/01/managing-alliances-with-the-balanced-scorecard`

16. Soliman, M. T. (2008). The use of DuPont analysis by market participants. *The Accounting Review, 83*(3), 823–853. `http://dx.doi.org/10.2308/accr.2008.83.3.823`

17. ASCM. (2022). The supply chain operations reference model, Version 14.0. Association for Supply Chain Management. scor.ascm.org

18. Smith-Daniels, V., Smith, D. J., Whitecotton, S., & Schneller, E. (2006). *Supply chain Metrics metrics and benchmarking: Estimating the foundaton for knowledge sharing and performance improvement across the health sector industry.* Arizona State University.

19. Leuschner, R., Rogers, D. S., & Charvet, F. F. (2013). A meta-analysis of supply chain integration and firm performance. *Journal of Supply Chain Management, 49*(2), 34–57.

20. Mackelprang, A. W., Robinson, J. L., Bernardes, E., & Webb, G. S. (2014). The relationship between strategic supply chain integration and performance: A meta-analytic evaluation and implications for supply chain management research. *Journal of Business Logistics, 35*(1), 71–96.

21. Van Der Meulen, R. (2017). *5 Stages of logistics maturity.* Gartner. `https://www.gartner.com/smarterwithgartner/5-stages-of-logistics-maturity`

22. The design for this table was carried out under contract number W81XWH-15-9-0001 and submitted to the Defense Logistics Agency and Advanced Technology International on March 7, 2019. This version does not include assessment of the FISCO levels of development for the Defense Health Agency.

23. Ansari, S. M., Fiss, P. C., & Zajac, E. J. (2010). Made to fit: how practices vary as they diffuse. *Academy of Management Review, 35*(1), 67–92.

24. Zajac, E.t., op. cit., p. 429.

25. Zajac, E.T., op. cit., p. 431.

26. Kaplan, R. S., & Norton, D. P. (2001). Transforming the balanced scorecard from performance measurement to strategic management: Part 1. *Accounting Horizons, 15*(1), 87–104.

8 Organization Design for Managing the Supply Chain—*A Well-designed Organization Makes It Easier to Succeed*

8.1 Introduction

Strategy, as was discussed in Chapter 2, requires management, and a core element of strategy is the organization's design. Peter Drucker[1] has written "that there is no one right or universal design but that each enterprise needs to design around the key activities appropriate to its mission and its strategies." This applies to healthcare organizations. Very different missions and strategies characterize hospitals and healthcare organizations. They are highly differentiated by market conditions, system complexity, access to financial and human resources, financial structure (e.g., investor-owned vs. not-for-profit), regulatory environment, and geographic location. Accordingly, the design of each institution's organization will differ.

System complexity, as is discussed in detail in the following pages, also pertains to the mix of hospitals and other delivery units within the system. Hospitals face a rather unstable environment because of governmental regulations, reimbursements (economic or financial conditions), and ever-changing technology. In addition, overall demand may be predictable (number of admissions), but the exact type of care is highly unpredictable on a daily basis. This instability or uncertainty means that decision-makers usually do not have sufficient information about environmental factors and have difficulty predicting external changes and impacts. Uncertainty increases the risk of failure for organizational responses and makes it challenging to compute costs and probabilities associated with decision alternatives.

Strategic management requires the formulation, implementation, and evaluation of managerial actions that enhance the value of a business enterprise.[2] Organizational design is a strategic management construct that consists of the building blocks for organizations to achieve their strategy, mission, objective, and goals.[3] It is best realized through self-reflection regarding the organization's sense of purpose of how to make a difference for the organization's clients, employees, and other stakeholders.[4] In the complex healthcare environment previously described, design decisions that do not achieve strategic goals are probably the wrong decisions. Whether a single hospital or a multi-hospital system aspires for a high degree of supply chain management maturity, it becomes clear that design must promote integration, especially as the design has an impact across the functions characterizing a fully integrated supply chain (FISCO). Finally, as is discussed in this chapter, design must have a "strategic fit" with the nature of the organization and the environment(s) in which it is positioned.[5]

The idea of "managerial frames" suggests that those who lead and bring about change in organizations rely on frames of action to carry out their work, especially as they work to bring change to their organizations.[6] This idea is relevant for those who engage in the design of supply chain work within the healthcare system. The last section of this chapter introduces the idea of managerial lenses as "frames" for supply design, transformation, and everyday work, including (a) supply management, (b) supply as strategy, (c) supply as transaction, (d) supply as service, (e) supply as orchestration, and (f) supply as transformation.

8.2 The Role of Organization Design

An effective organization design divides the tasks of supply chain requirements into manageable structures and specialized jobs, and coordinates the tasks, which interact with each other, for the firm to reap the benefits of the design.[7] It entails calculated components to manage a firm's internal and external environments to maximize the utilization of resources in relation to objectives.[8] Integral to success is the precise specification of goals and tactics that an organization will undertake. At its most fundamental level, it involves decisions around:

1. Division of work: enhancing individuals' proficiency in performing their work, and thus, improves the efficiency and effectiveness with which the work can be performed.
2. Departmentation: the grouping of work and workers into manageable units or departments.
3. Authority and responsibility relationships: individuals need to be assigned the responsibility and authority for the completion of work.
4. Span of control: the workers need to be grouped according to the number of subordinates reporting directly to a manager.
5. Coordination: how work is assembled and synchronized to function harmoniously in attaining organizing objectives.[9]

Design decisions should be attentive to the mission and vision, and flow from the organization's environment and goals.[10] Good design is also an enabler to implement the strategy efficiently and effectively.[11] Accordingly, the structural design of a supply chain management group requires the following:

1. An "extra" design element of the structure that interfaces with the outside world of suppliers and markets. "Extra" here means focusing outside the organization on the supplier relationship management function (SRM) and purchasing partner-related function (PPM) that is discussed in Chapter 1.
2. The "inter" design, or the structure that interfaces with internal units, sites, and projects. *Inter* here means interdepartmental across the organization, the internal supply management (ISM) function that is discussed in Chapter 1.
3. The "intra" design, or structure inside the organization that translates, coordinates, and integrates the extra and inter designs. *Intra* means within the supply organization,[12] including the ISM function that is discussed in Chapter 1.

In many ways, design refers to the overall look of the organization, including its formalization (the extent to which expectations regarding the means and end of work are specified and written), the centrality of authority and decision-making complexity, the number of distinctively different job titles or occupational groupings, and the number of distinctly different units or departments in an organization.[13]

8.3 Supply Chain Design for a Boundary Organization

Supply chain departments within a healthcare facility are "boundary organizations" that must manage supplies to support the operations and strategy of the hospital's internal organization (downstream to users/patients) and the various upstream trading partners. As boundary organizations, supply chain departments have a responsibility to internal organizations (e.g., clinicians) and external organizations (e.g., suppliers). Organization design for the supply chain must thus be responsive to the dilemmas of a boundary organization that interacts with the very different environments[14] of its internal and external customers and the broader health sector ecosystem. Such design is essential for health sector provision, as healthcare provision is highly resource-dependent, with provider organizations producing virtually none of the supplies necessary to carry out their work.

Supply chain design in a boundary organization must facilitate both the sourcing and purchasing of products and the orchestration of inventory and delivery of products to support operations;[15] assuring coordination of the major drivers of success which include (a) logistics synchronization, (b) information sharing, (c) incentive alignment, and (d) collective learning.[16] And it must do so while meeting the challenges of the health sector, including clinician preference and the differences in products needed to provide service.

Hospitals and healthcare systems are among the most resource dependent of any kinds of organizations.[17,18] They make little of they use. Critical is coordination and managing dependencies between entities and the joint effort of entities working together toward mutually defined goals[19] and to bring innovation and integration to a system.[20] It is a principal feature of organizational design. Coordination can be via human interaction, governance, the use of technology, or some combination of these three. One of the leading supply chain departments in the United States is Banner Health, an integrated delivery network (IDN) with over 30 hospitals and clinics. Banner explicitly recognizes the value in aligning with stakeholders across the supply chain service segments (Exhibit 8.1).

Aligning with stakeholders: **Supply Chain Services Segments**

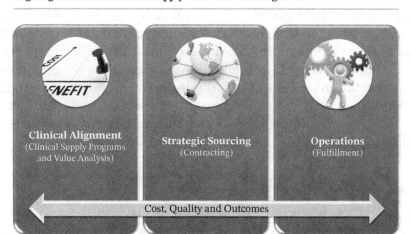

Exhibit 8.1: Supply chain services segment alignment.

For the supply chain function to mature, organizational design must transcend from a "mere" focus on contract management and moving goods through to the point of service to become an entity characterized by its ability to collaborate with stakeholders—both upstream to suppliers and downstream to those at the point of service. This is important as transaction costs in the supply chain range from 35% to 40% of supply chain costs.[21] This transformation is especially challenging for smaller hospitals where there may be insufficient resources for automating technology, spend volume, and the personnel with the skills necessary for engaging the marketplace.[22]

8.3.1 Design for Integration and Desired Outcomes

Supply chain integration, discussed in the introduction to this book, refers to the activities and mechanisms used to achieve unity of effort across organizations, externally and internally, across the different specialized areas.[23] When well positioned in a healthcare delivery system, the supply chain contributes to excellence in clinical outcomes, integration, and sustainability.[24,25]

Appropriate supply chain design is fundamental to achieving a FISCO.[26] Such integration is challenging, yet crucial, in the complex health delivery system characterized by (a) an extraordinary number of products needed to satisfy customer needs; (b) the role of clinicians and their influence in a professional organization; (c) the enormous costs associated with pharmaceuticals and medical supplies; (d) the impact of failure to perform (e.g., the consequences of stockouts); (e) the constraints imposed by regulations; (f) the challenges imposed by reimbursement schemes;[27] and (g) mergers and acquisitions that have brought together organizations, within a single hospital system, with different missions, technologies, and clinical staff characteristics and expectations.[28,29] Supply chain design occurs within a dynamic network of suppliers as those suppliers themselves select and de-select suppliers, move into new markets, and adopt new processes and strategies.[30]

8.3.2 Design for Strategic fit

Managerial decisions must meet the demands of the organizations in which they are employed. The idea of "strategic fit"[31] can be drawn upon to explain how different solutions may represent progressive practices in different organizations.

Strategic fit/misfit reflects the alignment of actions with the vision and values of a hospital or hospital system and its culture to enhance organizational performance. Exhibit 8.2 depicts the relationships among environment, strategy, structure, and the context of strategic fit for organizational performance. Importantly, strategic fit has been linked to achieving value for money in healthcare systems in the United States and abroad. The success of such actions should be judged by a variety of factors, including:

1. Contribution to successful clinical outcomes in the eyes of patients;
2. Contributions to successful clinical outcomes in the eyes of providers;
3. The extent to which the product results in increased utilization (e.g., as a result of emergency room turnover);
4. Improved access as a result of savings;
5. Improved safety for the patient;

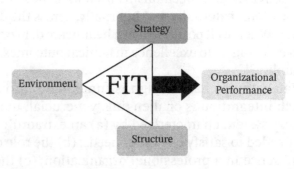

Exhibit 8.2: Elements of strategic fit.

6. Improved employee safety; and
7. Reduced total expenditure per admission.

For the hospital supply chain, the environment also includes the legal and regulatory structure that affects both the hospital and the supply and distribution channels upstream from the point of delivery. The external environment, which also determines standards relating to infection rates and the shielding of employees from dangerous materials, affects purchasing goods and services. Exhibit 8.2 recognizes that changes in the environment may well impact design and strategy and the impact of the exchange systems which would include group purchasing organizations (GPOs), distributors, IT vendors, and others.[32]

8.3.3 The Ecosystem of Healthcare Supply Chain Design

The design for the supply chain function must take place within an ecosystem of healthcare organizations that are themselves parts of large systems. Of the over 4,000 hospitals in the United States, over 3,500 are parts of a health system, many of which have grown through mergers and acquisitions.[33] Banner Health, Mayo Clinic, HCA Healthcare, and CommonSpirit Health are examples of large systems providing care facilities in multiple states and across large geographic regions. This is especially relevant as one considers supply distribution networks' design and ability to service multiple system members. While a system may operate within a single state, even those may be subject to a large geographic spread, which may influence design. Sometimes, a system may choose to develop a consolidated service center to meet its distribution goals. In other instances, it may utilize a distributor's services to distribute in areas with less concentration. This is fundamentally a strategic-fit decision around centralization based on the characteristics of an environment served. Ultimately, the decisions must meet the challenges of a highly resource dependent organization.

Exhibit 8.3 provides insight into the discussion. The largest health systems in the United States are highly divergent concerning their governance structure, ownership, number of hospitals, licensed beds, revenue, relationships with clinicians and degree of integration. And their range of services offered within and across the system can also be variable. HCA Healthcare is the most extensive for-profit health system in the United States, with over 200 hospitals in its network. Universal Health Services operates 179 hospitals and CommonSpirit Health has 164 hospitals. The 10 largest health systems in the United States collectively manage more than 1,300 hospitals—nearly 18% of active hospitals tracked in

Exhibit 8.3: Characteristics of the largest health systems (by number of hospitals, 2022).

Health System	Number of Hospitals	Staffed Beds	Net Patient Revenue	Total Med/Surg Supply Cost	Governance
HCA Healthcare	209	41,200	$48.0B	$7.49B	For-Profit
Universal Health Services	178	21,300	$9.87B	$0.88B	For-Profit
Common-Spirit Health	164	19,600	$30.4B	$5.22B	Non-Profit
Ascension Health	129	18,300	$23.50B	$4.04B	Non-Profit
Trinity Health	105	14,500	$20.19B	$3.93B	Non-Profit
Community Health Systems (CHS)	86	10,300	$10.77B	$1.84B	Non-Profit
Tenet Healthcare	83	14,200	$14.38B	$2.87B	For-Profit

Source: Definitive Healthcare data for FY2021

HospitalView. Large health systems keep patient referrals in-network to help improve care coordination, enhance the patient experience, and prevent revenue loss by referring outside a hospital's network. As these systems have grown, expectations for supply chain, significantly to reduce costs, have increased, as have expectations for supply to contribute to clinical outcomes. Thus, a focus on supply chain design is important and inevitable.

Clinical Services Considerations

Strategic fit for a supply chain system design must consider the number and types of services offered by individual hospitals and hospitals across a system. Hospitals offering "supply intensive services" (i.e., services where supply is a significant proportion of the total cost of an episode of care) such as cardiology, orthopedics, and spine require a more robust supply chain than a community hospital with only general surgery services. Hospitals also differ by focusing on specific populations (e.g., women's and children's hospitals) or disease entities (e.g., cardiac hospitals and cancer centers). Another category of hospitals is academic health centers. These organizations, with medical schools and other health profession education programs, engage in a large amount of research and teaching in addition to patient care. The supply chain function in these organizations must be balanced across these functions. Academic health centers, for example, are centers with a full range of services that aim to expose learners/students to many different approaches to care. They are characterized by a high-dollar supply spend.[34]

Healthcare System Structure Considerations

Supply chain design must have strategic fit with the span of control characteristics of the broader organization. As previously suggested, the degree of integration across large systems is variable. Some systems are best characterized as "holding systems," with relatively loose levels of control for individual hospitals or hospitals within a region. Others are best characterized as "operating systems," with significant control and standardization for many processes and functions, including the supply chain. The ability to make and implement system-wide supply chain guidelines, such as sourcing directives, may be much more difficult to achieve with a holding system with very different medical staff expectations for choice. Many hospitals remain associated with religious orders, which may strongly influence their service lines catering to women and populations in need and revenue mix.

Governance requires consideration in supply chain design for strategic fit. Approximately 25% of community hospitals in the United States were classified as for-profit and are expected to yield high earnings for investors. They are expected to manage their resources, including supply chain resources, in an organized and prudent manner. While such expectations are prevalent for all hospitals, supply chain design may have different dimensions of accountability, and thus, strategy. HCA Healthcare, the largest investor-owned system in the United States (working with its GPO, Health Trust Purchasing Group), is known for its low number of suppliers of equivalent products. It is also known for working with its hospitals and clinicians to consolidate spend. Nearly 20% of hospitals in the United States are controlled by state or local government. These organizations are frequently bound by state purchasing regulations, as are federal government hospitals bound by the Federal Acquisition Regulations (FAR).[35]

The supply chain environment that must be considered includes both the internal and external environment within the system. For instance, the market conditions of the physicians may affect the physicians' external and internal behavior. Market conditions may also include socio-cultural factors, such as a hospital's linkage to a religious order with a strong commitment to bringing healthcare to the marginalized. These environmental conditions should be considered along several dimensions. The simple-complex dimension refers to the degree of heterogeneity in an organization's operations. Healthcare generally operates in a more complex and less predictable environment than other industries as it involves many technologies and is a focal point for cultural and value changes (see Exhibit 8.4). It has a complex mix of human resources and interfaces. Hospitals, by their very nature, serve several diverse customers, unlike most other industries with scientific developments constantly updating their procedures and services.

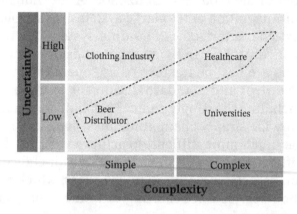

Exhibit 8.4: Industry complexity versus uncertainty matrix.

Clockspeed Considerations

Chapter 1 discussed the concept of clockspeed, as developed by Charles H. Fine, as a framework for understanding healthcare as a sector characterized by different rates of change in products, processes, and organization.[36] While organizational structure for healthcare has been relatively slow to change,[37] hospitals are increasingly characterized by rapid change—the proliferation of outpatient clinics, relationships with contracting partners for services, and increased use of technologies for service delivery (e.g., telemedicine) and communication (e.g., patient portals). Indeed, much has been accelerated by the Patient Protection and Affordable Care Act's incentives for hospitals to take responsibility for all of the episodes of patient care.[38] When the hospital becomes the focal point—with its various functions and services relating to the need for supply across a full set of settings, for both services and products, there is a very different view of the value of supply chain management, but also the need for a different set of designs for the supply chain function. Recognized is the need for revisiting design and its strategic fit with evolving and changed circumstances.

Centralization versus Decentralization Considerations

Centralization is not "merely" a decision around how or where to place supplies. It could be thought of as the proportion of the hospitals within a system reporting that the service was provided by the system even if it was also provided by the hospital, and *integration* refers to the extent to which the system assimilates the services and arrangements through direct ownership and direct provision or contract them out to other organizations.

Supply chain designers may assess their options as follows:

1. Decentralized and relatively differentiated;
2. Highly differentiated but relatively decentralized;
3. Highly centralized and highly differentiated; and
4. Those that are least differentiated and most centralized.

The centralized, complex, formalized organization does not fit all situations. However, the opposite of this, the decentralized, informal, or simple organization, does not fit all situations either. As a result, a hybrid form of supply chain organizational design is often more appropriate. This comprises some centralized and some decentralized elements. Consistent with research in other industries, the progressive hospitals, and systems we have studied over time reveal that a hybrid organizational design is the most effective.[39] In a hybrid supply organization, activities, responsibilities, and accountabilities are shared between operating units and the corporate supply chain leadership. Some activities and policies are centralized at the system level, while others are decentralized to individual hospital units and sub-units. In some situations, there may be extensive policies and procedures, while individual flexibility is fostered in others. Some aspects of the supply chain structure may be complex with many levels of hierarchy and rigid reporting relationships. Other parts of the organization may be flat with loose reporting relationships. Smeltzer's notion of "tight-loose-design," where a corporate entity specifies the parameters for accountability, such as dual sourcing, and a regional entity has latitude for product selection, is a good example of a hybrid supply chain design model.[40,41]

A review of the classic literature on organizational design indicates that both the centralized and decentralized structure has advantages and disadvantages within supply chain management. Facets of formalization and complexity characterize both centralized and decentralized structures. Managers contemplating design features will also see that trade-offs exist with each of the dimensions of organizational design. For instance:

1. With centralization, it may be easier to develop a larger spend volume by coordinating across hospitals, *but* individualized, specialized needs within a hospital may be lost.
2. As jobs become more complex, a greater level of specialization may develop, *but* flexibility is lost as personnel does not know how to adapt to a local supply need quickly.
3. Formalization may allow for a consistent way of recording and controlling costs, *but* understanding costs within a hospital unit may be complex.

Local reporting lines of authority and responsibility make it easier to relate to local internal and external customers. Still, taking advantage of leveraged buying across the hospitals is challenging.

A primary reason for these trade-offs is that systems seldom have the same organizational environment and goals/strategies across system members. An example provides clarification for this statement. Consider a large system with several large community hospitals, a small suburban community hospital specializing in oncology, another hospital focusing on children, and another with a significant cardiac care center. In addition, the system has an assisted care center and a community outpatient clinic. Each of these facilities operates in a distinctively different environment. Even the two large community hospitals have slightly different markets due to differing socio-cultural factors within their regions. In addition, each hospital has different technology and financial environments.

The preceding paragraph details a very complex system.[42] Because of the different environments, each hospital may craft a different strategy for meeting these goals. One of the community hospitals in a lower socio-economic region gains a strategic advantage by attempting to be the low-cost provider within the community. Meanwhile, the other community hospital attempts to differentiate itself through customer satisfaction. It emphasizes promotional campaigns designed to develop an image of providing patient convenience and comfort in addition to quality care. Cardiac care and oncology centers focus on providing specialized treatment.

Much research and case studies about organizational centralization and decentralization have been published in strategic management and operations management journals and textbooks. Exhibit 8.5 summarizes some advantages and disadvantages to best appreciate the design decision process.

Exhibit 8.5: Centralization/decentralization summary.

Centralization	Decentralization
Advantages	**Advantages**
▪ Greater specialization of the buying process: may specialize on a certain type of commodity, capital equipment or physical preference items, etc. ▪ Consolidation of supply requirements resulting in greater buying clout ▪ Bundling of suppliers so that fewer are required – improved administration of suppliers ▪ Primary decision-makers physically close to each other ▪ Ability to develop a critical mass of expertise in one location (economies of scale) ▪ Strong focus on strategy ▪ Improved control and universal policies and procedures ▪ Lower administrative cost of purchasing	▪ Easier coordination with hospital users ▪ Faster response to local needs ▪ Effective use of local sources ▪ Autonomy of local unit and pride in local efforts ▪ Simple reporting lines ▪ General job skills ▪ Better understanding of local cost structure
Disadvantages	**Disadvantages**
▪ Less ability to use generalized job skills across supply commodities or functions; greater propensity to become bored with the job ▪ May overlook specialized needs in different hospitals ▪ Smaller and unique suppliers required for specialized services may be overlooked ▪ May lose physical contact with users in different hospitals ▪ Critical mass may become psychologically isolated from users ▪ Less focus on individual needs within the hospital ▪ Individualized needs are lost to universal control as a result of universal policies and procedures	▪ More difficult to coordinate with other business units ▪ Become accustomed to responding on an ad hoc basis—little planning ▪ Focus on local sources with coordinating sources with other units ▪ Lack of commitment to the entire system's objectives ▪ Poor coordination with the system ▪ Functional complex specialization is more difficult ▪ Poor understanding of total cost across the system

8.4 Roles, Authority, and Responsibility

Supply chain design must encompass individuals' roles, authority, and responsibilities to achieve organizational goals. Determining the appropriate divisions of work, along with authority and responsibility between the supply management processes and the clinical process, is the first step in the organization's design. Important is understanding, 'What is the role of the clinical staff within the supply process? Should the clinical staff be part of the ongoing supply process, or should they be separated?' These strategic questions will, however, influence the design of the supply choice and contracting processes. The discussion of value-analysis processes in Chapter 4 provides insight into this issue.

Exhibit 8.6 can assist with the answer to this question. At one end of the continuum is the cost leadership strategy. To meet the objective of this strategy, professionals are required with a strong background in cost analysis, strategic sourcing, and logistics management. These highly specialized experts have significant authority and responsibility within the supply process. But in a focus strategy, the supply specializations should be shared to a greater extent with the clinical staff.

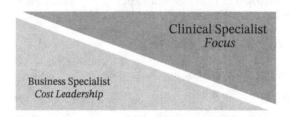

Exhibit 8.6: Division of work/authority and responsibility.

In neither case is total authority and responsibility with one party. Authority and responsibility are divided between the clinical and supply staff. Also, the division may vary within one hospital or throughout the system for different commodities and physician preference items. A hybrid organizational design is required to account for these differences.

Knowing the answers to these questions regarding cost and focus provides insight into the design of the supply chain as the orchestration of a set of facilities, suppliers, customers, products, and methods of controlling and using inventory, purchasing, and distribution to achieve the goals of provider organizations.[43]

8.5 Hybrid Organization Design

Hybrid organizational design comprises a combination of centralized and decentralized, formal and informal, and complex and simple. A hybrid design is an open system that does not seal itself off or exclude other possibilities. A hybrid system may be said to be a loose-tight fit. It has loose formalizations in some aspects of the organization while tight procedural controls in other parts. Some progressive systems, for example, have tight centralized control for the use of a GPO for commodity items, but lose control for physician preference items.

A hybrid system can continuously change and adapt to its environment.[44] Innovation is very difficult in the health sector, but hybrid systems consistently demonstrate the ability to innovate.[45] The challenge with the hybrid organization is combining organizational design elements with agility across parts of the system. Combining elements is problematic because ambiguous parameters may exist when considering control, responsibility, and accountability. A hybrid organizational design also requires communication and coordination, where roles are not always clear. Perhaps most important is that the management of the supply chain design cannot be relegated to the hospital's tacticians; "rather it must be part and parcel of the organization's key strategic thinking."[46] Fine advises, however, that to accomplish the design, "you need to have a clear image of what our supply chain design looks like, who is doing what for whom, and where the 'clockspeed bottle-necks' are occurring."[47] Progressive hospital supply leaders monitor the different hospital environments by employing clinical resource specialists to act in linking pin roles between the supply chain department and other operational units.

8.5.1 Requirements of an Effective Hybrid Organizational Design

Important attributes are necessary for an effective hybrid organizational design in healthcare. These include an open systems approach in which roles and responsibilities are flexible and accompanied by clarity of goals and high levels of employee communication and coordinator.

Open systems approach. This approach requires a combination of external focus, operational flexibility, and interaction. The entire organization is seen as interacting systems open to the inputs and outputs of each other. This interaction requires that employees understand the importance of interaction and mutual dependency.

In an open system, one unit's goals and outcomes depend on another unit's goals. They are not exclusive of each other. In operational terms, a physician, a quality control manager, and a supply manager would depend on each other to meet individual and organizational goals. In contrast, in a closed system, supply managers may meet their goals by reducing the purchase price for an item such as a stent, which may ultimately affect quality or physician satisfaction. Supply managers work to maximize their own goals without regard for others in the organization.

The open system in healthcare is related to chaos theory, an approach in which participants live in a complex world full of randomness and uncertainty.[48] Healthcare environments are characterized by surprise, rapid change, and confusion caused by uncertainty. As a result, managers cannot measure, predict, or control the unfolding drama inside or outside the organization in traditional ways.[49] The open, hybrid organization recognizes this randomness and disorder, and attempts to adapt to the chaos rather than completely change.[50] Necessary, as detailed in the following, are (a) flexible roles, responsibilities, authority, and clarity of goals; (b) employee community and coordination skills; and (c) teams designed to meet the contingencies of hybrid organizations.

Flexible roles, responsibilities, authority, and clarity of goals. A supply chain executive in a large integrated health system pointed to the importance of flexibility, agility, responsibility, and clarity of goals. "In the past, we defined ourselves by who we reported to. This is no longer the case. Now the important thing is to meet your individual, organizational, and project goals."[51] This individual expressed the importance of goals rather than adherence to highly defined roles and just keeping their superiors happy. In an open system, goals dominate, and roles and responsibilities must remain flexible to remain consistent with organizational culture. Additionally, flexibility in reporting is an important attribute, albeit one that can lead to employee confusion. An instance observed was a supply manager who reported to the facilities manager when the hospital was refurbishing the birthing center. Then, on the next project, in which the hospital was reconfiguring the storage areas and receiving docks, the same facility manager reported to the supply chain manager. Responsibilities were reversed from one project to another.

Some of the confusion associated with such reporting is expressed by a nurse who worked on standardization projects but reported to the supply management group. She had said, "To whom I report is not important, and those who think that, will have trouble in this system."[52] She went on to say, "When someone starts to ask me about my credentials, I know that they do not get it. And not everyone does at this point!" Supply chain management aims to meet organizational expectations for clinical and business performance.

Employee communication and coordination skills. Greater communication skills are required in an open system than in a closed system because it is necessary to be able to influence others without line authority. In the traditional bureaucratic organization, the influence was based on rules and procedures in addition to the hierarchy of authority. In the hybrid system, authority is more likely based on technical knowledge, motivational abilities, and charismatic leadership.

A senior manager who earned a Master's degree before entering the workforce provided an interesting and humorous quote during one of our research projects:

> *"I was fortunate to be well educated and join the workforce at a relatively high level back in the 1970s. It was great because people would listen to me. But now I realize they only listened to me because of my position. Now I have to convince them that what I am saying has merit. That is not always easy!! It has probably forced me to be a much better communicator."*[53]

Communication and coordination are vital for both vertical and horizontal linkages. As one supply executive of a large system commented:

"Sometimes I wonder what keeps this place together. Not long ago, I realized that it was the communication that kept us stuck together—the glue that keeps the ship together—and sometimes it seems pretty wobbly!"[54]

8.5.2 Team Design to Meet Contingences of a Hybrid Organization

The use of teams that are made up of a broad spectrum of professionals is vital in a hybrid organization and is discussed in Chapter 4 in the section of value analysis teams (VATs). VATs and other team efforts are generally characterized by membership heterogeneity and are "cross-functional teams." Such teams, which are essential for both horizontal and vertical coordination and implementation of strategy, require careful design around factors that include:[55,56]

Team size. First, the correct members must be included. For instance, a standardization committee on orthopedic implants without key users such as an orthopedic surgeon would have limited effectiveness.

Team skills. The team members must have sufficient team skills. This was a particularly intense issue in several of the case studies. Unfortunately, many of the participants had a difficult time separating individual perspectives and the team goal. This is a particular healthcare issue because many key decision-makers have had limited team-building training experience. On the other hand, the success of cross-functional teams could be primarily attributed to the superior team and leadership skills of everyone involved.

Team incentives. The third characteristic of effective teams is highly related to the other two characteristics. For individual and team contributions and clinical and business contributors, the correct incentives must be in place. This is not an easy task but an essential one.

8.5.3 Frames for Supply Chain Managerial Action

Organizational design is not a perspective neutral activity. Managers tend to assess their work by employing, whether knowingly or not, one or more managerial frames. A managerial "frame" is a lens or set of lenses employed by individuals to better understand the world of how to view the supply chain[57] and serve as a basis for managerial action. A manager who tends to look at problems through a human resources frame will operationalize problems differently from a manager who sees the issues through a frame grounded in an organization's culture. The challenge of finding the right way to frame the healthcare supply system has always been difficult, but the need to do so has become overwhelming in the turbulent and complicated world of the twenty-first century. Approaches to management and organization that proved effective for healthcare organizations in the past, especially as they have grown in size and complexity, are now superseded.[58] Supply chain managers draw on a number of rather specialized frames for assessing their environment and world of work.

Supply Chain Assessment Frames

In this section, we present the six frames from which supply chain management can be viewed. These are illustrated in Exhibit 8.7. The more significant ways of framing supply chain management (lenses) are described in detail.

Supply Chain as Transaction   Employing a transactional frame leads a manager to judge activities, actions, and actors (individuals) on the

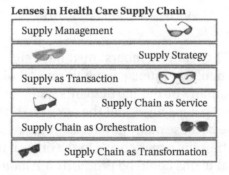

Lenses in Health Care Supply Chain

Supply Management	
	Supply Strategy
Supply as Transaction	
	Supply Chain as Service
Supply Chain as Orchestration	
	Supply Chain as Transformation

Exhibit 8.7: Lenses in health care supply chain.

basis of their ability to facilitate the movement of goods and services from manufacturer to the point of service. This frame lends itself to quantitative analysis and benchmarking that tracks products over time and workers on the basis of completed contracts, goods received, and procedures completed. Ease of access and price, rather than contribution to the larger enterprise, is key to transaction analysis. Transaction, as a frame, requires the supply chain manager to think strongly in terms of tactics and the need to complete the job at hand. While such a frame is important to assume, it can impair the goal of achieving value.

Supply Chain as Service A service frame, which is dependent on the transactional frame, aligns the supply function with assuring satisfaction for internal customers (e.g., clinicians) across the hospital and the system. Products in this scenario are satisfiers for highly valued processes—that could not be undertaken without products. They also provide satisfaction to workers by meeting their preferences and assuring few inconveniences to workforce participants. A not infrequent complaint by nurses, for example, is the inordinate amount of time they spend seeking a product for a patient. This constrains their ability to do their jobs. In the most progressive supply chains, supply chain teams act proactively—they focus on the larger, system's goals, such as improving patient satisfaction through purchasing better materials to increase service quality.

Supply Chain as Orchestration The supply chain function in the modern hospital and hospital systems represents the intersection of many customer demands and broader system requirements for knowledge. Success requires orchestration—working to bring together, through sourcing decisions, contracting, logistics, and combinations of products that enhance performance. Successful value analysis processes, as were discussed in Chapter 3, require expertise in orchestration. An "orchestration" frame is operational when supply chain executives can channel their decisions to support organizational goals that transcend a single procurement order or that impact multiple stakeholders. A focus on safety, for example, might lead supply chain managers to prefer "sharps" products that work well together to avoid needle sticks, or when used together, promote reduced length of stay (which is associated with reduced patient injuries). The orchestrator must intimately know all aspects of the enterprise and just as a musical orchestra leader can detect when one section is out of tune or off the beat, the SCM orchestrator must be sensitive to disconnects and respond to them.

Orchestration requires working closely with physicians, nurses, technicians, and a wide range of non-clinically trained professionals to manage the products and the technological innovation that characterizes modern hospital practice. And as in other industries, the management of such an environment requires skills associated with motivating and leading with technical professionals, the management of innovation, providing leadership in the innovation process, managing knowledge as it relates to work, and designing organizational processes for innovation.[59]

Increasingly, orchestration requires understanding of the challenges associated with managing within a complex network.[60] Necessary is the development of trust among buyers, suppliers, and end users. Successful network managers utilize their resources to effectively coordinate the efforts, develop risk and benefit sharing, and effectively deal with conflict resolutions.[61] Harland and Knight[62] identify six key roles that one can assume in orchestrating networks:

- Network structuring agent—Monitors and influences the competitiveness of supply markets. Acts to protect critical suppliers from the detrimental consequences of fragmented purchasing. Restructures supply routes to interface directly with manufacturers rather than wholesalers.
- Coordinator—Acts to manage both ongoing and completed projects with network partners.
- Advisor—Provides advice on supply policy and strategy matters to internal network partners.
- Information broker—Collects, analyses, and disseminates information to network partners in order to better manage the interests of the relationship as well as focus on key issues and performance metrics.
- Relationship broker—Facilitates inter-network communication and negotiation as well as encourage change to deal with specific performance related issues.
- Innovation sponsor—Promotes and facilitates product and process innovation.

These roles demand skills that create and help establish a sense of trust and of collaboration among the various parties involved with the network. Managing within a network means having the knowledge and skill to be able to introduce and connect people—clinicians, GPO, distributor, manufacturer, and IT—in such a way as to enable both sides of the relationship to benefit. On a more subtle level, managing network relationships involves the utilization of information—how to gather it and how to use it.

With the establishment of measurable metrics and through the use of the data that IT solutions provide, managers are able to view their own progress, clarify responsibilities of partners and establish accountability for all members of the network. For example, by working with suppliers to implement long-term solutions, both parties can benefit from captured efficiencies such as a reduction in the number of orders handled, an improvement in on-time delivery, or a reduced number of order mistakes. The true meaning of orchestration in a working network lies in the fact that the members can act together in order to produce the greatest benefit for everyone involved.

Supply Chain as Transformation A transformational frame judges products on the basis of their contribution to some organizational/clinical goal (e.g., improved safety) and individuals on the basis of their ability to advance the goals of the organization. The transformational frame considers materials as one input into improving organizational performance. It assists managers to see resources as assets—not just a pass-through or potential liabilities. In this scenario, materials are synergistic. They allow procedures and processes to be completed more effectively. Materials in the transformational model are selected because they lead to better services, outcomes, and new ways of doing things. Materials and processes are selected on the basis of their sustaining the hospital's agility and adaptability in a quickly changing environment. The transformational lens is sensitive to both the changes in the healthcare delivery environment and the ongoing changes in the supply chain environment.

8.6 Chapter Summary

Following Drucker's contention that organizational design begins with building blocks, this discussion has reviewed these building blocks. Careful design of the building blocks is critical for a highly resource dependent organization subject to a great deal of uncertainty, such as a hospital or hospital system. Based on the current literature and the results of the case studies, a hybrid organizational design is recommended for most situations.

The hybrid design is recommended because of the variety of environmental issues faced within individual hospitals and across an IDN, which may be composed of a variety of hospitals, clinics and other points for providing care. Because of the environmental complexity, differences in strategies exist from one unit to another within a system. The idea of a hospital as an organization with units affected by various "clockspeeds" further supports the need for a hybrid system with an open, flexible approach to organizational design.

The idea of clockspeeds leads to the recognition that it is difficult for supply chain and other healthcare executives to shape their organizations in an environment where there is no simple or universal answer for organizational design. Organizations at different stages in their life-cycles require different kinds of management.[63] Hospitals are a curious combination of continually growing and aging departments, processes, procedures, and technologies. New kinds of laboratories emerge to meet new technologies, and processes are outsourced due to changing time demands by patients and payors. No one supply design or strategy will fit all of a hospital's units.

The progressive supply manager must be prepared to assess not only the best strategy for the overall supply function, but the strategy necessary to meet the demands of a variety of internal and external customers. In each case, the supply chain manager will find it necessary to determine the centralization, formalization, and complexity that is required within each unit.

Importantly, the organization of the supply chain function is not "merely" designed to manage the everyday aspects of bringing products to patients, but it must also be designed to assure the sustainability of operations under times of stress, such as an accident that impacts multiple people, hurricane, or, as we witnessed, severe shortages during the COVID-19 pandemic. How the organization assures "readiness" or "business continuity," that was discussed in Chapter 3, requires mention here—since the organization that is only focused on today's requirements, and overly relies on others to investigate achievement of a "just-in-case" environment, will find itself wanting.

Notes

1. Drucker, P. F. (1993). *Management: Tasks, responsibilities, practices* (Reprint edition),. Harper Business.
2. Teece D. J. (1990) Contributions and impediments of economic analysis to the study of strategic management, Produced and distributed by Center for Research in Management, University of California, Berkeley Business School.
3. Drucker, P. F. (1993). *Management: Tasks, responsibilities, practices* (Reprint edition),. Harper Business.
4. Caplow, T., Merton, R. K., & Merton, R. K. (1964). *Principles of organization* (pp. 119–124). Harcourt, Brace & World.
5. Zajac, E. J., Kraatz, M. S., & Bressler, R. K. F. (2000). Modeling the dynamics of strategic fit: A normative approach to strategic change. *Strategic Management Journal*, 21(4), 429–453.
6. Kanter, R. M. (1985). *The change masters: Innovation and entrepreneurship in the American Corporation*. Free Press.
7. Rivkin, J. W., & Siggelkow, N. (2003). Balancing search and stability: Interdependencies among elements of organizational design. *Management Science*, 49(3), 290–311.
8. Bracker, J. (1980). The historical development of the strategic management concept. *The Academy of Management Review*, 5(2), 219–224.
9. Blackburn, R. S. (1982). Dimensions of structure: A review and reappraisal. *The Academy of Management Review*, 7(1), 59–66.

10. Galbraith, J. (1977). *Organization design*. Addison-Wesley.
11. Rodgers, S. (2004). Supply management: Six elements of superior design. *Supply Chain Management Review, 19*(03), 48–54.
12. Ibid.
13. Blackburn, R. S. (1982). Dimensions of structure: A review and reappraisal. *The Academy of Management Review, 7*(1), 59–66.
14. Rodgers, op. cit.
15. Fine, C. H. (2000). Clockspeed-based strategies for supply chain design. *Production and Operations Management, 9*(3), 213–221.
16. Chen, D. Q., Preston, D. S., & Xia, W. (2013). Enhancing hospital supply chain performance: A relational view and empirical test. *Journal of Operations Management, 31*(6), 391–408.
17. Hillman, A. J., Withers, M. C., & Collins, B. J. (2009). Resource dependence theory: A review. *Journal of management, 35*(6), 1404–1427.
18. Montgomery, K., & Schneller, E. S. (2007). Hospitals' strategies for orchestrating selection of physician preference items. *The Milbank Quarterly, 85*(2), 307–335.
19. Malone, T. W., & Crowston, K. (1994). The interdisciplinary study of coordination. *ACM Computing Surveys, 26*(1), 87–119.
20. Fisher, E. S., Shortell, S. M., Kreindler, S. A., Van Citters, A. D., & Larson, B. K. (2012). A framework for evaluating the formation, implementation, and performance of accountable care organizations. *Health affairs, 31*(11), 2368–2378.
21. Kwon, I.-W., & Kim, S.-H. (2018). Framework for successful supply chain implementation in healthcare area from provider's prospective. *Asia Pacific Journal of Innovation and Entrepreneurship, 12*(2), 135–145.
22. Ibid.
23. Bazzoli, G. J., Shortell, S. M., Dubbs, N., Chan, C., & Kralovec, P. (1999). A taxonomy of health networks and systems: Bringing order out of chaos. *Health Services Research, 33*(6), 1683–1717.
24. Nabelsi, V., & Gagnon, S. (2017). Information technology strategy for a patient-oriented, lean, and agile integration of hospital pharmacy and medical equipment supply chains. *International Journal of Production Research, 55*(14), 3929–3945.
25. Foerstl, K., Hartmann, E., Wynstra, F., & Moser, R. (2013). Cross-functional integration and functional coordination in purchasing and supply management: Antecedents and effects on purchasing and firm performance. *International Journal of Operations & Production Management, 33*(6), 689–721.
26. Lee, S. M., Lee, D., & Schniederjans, M. J. (2011). Supply chain innovation and organizational performance in the healthcare industry. *International Journal of Operations & Production Management, 31*(11), 1193–1214.
27. Rego, N., & de Sousa, J. P. (2009). Supply chain coordination in hospitals. In L. M. Camarinha-Matos, I. Paraskakis, & H. Afsarmanesh (Eds.), *Leveraging knowledge for innovation in collaborative networks* (pp. 117–127). Springer.

28. Montgomery, K., & Schneller, E. S. (2007). Hospitals' strategies for orchestrating selection of physician preference items. *The Milbank Quarterly*, *85*(2), 307–335.

29. Abdulsalam, Y., Gopalakrishnan, M., Maltz, A., & Schneller, E. (2018). The impact of physician-hospital integration on hospital supply management. *Journal of Operations Management*, *57*(1), 11–22.

30. Choi, T. Y., Dooley, K. J., & Rungtusanatham, M. (2001). Supply networks and complex adaptive systems: Control versus emergence. *Journal of Operations Management*, *19*(3), 351–366.

31. For a better understanding of the concept "strategic fit" see:Venkatraman, N., et al. (1989). The concept of fit in strategy research: Toward verbal and statistical correspondence. *Academy of Management Review*, *14*(3), 423–444.Venkatraman, N., & Camillis, J. C. (1984). Exploring the concept of fit in strategic management. *Academy of Management Review*, *9*(3), 513–525; andZajac, E. J., Kraatz, M. S., & Bressler, R. K. F. (2000). Modeling the dynamics of strategic fit: A normative approach to strategic change. *Strategic Management Journal*, *21*(4), 429–453.

32. Alexander, J. A., & Morrisey, M. A. (1989). A resource-dependence model of hospital contract management. *Health Services Research*, *24*(2), 259.

33. Schwartz, K., Lopez, E., Rae, M., & Neuman, T. (2020) What we know about provider consolidation, Kaiser Family Foundation. https://www.kff.org/health-costs/issue-brief/what-we-know-about-provider-consolidation

34. Abdulsalam, Y., & Schneller, E. (2019). Hospital supply expenses: An important ingredient in health services research. *Medical Care Research and Review: MCRR*, *76*(2), 240–252.

35. U.S. General Services Administration. Federal Acquisition Regulation. https://www.gsa.gov/policy-regulations/regulations/federal-acquisition-regulation-far

36. Fine, C. H. (1999). *Clockspeed: Winning industry control in the age of temporary advantage* (Revised edition). Basic Books.

37. Ibid.

38 Patient Protection and Affordable Care Act. (2010) Public Law 111–148. 111 Congress. March 23, 2010.

39. Such observations for other industries have been made by Leenders, M., & Fraser Johnson, P. F. (2000). *Major Structural Changes in Supply Organizations*. CAPS Research. andJohnson, P. F., Leenders, M., & Fearon, H. (1998, Winter). Evolving roles, and responsibilities of purchasing organizations, *International Journal of Purchasing and Materials Management*, 2–11.

40. Smeltzer, L. R. (1997). *Conditions that create influence for purchasing in corporate strategic planning.* Center for Advanced Purchasing Studies.

41. Vähätalo, M., & Kallio, T. J. (2019). Managing health services–tight integration or loose coupling. *Nordic Journal of Business*, *68*(4), 5–24.

42. Dooley, K. (2002). Organizational complexity. *International Encyclopedia of Business and Management*, *6*, 5013–5022.

43. Altiparmak, F., Gen, M., Lin, L., & Paksoy, T. (2006). A genetic algorithm approach for multi-objective optimization of supply chain networks. *Computers & Industrial Engineering, 51*(1), 196–215.

44. Aldrich, H. (2008). *Organizations and environments.* Stanford University Press.

45. Abdulsalam, Y., Gopalakrishnan, M., Maltz, A., & Schneller, E. (2015). Health care matters: Supply chains in and of the health sector. *Journal of Business Logistics, 36*(4), 335–339.

46. Fine, op. cit.

47. Ibid.

48. Begun, J. W., Zimmerman, B., & Dooley, K. (2003). Health care organizations as complex adaptive systems. *Advances in Health Care Organization Theory, 253*, 288.

49. Huey, J. ((1993). Managing in the midst of chaos. *Fortune, 127*(7), 38.

50. Straub, K. (1997). Chaos theory. *Health Management Technology, 18*(10), 12–15.

51. Schneller, E., & Smeltzer, L. (2007). *Strategic management of the health supply chain* (pp. 170). Jossey Bass.

52. Ibid.

53. Ibid.

54. Ibid.

55. Manz, C. C., Keating, D. E., & Donnellon, A. (1990). Preparing for an organizational change to employee self-management: The managerial transition. *Organizational Dynamics, 19*(2), 15–26.

56. Monczka, R., & t Trent, R. (1993). *Cross-functional sourcing team effectiveness.* CAPS Research.

57. Bolman, L. G., & Deal, T. E. (2013). *Reframing organizations: Artistry, choice, and leadership* (5th ed.). Jossey-Bass.

58. Arndt, M., & Bigelow, B. (2000). The transfer of business practices into hospitals: History and implications. In *Advances in health care management* (Vol. 1, pp. 339–368). Emerald Group Publishing Limited.

59. Wallace, M., & Schneller, E. (2008). Orchestrating emergent change: the 'hospitalist movement' in US Healthcare. *Public Administration, 86*(3), 761–778.

60. Choi, op. cit.

61. Johnsen, T., Wynstra, F., Zheng, J., Harland, C., & Lamming, R. (2000). Networking activities in supply networks. *Journal of Strategic Marketing, 8*(2), 161–181.

62. Harland, C. M., & Knight, L. A. (2001). Supply network strategy: Role and competence requirements. *International Journal of Operations & Production Management, 21*(4), 476–489.

63. Adizes, I. (1990). *Corporate lifecycles: How and why corporations Grow and Die and what to do about it* (1st ed.). The Adizes Institute.

9

Information Technology (IT) Strategies— *Information Is the Glue that Binds*

Supply chain management (SCM) is complex, sometimes involving the processing of thousands of data points. Such processing is well beyond the capability of mortal humans. Powerful technology to manage the many transactions and associated data is necessary. This chapter describes how and what technology is used by healthcare organizations to support these needs. The discussed technology can transform the myriad data points into useable information to help supply chain professionals and clinicians better perform their jobs. As we say in the subtitle, "Information Is the Glue that Binds."

This chapter begins by explaining how value is derived from technology—through automation and digitization. It then proceeds, step-by-step, through the supply chain processes, describing the typical ways that organizations use technology to manage transactions; automate processes; and store, access, analyze, and utilize data. The chapter concludes with a discussion about how organizations drive higher performance through the use of technology today and the directions that technology will evolve in the future (recognizing that any printed discussion of this is at risk of becoming outdated given the rapid rate of technological innovation). We will begin by focusing on the foundational value proposition from technology.

9.1 The Value of Supply Chain Technology

As with other endeavors in life, technology adds material value to human endeavors, and in this case, to the management of the healthcare supply chain. Many of the capabilities used to manage supply chains and the resulting accomplishments could not be possible without the underlying technology supporting SCM organizations. Information technology (IT) has been employed across the functions in the Fully Integrated Supply Chain Organization (FISCO) model to support many of the most important challenges faced by healthcare delivery systems. A mature FISCO, as described in Chapter 1, extensively employs IT to integrate systems across the enterprise, creating interfaces among the enterprise resource planning (ERP) systems, the electronic healthcare record (EHR) systems, and the general ledgers. Together, these systems can help capture data on products used in patient care, calculate supply expense per procedure or episode of care, and support supply decisions based on clinical pathway standards. After the fact, analytics can further support patient care and supply decisions by understanding the relationship between products used and outcomes achieved. Opportunities for advancement result with continued technological innovation that further optimizes operations of supply chains.

Technology solutions support SCM in two ways: (a) automating processes, and (b) digitizing the vast amounts of data needed to manage the multitude of products purchased and used by healthcare systems. The following sections discuss the two underlying value streams created by each of these tools.

9.1.1 Automating the Processes

Typical healthcare organizations source tens of thousands of products globally to support thousands of clinicians and other workers essential to clinical and administrative operations. To support this level of effort and complexity, supply chain managers need support; they cannot manually manage the complexity. Technology solutions are available to automate almost all supply chain processes. Most orders for products can be created electronically, and if not, they can be manually entered by the requesting clinician or end user and forwarded to the supply chain team to send electronically to suppliers. For example, standard medical supplies such as intravenous fluids and personal protection equipment (PPE) that are stored in cabinets and storage rooms on patient floors typically have replenishment orders created automatically as consumption is recorded. In more complex settings, such as surgical units, nurses must often create purchase orders for consignment or other products (often implantable devices) that are purchased after they have been used in a procedure. Many of these orders are still handled manually, although there have been recent advancement in tools to automate the ordering and replenishment process for such devices. Nurses or supply chain personnel help prepare for a surgical case by gathering the products that individual physicians have indicated they want to use in specific types of procedures.

Identifying the quantity and locations of inventoried products across a large medical campus is more easily handled through the use of technology that specifies details about specific products, including standardized identifiers (with batch/lot/serial numbers and expiration dates), units of measure, quantities of each, and even price. The medications administered and products used (especially implants) are documented in the EHR, which serves as a personalized inventory record of products used in a particular patient's care.

Automation tools add significant value to the operation of a healthcare system. Requests are handled quicker and with more accuracy. Product deliveries are made more efficiently. Costs are lower. Quality is higher. In summary, automation improves process performance by:

- Standardizing processes;
- Speeding up processes;
- Making correct decisions without human intervention;
- Reducing labor requirements; and
- Being available 24 hours a day, 7 days a week.

Value through technology automation eventually trickles through to value for patients and clinicians. For example, technology can free up clinical staff from the burden of clerical tasks and allow them to spend more time focused on patients and their care. Automation can also improve many SCM processes from the point of procurement through to payment for goods, or what is known as the procure-to-pay (P2P) cycle. The key subprocesses are depicted in Exhibit 9.1.

Underlying many of these processes are the data elements held within the item master. The item master, housed as a part of the ERP system, either on premise or in the cloud, holds standardized and normalized data on the products purchased regularly by a hospital or health system and is structured to support clinical, financial, and supply chain processes. The management of item master data is a key function within the FISCO.

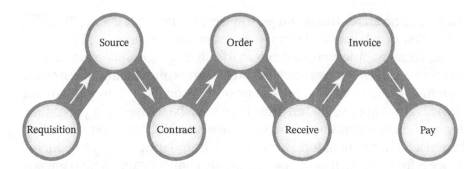

Exhibit 9.1: The P2P cycle.

We cannot overstate the value of automation to improve efficiency and effectiveness in healthcare delivery. With the thousands of products used by clinicians and other healthcare workers, automation is an essential component of SCM. Automation of supply chain processes between providers and suppliers has also grown significantly with the advent of business-to-business (B2B) marketplaces and exchanges, first introduced in the late 1990s. Today, most hospital and healthcare systems use commercial exchanges, which provide technology platforms to place purchase orders, and to receive confirmations, advanced ship notices, and invoices from their suppliers. As technology continues to develop (particularly with artificial intelligence), greater benefits from automation will accrue.

9.1.2 Digitizing the Supply Chain

Commonly discussed and advocated is the automation and digitization of the supply chain. The two activities, in fact, are separate but related functions. In order to successfully automate processes, the data used must be clean, accurate, and synchronized with other parties, including suppliers. Automation of processes, meanwhile, helps create a digital record of transactions.

The digitization of the supply chain materially aids information flow, both inside the hospital as well as outside with supply partners. By making all of the information about supplies, including their location, the amount of inventory on hand, the acquisition price, and the status of transactions, supply chain professionals and clinicians can ensure products are available when needed or take corrective action as necessary. Digitization also supports analytics to understand how products contribute to better outcomes as well as opportunities to improve pricing through contracting. Digitization offers a range of benefits in how product data is managed, including:

- Accuracy—Use of standard identifiers provides clarity as to product identification;

- Consistency—The same information is available to all authorized users;
- Immediacy—Authorized individuals have access as soon as the data is published;
- Accessibility—Data can be retrieved by any authorized user; and
- Security—Information is protected through complex authorization algorithms.

Bottom line, digitization greatly simplifies and enhances the sharing and analysis of fundamental information, which helps generate value for clinicians and patients. Every step in the P2P process benefits from digitization.

Maximizing the effectiveness of digitization requires digital records for all elements of the supply chain, including:

- Supplier data;
- Contract terms and conditions;
- Product data:
    - Industry standard identifiers;
    - Physical descriptions (weight, size, special handling or regulatory requirements); and
    - Units of measure;
- Packaging size
    - Batch/lot/serial numbers, and
    - Expiration dates;
- Order information;
- Contract price;
- Shipment status; and
- Adverse event and recall data.

The resulting database for these records quickly becomes very large, but managing large databases is much easier with advancements in cloud technology, discussed in more detail later. Required is careful consideration of the security rules for regulating who has access to the data. Typically, well-designed systems that manage these databases have mechanisms for assigning secure access to the appropriate fields. These need to be carefully designed and implemented.

Another important role for technology is management of the provenance of medical products. Supply chain managers need to be assured that the products they receive are exactly as they were intended and represented. Was it fabricated at a reputable manufacturing site? Was it appropriately protected during its transport from the point of manufacturer to the point of use? Did the shipments maintain proper storage and handling requirements? Are any of the products subject to recall or expired? Distributed ledger technologies, such as blockchain, can create a chain of custody for products are increasingly being used to track and monitor movement and condition of products from the manufacturing site to the point of use in patient care.[1]

Regulation to track and trace the movement of pharmaceutical products is further developed than it is for medical device products, although steps have been taken to create similar capabilities for devices. The U.S. FDA Unique Device Identification rule, which requires manufacturers to assign and label their devices with unique device identifiers (UDIs) in both human and machine readable (e.g., scannable) formats, is a foundational step.[2,3] The UDI includes both a product's standardized device identifier, as well as the information used by the manufacturer to control its production, such as the batch, lot, or serial number and expiry date. Capturing this level of information in a digital record plays an important role in patient care. Providers are increasingly incorporating improved product management through UDI integration.[4]

9.2 Technology Framework and Systems for Supply Chain Management

Because the supply chain extends beyond the four walls of the hospital or healthcare system, upstream to manufacturers and downstream to patients and the various providers who care for them, SCM requires intensive information collection, sharing, and processing. Accordingly, the technology and information processing systems that support SCM are of critical importance. In healthcare, the IT environment is composed of two interrelated sets of systems—clinical and business systems. Both are critical to the effective functioning of a modern healthcare system. Exhibit 9.2 displays their interaction with each other, which is critical to the success of their deployment. Much information is shared and passed between each other. Together, these systems constitute the information backbone for a healthcare organization.

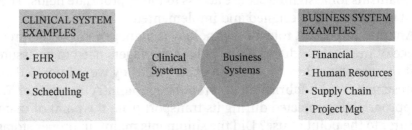

Exhibit 9.2: Business versus clinical systems.

Clinical systems support clinicians by managing a wide array of activities through the control of patient records and clinical protocols. The centerpiece of these clinical systems are electronic health records (EHRs) that are essentially databases of clinical records for patients. The two largest and most widely adopted EHR platforms are operated by EPIC and Cerner (the latter acquired in 2022 by Oracle, which also offers ERP systems).

The key business systems deployed by hospitals and healthcare systems are the ERP solutions, which support all of the financial and operating processes of a healthcare organization. A key part of these systems is the SCM component, which controls both order and inventory management processes. Major ERP system vendors are Oracle, Infor, Workday, SAP, and Meditech.

Before delving into the specifics of these core systems, it is important to maintain a focus on the primary objectives for the use of supply chain information. All supply chains use information for two primary reasons—processing transactions (controlling) and knowing information (sharing)—as outlined in the following:

- Processing transactions:
    - Clinical orders,
    - Requisitions from users (internal customers),
    - Supplier contracts,
    - Purchase orders,
    - Shipment transactions, and
    - Invoices.
- Knowing information:
    - Clinical records,
    - Customer requirements,
    - Supplier capabilities,
    - Contracts and pricing,
    - Network capabilities,
    - Quantity of inventory available at each location,
    - Status of all orders in progress, and
    - Performance measurement.

9.2.1 ERPs

The four core functions of SCM (sourcing, contracting, order management, and inventory management) are supported by the main modules of an ERP system. These systems have four to five distinct specialized business support modules that are integrated with each other. These modules are typically finance, human resources, customer relationship management, SCM, and (when applicable) manufacturing, as illustrated in Exhibit 9.3.

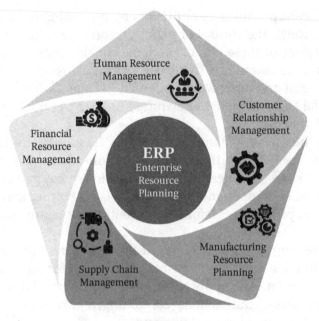

Exhibit 9.3: The main modules of an ERP system.

The advantage of integrating these modules is that if anything happens in one part of the business, all of the relevant functions throughout the business will accurately and comprehensively reflect that event's specifics. For example, when an order is placed for a particular medical product, many other areas (such as inventory, contract management, accounts payable, and warehouse receiving) are impacted and correctly updated. This helps ensure that business decisions are made with a full understanding and appreciation of other activities that impact business and clinical operations.

When we unpack the elements of SCM within an ERP environment, we find subprocesses that align with the business processes discussed earlier in this book. The standard subprocesses for SCM within an ERP environment are:

- Order management,
- Materials management,
- Sourcing,
- Contracting,
- Purchasing,
- Accounts payable,
- Manufacturing management,
- Warehouse management, and
- Transportation management.

By having all of these processes operate in a synchronized manner, all business decisions, from strategic to operational, are made faster with fewer errors and greater efficiency. For healthcare, this directly supports the triple aim of lower costs, improved experience, and better patient outcomes. In today's healthcare environment, it is difficult, if not impossible, to operate a successful provider operation without an ERP solution.

9.2.2 EHRs

In a healthcare system, clinicians spend considerable time with EHRs, which provide critical data to support clinical workflows and advise on patients' conditions.[5] On a patient-by-patient basis, these systems track the protocols followed, control and record the medications dispensed, store all laboratory results, schedule patient procedures, and even advise the clinician on evidence-based treatment plans.

The EHR creates a form of inventory record of sorts for the patients by identifying a wide range of homeostatic conditions:

- Medical condition,
- Past procedures,
- Diagnoses,
- Protocols applied,
- Medication prescribed,
- Procedures prescribed and delivered, and
- Diagnostic tests.

With digital records, the history of the patient, along with current protocols, can be shared with other clinicians caring for the same patient. Once again, the system gains accuracy and speed.

While the concept may appear simple, its implementation is not. Medical records appear in many locations, created by a widespread set of clinicians, and with both structured and unstructured data, the latter of which requires natural language processing (NLP) to support computer-driven analytics. Consequently, additional technology programs are required to read, translate, and format these records into common data sets that can be accessed by healthcare organization information technology systems. A hallmark of many EHR implementations has been the ability for the hospital or healthcare system to customize the technology, which has made it far more difficult to create interoperability between EHRs even if they are provided by the same company and have been configured similarly. As a result, EHRs can operate in a "Tower of Babel world," with different languages, different ways to say similar things, and different protocols.[6] A digitized record is of no use unless it can be read and interpreted by other digitized systems.

When implemented well, these records have the potential to provide substantial benefits to physicians, clinical practices, healthcare organizations and patients. These systems can facilitate workflow and improve the quality of patient care and patient safety. Between 2011 and 2021, adoption of EHRs by both physician practices and hospitals increased substantially, from 34% to 78% and 28% to 96%, respectively.[7] Still, doctors have expressed frustration with systems that they say take time away from actual patient care.

The benefits that healthcare organizations derive from EHRs are substantial and broad based. The Agency for Healthcare Research and Quality (AHRQ)[8] has listed the following benefits:

- Physician access to patient information, such as diagnoses, allergies, lab results, and medications.
- Access to new and past test results among providers in multiple care settings.
- Computerized provider order entry.
- Computerized decision-support systems to prevent drug interactions and improve compliance with best practices.
- Secure electronic communication among providers and patients.
- Patient access to health records, disease management tools, and health information resources.
- Computerized administration processes, such as scheduling systems.
- Standards-based electronic data storage and reporting for patient safety and disease surveillance efforts.

Given the sensitive nature of data held in EHRs, some have expressed concerns about the risk of hacking. There has been an uptick in cyber-attacks on hospitals and health systems, given that patient data is considered more valuable on the black market than even financial data exposed in other incidents. On the other hand, digital records have been shown to be safer and more secure than maintaining data on paper or in local computers, laptops, or mobile devices that can be comprised and/or removed. For example, leaving workstations unattended may leave them open to unauthorized access. Anyone concerned that digital records are not as secure should visit a hospital ward and look at the many charts and files laying on unattended desks and shelves. To overcome this security gap, certified EHRs have built-in security measures, and as is discussed in the section on cloud technology, the certified vendors hosting the applications and data are experts in data encryption and must stay on top of the latest security measures to protect their entire customer base.

Notwithstanding these risks, many physicians and other clinicians who have adopted EHRs within their practice have reported that the benefits are real and that their patients can receive better medical care as a result.

It has been pointed out that while it makes sense that the item master (discussed previously) should also feed the EHR to support documentation of the products used in patient care, and thus, improve safety and access to information on product efficacy, using the item master to feed standardized product data to the EHR has continued to be a challenge[9] except in the most mature healthcare systems.[10] This has been an important consideration and priority with the increasing adoption of cloud-based ERPs and EHRs.

9.2.3 Cloud Technology

The use of cloud technology has proven successful for multiple industries and purposes, including healthcare. Cloud-based systems provide access to applications and data hosted in the cloud, as opposed to more traditional on-premise technology installations where the applications and associated data are housed on site and the organization using the technology—in this case, the hospital or health system—is responsible for the hardware, data servers, and software upgrades. To the user, the experience is almost the same as interfacing with servers that are in the next room, although cloud technology can also be accessed through a variety of desktop and mobile devices. Exhibit 9.4 indicates the array of cloud-supported services that an organization might employ. In 2021, Gartner reported that 75% of healthcare providers responding to its

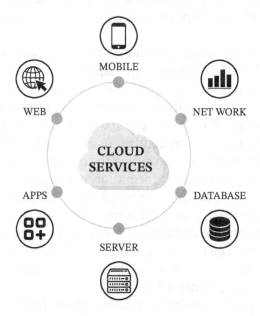

Exhibit 9.4: The cloud service ecosystem.

cloud end-user buyer behavior study said they planned to increase their spending on cloud technology.[11]

According to IBM, one of pioneers in cloud technology, there are three key benefits to cloud technology:[12]

- **Flexibility:** Users can scale services to fit their needs, customize applications, and access cloud services from anywhere with an internet connection.
- **Efficiency:** Enterprise users can deliver applications to market quickly without worrying about underlying infrastructure costs or maintenance.
- **Strategic value:** Cloud-based services give enterprises a competitive advantage by providing the most innovative technology available.

The biggest impact on the healthcare supply chain is the growing migration to cloud-based ERP[13] systems by hospitals and health systems that seek lower installation costs, automatic software upgrades, and according to analyst firm International Data Corporation (IDC), the "ability to access and analyze massive amounts of data in near real time."[14] This latter point is particularly important to integrate supply chain, financial, and clinical data to optimize the cost and quality of healthcare delivery. By storing data in the cloud, hospitals and healthcare systems also face less risk of losing critical data as the result of fires or other natural disasters. Gartner has also stated that "The rapid pace of innovation in cloud infrastructure and platform services (CIPS) makes cloud the de facto platform for new digital services and existing traditional workloads."[15]

With the move to cloud, hospitals and healthcare systems can outsource many of the IT management responsibilities to the ERP vendor, which are delivered in a software-as-a-service (SaaS) model. By outsourcing these duties, healthcare systems can focus on their core competencies. That said, it is critical to choose a vendor that not only offers the necessary business functionality but also can also meet the demands of a mission critical service such as healthcare. This is particularly important given the sensitivity of information managed by health systems, including the confidentiality of patient data. While some have expressed concerns about allowing an outside party to manage their data, cloud-based ERP vendors are considered far more equipped to monitor for security risks and keep security protocols updated as a core competency compared to most hospitals that face increasing financial constraints and are not, at their core, IT organizations.[7]

For the management of the healthcare supply chain, cloud technology has opened up a realm of new value creation possibilities. Many steps are taken out of the process, more users (including those working in remote or disparate locations) have direct access to relevant and accurate data, and the timeliness of the available data is enhanced. This improves the efficiency of supply chain processes and, more importantly, enables supply chain managers to add capabilities that support greater effectiveness from their actions. Such tools include:

- Directly engaging clinicians in supply chain decisions;
- Expanding the breadth of the relationship with suppliers to include their upstream product maps; and
- Developing advanced performance metrics by linking clinical and supply chain data.

Switching to cloud-based ERP systems has critical implications for how supply chain data is managed and utilized. While a cloud-based ERP system can support the integration of clinical, financial, and operational data, the health system must ensure the data feeding the ERP, and on which downstream operations depend, is accurate. Mechanisms should also be in place to address the continual changes in products, vendors, price, and so on.

Advances in ERP systems, especially cloud-based systems that can be more easily upgraded, are supporting more and more business functionality. Depending on the version of the ERP (on-premise or cloud-based), there are still times when a hospital or healthcare system needs to add additional technology.

One of the areas where technology enhancements are sought is in warehouse management tools. While most ERPs have a warehouse management system (WMS) module, it may not be sufficiently robust for a large, complex operation with significant and dynamic needs. For example, a complex warehouse with a large workforce would want to have a sophisticated productivity management system embedded in its WMS. Such organizations would seek a best-in-class solution rather than a limited solution integrated within the ERP. This is not a simple decision to make, for example, considering the trade-off of greater functionality (best-in-class) versus the value of managing all transactions within a single system.

ERP systems generally have the ability to send the electronic interchange of business documents/transactions (EDI) to individual suppliers, although most health systems have opted to use B2B exchanges in order to create a single connection through which they can do business with multiple suppliers. Those exchanges offer the capability of integrating directly with the ERP system, whether on-premise or in the cloud.

In some cases, all required functionality may not be available in the ERP. Advanced procurement solutions that analyze and portray spending patterns are valuable to high performing SCM organizations. Some of these products will interface with the ERP to provide added functionality. Exhibit 9.5 illustrates how an intermediary can integrate and support an ERP in the P2P process, which is similar to the role played by other spend management and B2B exchange solutions on the market.

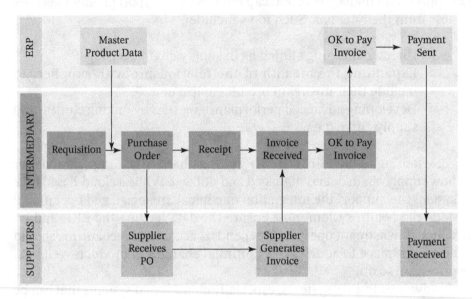

Exhibit 9.5: The ERP's role in the P2P cycle.

In other cases, supply chain teams may need additional financial analytics capabilities to analyze and portray spending patterns.

Other specialized applications may be acquired to support the collection and dissemination of performance metrics that drive predictive analytics. As an organization begins to leverage developments in artificial intelligence (AI), specialized systems are available to drive decision-making. Areas that are evolving quickly in their utilization of AI, and therefore require careful tracking, include supply chain network design, supplier selection, supply chain sustainability, inventory planning, and demand planning.[16,17]

9.3 IT as a Strategy for High Performance

While well-designed advanced technology can provide competitive advantage, IT is not always viewed as a core strategic competency in hospital and healthcare systems. However, FISCOs recognize that IT solutions will play a critical role in their future clinical and business performance. Hence, IT development and implementation is a key part of organizational strategy and maturity. These more progressive organizations have a vision for how the various functions of the health-care organization—from clinical to administrative—can be enhanced to benefit patients and their care. Such organizations view digitized health-care as the future of their services and an enabler of high performance. The following sections describe the elements of a high-performance strategy for IT.

9.3.1 The Primary Value Drivers

Through a well-architected IT framework and the use of advanced auto-mation and digitization tools, SCM organizations can add significant value to the entire healthcare organization. Automation programs, a key driver of value, generate benefits through:

- Productivity:
  - Streamlining physical flows of products from the source through to the bedside;
  - Simplifying transaction processing through algorithms that make decisions based on human decision patterns;
    - Invoice processing;
    - Inventory replenishment;
    - Contract compliance monitoring.
  - Assisting clinicians in product ordering decisions by providing detailed information on product characteristics and usage.
- Robotic Process Automation:
  - Streamlines operations for highly repeatable processes in the supply chain, removing both clerical burden on staff and human error;
  - Incorporates machine learning tools to aid decision-making; and
  - Standardizes processes among a large number of users to provide consistent high-quality service within the system.

The second major value driver through SCM technology is the dig-itization of all manual records and the sharing of data extracted from business and clinical applications, such as ERP and EHR systems. Sub-ject to appropriate access rights, this enables virtual access to all relevant records by any authorized user at any time, in any place. As a result, benefits arise by linking a broad set of data elements for analysis and understanding. Such capabilities enable:

- Information sharing:
  - Easily access all information required for supply chain decision-making;

- Collect and report supply performance at the point of care/use;
- Correlate EHR data with supply chain data to better understand how medical outcomes relate to product usage; and
- Analyze large amounts of data, previously only manually accessible, to better understand product and clinical performance issues.
- Clinical case costing:
  - Link operating costs with clinical case outcomes; and
  - Identify clinical products that correlate with better patient outcomes.
- Contract management:
  - Monitor and assess contract performance;
  - Develop optimization strategies for better sourcing; and
  - Identify new standardization and contracting opportunities.

9.3.2 Technology Evolution and Developments

The nature of technology is that it will continue to evolve. This certainly applies with SCM. At the risk of being outdated as soon as it is published, we describe three main areas of technology development that are, and will continue to have, a profound impact on the practice of SCM in healthcare systems—machine learning (ML), the Internet of Things (IoT), and AI Chatbots.

ML Tools

The goal of ML tools is to attain humanlike AI. These cognitive architectures are platforms that can reason about problems across multiple domains, develop new insights, adapt to unknown situations, and reflect on their new reality.

Cognitive functions allow computers to perceive the world, analyze and understand the information gathered, and behave in an informed manner. When working in combination with business expertise, these IT solutions lead to a variety of valuable options, including ML, NLP to access and utilize unstructured data, and intelligent virtual assistants.

When cognitive computing is applied to procurement solutions, the result is cognitive procurement, a process in which computers use data mining, pattern recognition, and NLP to mimic human activity concerning procurement processes. This cuts down on a great deal of manual work that would otherwise be required, improving efficiency and cutting costs for the procurement team. This can allow supply managers to undertake other value-adding and strategic initiatives.

With the increasing role of information in today's business environment, managers need effective methods to uncover meaning from vast amounts of data. AI and ML offer a powerful set of methods that enable computers to find the hidden structure of data and obtain invaluable insights.

IoT

The IoT is a network of physical objects (things) embedded with sensors, software, and other technologies to connect and exchange data with other devices and systems over the Internet. These are often located in remote locations, transferring data to central (often cloud-based) databases for processing and analyzing. In SCM, IoT is used to connect various data points (devices used to monitor the supply chain) to provide information that will lead to higher operational efficiency and better awareness of product status. IoT provides managers with a coherent stream of real-time data regarding the location of the product and the transportation environment. Managers are alerted if the product is shipped in the wrong direction and will be able to monitor the delivery of ready goods and raw materials.

While IoT is a revolutionary technology in almost every major industry—retail, transportation, finance, healthcare, and energy—IoT shows its potential to the fullest in processes like supply chain management. Forecasting and oversight applications with input from remote devices help product managers improve the operational efficiency of distribution and add transparency to decision-making. Some examples of IoT applications in SCM include:

- Real-time location tracking;
- Storage condition monitoring;
- Forecasting the movement and the arrival of the product;
- Locating goods in the warehouse;
- Providing alerts when components need servicing or replacement; and
- Planning routes, considering traffic, weather, possible accidents, or other delay-inducing occurrences that happen on the way.

In healthcare, IoT offers considerable opportunity for creating tangible benefits. In a 2022 report, the National Institute of Standards and Technology (NIST) has identified that IoT has the potential to create a pervasive environment for monitoring patient health and safety, as well as improving how physicians deliver care.[18,19]

IoT technology is commonly used in healthcare today in energy meters, in-patient monitors, x-rays, and imaging devices. Patient monitoring for cardiac and diabetic care is common for linking patients to providers. During COVID-19, IoT devices were utilized extensively to monitor patients within their homes. As the hospital-at-home movement continues to expand, there will be an increasing need to monitor myriad medical devices at the point of service other than the hospital.[20, 21]

The proliferation of IoT brings new challenges to the healthcare manager. Products must now be sourced that are suitable for use in multiple settings and brought to these settings as required. An understanding of the home setting is quite different from the highly controlled hospital environment. With the proliferation of new medical devices and other IoT products introduced to the healthcare market at an all-time high, associated cybersecurity threats and other risks are a potential threat and need to be thoroughly assessed.

AI Chatbots

The promise of AI chatbots, such as ChatGPT, have created both anticipation and fear among healthcare professionals. Doctors have been impressed with the ability of the technology to perform tasks such as preparing patient charts and offering potential diagnoses based on patient clinical factors provided to the AI system. From a supply chain perspective, such tools could be used when planning or even at the point of patient care to help select the most appropriate products for such care. As advances are also made in the ability to predict future health needs, such as a patient's likelihood of acquiring a chronic condition or needing a total joint replacement, AI could also be used to support demand planning and forecasting. To realize this potential, more work needs to be done to ensure the accuracy and even authenticity of the data on which the chatbots make recommendations.[22]

9.4 Chapter Summary

This chapter has provided a broad overview of the use of IT as it applies to SCM to aid clinicians, administrators, and supply chain teams in performing their jobs. By automating the complex supply chain processes from sourcing to delivery, products are made available on a more reliable and timely basis. Further, automation helps manage expenses by efficiently processing and monitoring the transactions, and ideally creating more accurate (touchless) orders that do not require human intervention. IT also aids clinicians and administrators by making all documents available in digitized form, providing quick, searchable access at any location required.

The chapter also provided insights into how healthcare organizations are improving their performance through new, emerging technologies. Leading healthcare organizations are applying these technologies to advance their capabilities to better serve patients and to aid clinicians and administrators in providing quality care.

Notes

1. For example, Oracle's approach to block chain integration in ERP solutions. `https://www.oracle.com/in/blockchain/what-is-blockchain/blockchain-in-healthcare`

2. Rising, J., & Moscovitch, B. (2014). The Food and Drug Administration's unique device identification system: Better postmarket data on the safety and effectiveness of medical devices. *JAMA Internal Medicine, 174*(11), 1719–1720.

3. Department of Health and Human Services. (2013, Sept. 24). Unique device identification system. *Federal Register, 78*(185)). `https://www.govinfo.gov/content/pkg/FR-2013-09-24/pdf/2013-23059.pdf`

4. Tcheng, J. E., Nguyen, M. V., Brann, H. W., Clarke, P. A., Pfeiffer, M., Pleasants, J. R., Shelton, G. W., Kelly, J. F. (2021). The medical device unique device identifier as the single source of truth in healthcare enterprises-roadmap for implementation of the clinically integrated supply chain. *Medical Devices: Evidence and Research*, 459–467.

5. Overhage, J. M., & McCallie, D., Jr. (2020). Physician time spent using the electronic health record during outpatient encounters: A descriptive study. *Annals of Internal Medicine, 172*(3), 169–174. `https://www.acpjournals.org/doi/abs/10.7326/M18-3684`

6. Kush, R. D., Helton, E., Rockhold, F. W., & Hardison, C. D. (2008). Electronic health records, medical research, and the Tower of Babel. *The New England Journal of Medicine, 358*(16), 1738–1740. `https://dukespace.lib.duke.edu/dspace/bitstream/handle/10161/11023/NEJM%20EMR%20Standards.pdf;sequence=1`

7. HealthIT. (2021). National trends in hospital and physician adoption of electronic health records. HealthIT website. Retrieved December 11, 2022, from `https://www.healthit.gov/data/quickstats/national-trends-hospital-and-physician-adoption-electronic-health-records`

8. Agency for Healthcare Research and Quality. `https://digital.ahrq.gov/electronic-medical-record-systems#:~:text=%20Electronic%20Medical%20Record%20Systems%20%201%20Background.,the%20country%20that%20are%20implementing%20and...%20More%20`

9. Conway, K. (2014, Nov. 18). EHR Supply Chain Fusion. Healthcare Innovation. `https://www.hcinnovationgroup.com/policy-value-based-care/meaningful-use/article/13006989/ehr-supply-chain-fusion`

10. Trajkovski, O. (2021, Sept.) A supply chain management system completes the digital transformation in healthcare journey, Tecsys Blog. `https://www.tecsys.com/blog/2021/09/a-supply-chain-management-system-completes-the-digital-transformation-in-healthcare-journey`

11. Gartner. (2021). Market trends: The rapidly growing cloud opportunity in healthcare providers. Gartner website. `https://www.gartner.com/document/3999788?ref=sendres_email&refval=77843348`

12. IBM. website. `https://www.ibm.com/cloud/learn/benefits-of-cloud-computing`

13. GHX. (2022). GHX helps advance healthcare digital transformation by fueling cloud ERP adoption and ROI. GHX website. Retrieved December 11, 2022, from https://www.prnewswire.com/news-releases/ghx-helps-advance-healthcare-digital-transformation-by-fueling-cloud-erp-adoption-and-roi-301586358.html

14. Oracle NetSuite. (2022). What is cloud ERP and how does it work? NetSuite, Oracle NetSuite website. Retrieved December 11, 2022, https://www.netsuite.com/portal/resource/articles/erp/cloud-erp.shtml

15. Gartner. (2021). Gartner predicts the future of cloud and edge infrastructure. Gartner website. https://www.gartner.com/smarterwithgartner/gartner-predicts-the-future-of-cloud-and-edge-infrastructure

16. Sharma, R., Shishodia, A., Gunasekaran, A., Min, H., & Munim, Z. H. (2022). The role of artificial intelligence in supply chain management: Mapping the territory. *International Journal of Production Research*, *60*(24), 7527–7550. https://www.tandfonline.com/doi/full/10.1080/00207543.2022.2029611

17. Kumar, A., Mani, V., Jain, V., Gupta, H., & Venkatesh, V. G. (2023). Managing healthcare supply chain through artificial intelligence (AI): A study of critical success factors. *Computers & Industrial Engineering*, *175*, 108815. https://www.sciencedirect.com/science/article/pii/S0360835222008038?casa_token=XRli5EyOXLcAAAAA:GuZ-t6FPjcKQ4Ssd470r1sB-dEGyrGuO51nj_GieJ4-_Xbnagg4Utl1UdL7LWAxco65QA5A

18. National Institute of Standards and Technology (NIST). (2022). Internet-of-Things in healthcare (IOT-Health). https://www.nist.gov/programs-projects/internet-things-healthcare-iot-health

19. Fernandez, F., & Pallis, G. C. (2014). Opportunities and challenges of the Internet of Things for healthcare: Systems engineering perspective. In 2014 4th international conference on wireless mobile communication and healthcare-transforming healthcare through innovations in mobile and wireless technologies (MOBIHEALTH) (pp. 263–266). IEEE. chrome-extension://efaidnbmnnnibpcajpcglclefindmkaj/https://eudl.eu/pdf/10.4108/icst.mobihealth.2014.257276

20. Carroll, C. (2022, March 14). At-home monitoring creates virtual hospital for UCI Health, California Health Foundation Blog. https://www.chcf.org/blog/at-home-monitoring-creates-virtual-hospital-uci-health

21. Laplante, P. A., & Laplante, N. (2016). The internet of things in healthcare: Potential applications and challenges. *IT Professional*, *18*(3), 2–4. https://ieeexplore.ieee.org/abstract/document/7478533

22. Conway K. (2023, Feb. 23). Artificial intelligence and fake news: Imagining the potential for AI chatbots, Healthcare Purchasing News website. Retrieved February 25, 2023, from https://www.hpnonline.com/sourcing-logistics/article/21294816/artificial-intelligence-and-fake-news-imagining-the-potential-for-ai-chatbots

10 The Fully Integrated Supply Chain Organization (FISCO)—*Tying It Together and Looking Forward*

10.1 Introduction

Supply chain management (SCM) practitioners in the healthcare industry continually seek to deliver maximum value from their efforts. In doing so, they are extremely conscious of the requirement to meet clinical needs while also supporting administrative obligations. This becomes a classic cost and service optimization challenge. Consequently, in the healthcare industry, standards and policies are increasingly driving the supply chain to develop what is referred to as a clinically integrated supply chain strategy in the context of sustaining a financially responsible enterprise.

Just as clinicians are patient focused, SCM practitioners within provider systems must start with the patient and work backward as they develop solutions. This requires system processes that allow for data analytics and outcome analysis, down to the procedure, patient, physician, and supply and equipment utilization levels.

In support of this value acquisition effort, clinician involvement in SCM decision-making has expanded greatly in the past few years. Best practice supply chain processes and structures are now designed from the perspective of a clinically integrated supply chain that considers more than the acquisition price of products to include quality and patient outcome goals.

Throughout this book, we have proffered the Fully Integrated Supply Chain Organization (FISCO) concept to depict the characteristics of the most progressive supply chain organizations in the provider health sector. A full detailing of the FISCO concept is found in Appendix 1. FISCOs are generally characterized by a centralized sourcing and purchasing platform—including purchasing, a standardized value analysis process, integrated order and inventory management systems, and distribution processes. These FISCOs require system-managed materials personnel operating throughout all care settings, integrated quality management and standardization programs, and centralization of accounts payable and other financial systems managed by supply chain. The hallmark of a FISCO is the reduction of complexity[1] in an organization characterized by resource dependency.[2,3] While FISCOs may outsource some functions to commercial distributors and group purchasing organizations (GPOs), selection of such intermediaries and their management by the system is based on a collaborative approach to meeting provider-defined organizational goals.

The COVID-19 pandemic had an immense impact on the healthcare supply chain. Healthcare provider organizations, their intermediaries, suppliers, and the government proved to be unprepared for a disruption with the depth, breadth, and uncertainty in recovery patterns that characterized the pandemic. In the highly competitive U.S. healthcare delivery system, provider organizations scrambled to secure the supplies that were necessary to protect their patients, workers, and others operating in their facilities. Many were successful in managing through the disruption without significant patient impact, but it was not without herculean efforts.

In many ways, the historic and often over-arching drive toward greater efficiencies, including shifting manufacturing off-shore and reducing on-site inventories, had discounted the eventualities of a severe, long-lasting, and extensive disruption. As a result, the nature and degree of supply chain risk, especially risks associated with disruptions leading to the inability to access needed products, as discussed in Chapter 3, came to the forefront. How to manage to avert such risks, in both the short and long term, remains a topic of much discussion by provider organizations, intermediaries, and government.

In this final chapter, we elaborate on four overarching themes that have been mentioned throughout the book, often within the context of the lasting influence of the COVID-19 pandemic. We consider:

- The drive toward excellence in provider health sector supply chain design and performance within the context to reduce resource dependency;
- The need for integration between supply chain and clinical care;
- The achievement of value through driven investments in supplies and supply management; and
- Leadership and managerial challenges in a resource dependent and complex network.

Each of the overarching themes is reviewed in the following section.

10.2 Overarching Themes

10.2.1 The Drive toward Excellence

While purchasing and supply management departments continue to be under constant pressure to reduce costs,[4] the persistent drive for excellence in supply chain performance can be attributed to a more holistic view of cost effectiveness, quality, and outcomes.[5,6,7] Supply chain practice has sought to transform its traditional transactional role by demonstrating value through its contribution to both clinical and financial performance. Such transformation is facilitated by: (a) the decision by upper management to be world-class in purchasing and supply management; (b) an elevation of the supply function's visibility and strategic contribution to the organization's mission by its repositioning at the "C" level; and (c) recognition of the need for supply chain to be a critical part of the response to industry competition and disruption. Contributing to this transformation, and relevant to supply, are changes in how healthcare provider organizations are reimbursed, regulated, and evaluated. For example, under the Affordable Care Act (ACA) hospitals are:

- Financially penalized for having a relatively high number of hospital-acquired conditions, such as infections and falls. Supply chain is central in securing products that help control inflections and prevent falls, as well as other so-called never events.
- Financially penalized for 30-day unplanned patient readmissions. An effective value analysis program, as is described in Chapter 4, can contribute to the selection of devices that evidence has shown to contribute to better outcomes.[8]

- Increasingly accountable for total costs of care, including the role of product utilization in an episode of care, and in some cases, for the overall care of patients within a covered population over a specified period of time. Such accountability for managing costs, beyond the acquisition price of a product, provides a new rationale for healthcare system supply chain executives to identify critical items and reduce, if not eliminate, the use of products that fail to contribute to successful outcomes. Investments in technology, such as artificial intelligence (AI), as discussed in Chapter 9, can help guide decisions to meet the need to reduce costs while maintaining or improving quality.

All of these challenges are associated with the need for excellence in supply chain practice.

The critical role for excellence in SCM came to the forefront during the COVID-19 pandemic, specifically as to its centrality for assuring patient care and supporting preparedness and resilience. Supply chain disruptions and failures to prepare for such events led to heightened risk to patients, providers, and the general public.[9] Notably, requirements for resilience and preparedness were not previously built into the mission statements nor into sourcing and contracting processes in provider, intermediary, or supplier organizations. Markedly, government emergency backups, such as the Strategic National Stockpile (SNS), were insufficient and unprepared—especially around the provision of personal protective equipment (PPE) necessary for the protection of patients and clinicians in the event of a disruption of the magnitude of the pandemic.[10] Consequently, there was intense competition among healthcare providers, businesses, individuals, and governments to acquire such products, leading to escalation in costs (See Sidebar 10.1).[11,12]

Preparedness and resilience are now an expectation for excellence in supply chain practice across multiple industry sectors, including but not limited to healthcare. How is an expectation for preparedness and resilience best achieved? A 2008 CAPS Research study, pointing to the value of organizations considering supply chain as a center of excellence (COE), which is characterized by a pool of experts providing specific execution in support of multiple functions, is instructive. COEs are designed around the multiple supply chain functions discussed throughout this book—grounded in the proposition that no one individual and/or organization can be effective in managing all key supply chain functions—from supply market analysis through to sourcing, negotiation, implementation, and supplier management.

An insightful response by an organization outside of the health sector (as is described in Side Bar 10.2) suggests the development of two

Side Bar 10.1

Factors Contributing to PPE Shortage

First, a dysfunctional budgeting model in healthcare operations incentivizes hospitals to minimize costs rather than maintain adequate inventories of PPE.

Second, a major demand shock triggered by extensive healthcare system needs, aggravated by panicked marketplace behavior, quickly depleted PPE inventories.

Third, the federal government failure to effectively maintain and distribute domestic inventories of PPE.

Finally, global increases in demand and supply chain disruptions led to a sharp reduction in PPE exported to the United States, which was already highly dependent on offshore sources.

Market and government failures thus led PPE procurement by hospitals, healthcare providers, businesses, individuals, and governments to become competitive and costly in terms of time and money. . .because health is a public good, markets are not suitable mechanisms for rationing the resources necessary for health, and transformative changes are necessary to better protect healthcare practitioners.

Source: Cohen, J., & van der Meulen Rodgers, Y. (2020). Contributing factors to personal protective equipment shortages during the COVID-19 pandemic. *Preventive Medicine, 141*(106), 263.

COE components—a Supply Chain Management Strategies Group and a Supply Chain Management Infrastructure Group.[13] When it comes to assuring resilience and preparedness for uncertainties, we suggest a different skill set is necessary. Thus, we propose a third COE group, a Supply Chain Management Resilience and Preparedness Group, populated by individuals with multiple function skills related to preparation and management for disruptions.[14]

10.2.2 Integration between Supply Chain, Clinical Practice, and Suppliers

In Chapter 1, *integration* is defined as the degree to which an organization strategically brings together internal functions and external supply chain members to manage the intra- and inter-organizational processes. In healthcare, the integration between supply chain practice and clinical practice, which is elaborated on in Chapter 4, is the hallmark

Side Bar 10.2

Development of a SCM Strategies and Infrastructure Group

Responses by a CEO to a CAPS Research 2008 Study

"We have two groups of dedicated Supply Chain Management (SCM) experts who are focused on enabling the application of SCM concepts, techniques, and tools to meet strategic supply chain goals.

The SCM Strategies and SCM infrastructure groups focus on benchmarking best practices; process redesign, standardization, and automation; developing tool kits; and sharing business intelligence and knowledge."

The SCM strategies group is responsible for developing strategies, processes, technology, and enabling adoption of SCM best practices through internal consultants and strategic change management/communication processes and tools. The group also tracks and reports results.

The SCM infrastructure group is responsible for developing and overseeing compliance with Supplier Management policies and procedures and for designing and implementing professional development programs.

In addition, we used the COE concept to organize cross-functional commodity teams consisting of market analysts, cost-price analysts, item managers, buyers, contracting officers, and project managers. The teams develop Commodity Sourcing Strategy Plans for key categories that are aligned to internal business owner strategies. Individual sourcing events are executed according to the commodity strategies. These teams also commit resources to support cross-functional teams that are responsible for implementing broader strategic initiatives consistent with our Supply Management Three-Year Strategic Plan.

The SCM Preparedness and Resilience Group is responsible for meeting supply chain needs across a variety of disruptions of variable levels of uncertainty. The group continually updates the business continuity plan, working in conjunction with the government, suppliers, and intermediaries.

Source: Adapted from: CAPS Research: Extent of and Experiences with Centers of Excellence (COEs). (2008, Apr. 3). And CAPS Research, Extent of and Experiences with Centers of Excellence (COEs). (2019, Nov.). file:///C:/Users/cinnabar/Downloads/2019-12-04_centers-of-excellence-in-supply-management%20(1).pdf.

Side Bar 10.3

Clinical Integration in the Healthcare Supply Chain

"Clinical Integration in health care supply chain is an interdisciplinary partnership to deliver patient care with the highest value (high quality, best outcomes, and minimal waste at the lowest cost of care) that is achieved through assimilation and coordination of clinical and supply chain knowledge, data and leadership toward care across the continuum that is safe, timely, evidenced-based, efficient, equitable, and patient-focused."

Source: AHRMM. 2018 AHRMM Cost, Quality, and Outcomes (CQO). Also reported in: Taylor, B and Chung, C. Clinical Supply Chain Integration in a Data-Driven Health Care Environment, AHRMM Clinical Integration Taskforce. HiMSS19 Global Conference & Exhibition Presentation. Orlando, 2, 2019. Slide 21. https://365.himss.org/sites/himss365/files/365/handouts/552786184/handout-222.pdf

The purpose of integrating supply chain and clinical processes is to support safe, cost-effective care with the best outcomes possible. With the support of a clinically integrated supply chain, health systems can drive toward this goal—empowering various stakeholder teams and departments within a health system to work together to improve costs and care quality without compromise.

Source: Cardinal Healthcare. Optimizing supply chain in the wake of the pandemic. https://ww3.cardinalhealth.com/l/104412/2021-07-06/5df9bk

of a high-performing supply chain organization. There are new demands along with new opportunities.

Beyond a focus on strategies and infrastructure, achieving clinical integration requires:

- Strong clinician champions, evidence-based decision-making, outcomes review, and standardization;
- Process reviews and change management to reduce unnecessary variation; and
- Value analysis and sourcing processes to reduce variation, and alignment among clinical, financial, and operations.

From a supply chain perspective, clinical integration is characterized by its emphasis on clinical outcomes as achieved by moving toward a formulary or standardization of supply; improving supply chain processes; managing product stockouts, recalls, and expiration; and employing standardized data to track and trace products, and continually assess product contribution to outcomes.[15]

Integration is also associated with meeting industry best practices across various functions needed to achieve its goals. The functions assessed within maturity models, such as the FISCO (see Chapter 7), support an assessment of how well a healthcare system is moving toward excellence within and across functions (Exhibit 1.4) and embedded in FISCO characteristics (Side Bar 10.4).

Too often, integration focuses only on internal functions. An important FISCO function, requiring greater attention, is supplier relationship management (SRM). The hallmark of a FISCO is its ability to achieve standardization for both cost reduction and risk management, and through a more proactive approach across procurement and distribution functions to assure efficiency, effectiveness, and resilience.

In a highly resource dependent environment, such as the hospital, complexity reduction cannot occur without suppliers and providers working together to achieve organizational goals. Integration within the context of a FISCO is not merely an internal concept; it is reliant on the effective management of externalities—especially given the dynamic environment previously discussed. Indeed, SRM issues became clearer during COVID-19 as major suppliers experienced challenges in securing and allocating products to meet both demand and need.

Side Bar 10.4

FISCO Characteristics

- A FISCO is characterized by a robust effort to gain control over related organizational processes and to meet critical operational and strategic goals. It achieves effective and efficient flows of products, services, information, money, and decisions with the objective of providing maximum value to the customer.
- A FISCO evolves from decisions enabling control and alignment of internal, external, and outsourced functions. The hallmark of a FISCO is the reduction of complexity.
- FISCOs are judged by the extent to which they make significant contributions to the success of the enterprise. Current trends in healthcare are to integrate clinical requirements, patient outcomes, and supply chain performance.

10.2.3 Achieving Value for Investments

Purchasing to support the provision of healthcare is the process through which healthcare providers select and contract for supplies, while managing relationships with vendors.[16] An important impetus for value-based purchasing is the aim to move away from maximizing the volume of care provided to instead focusing on optimizing the value delivered to the patient. This idea is inherent in the value equation that is presented in Chapter 1 (Exhibit 1.1) and reproduced in Exhibit 10.1. Recognized is the need to align incentives between those who provide care and those who are paying for care—including government and commercial payors, employers, and patients themselves. The bundling of products and services, performance-based payments, shared risk and savings arrangements, and capitated payments have all contributed to the move toward value-based procurement.[17]

$$Value = \frac{Quality + Outcomes + Patient\ Experience}{All\ Resources\ Consumed\ in\ Care\ Delivery}$$

Exhibit 10.1: Healthcare value equation.

The value equation in Exhibit 10.1 brings conceptual clarity to the notion of value in a patient-and/or services-focused environment. On face value, the components of value appear straightforward, when in reality, value is an enormously complex concept. The supply chain manager may have a level of comfort exercising judgment in the purchase of linen. However, the purchase of more sophisticated medical devices requires close attention to clinician sensitivities, technological advancements, clinical data, and technical/service requirements.

The evidence regarding the ability to reduce procedural costs as a result of value-based purchasing for different episodes of care is uneven. However, for supply-intensive procedures, where the cost of an implant and other resources consumed can be as high as 40% of the total procedure,[18] savings are considerable with evidence of equivalent if not improved quality and outcomes.[19] A 2018 multi-country survey carried out by the consulting company Deloitte revealed that healthcare procurement for value across the globe is growing in maturity, and there is an emphasis toward buying services and solutions to support such initiatives.[20] Purchasing professionals should consider the bearing of their work on the quality and cost of patient care through attention to: (a) cost reduction, (b) risk reduction, (c) improved solution offerings from suppliers, and (d) meeting stricter quality and safety requirements from regulators.

Notably, new technologies, such as point of service diagnostic testing devices, have the potential to significantly affect the nature and flow of supplies away from laboratories to the point of care. Value accrues from this kind of change by reducing the time and number of visits required before the patient can be appropriately treated. Different supplies derive a different value for the hospital. As such technologies are considered for procurement, supply chain managers must recognize the impact of the technology, on both services and on the materials requirements for the organization.

Notably, much of our discussion has focused on the purchase of products and the value of products as assets to be employed for achieving the goals of the organization, while there is growing interest in the purchasing of services.[21] A contracted facility maintenance service, such as housekeeping, differs from temporary nursing services where there must be great vigilance in the selection of individuals who have the proper credentials and expertise to support the expected levels of clinical outcomes. The risk of poor housekeeping may be limited to low customer satisfaction, but can also increase the chance for infections. Correcting such risk for services, which are among the major costs to a hospital, requires relatively minimal efforts. The risk of poor nursing can be disastrous to the well-being of a patient.

10.3 Leadership and Organizational Challenges in a Complex Network

Supply chain leadership and management, given the complexity of the healthcare system, requires agility in moving between the different frames we introduced in Chapter 8. This is a part of the transformation of the supply chain to enhance clinical performance, which is a never-ending aspiration and a challenge. As the cliché states—it is a journey, not a destination!

Achieving the maturity of a FISCO requires acting within multiple frames, sometimes sequentially, but frequently in concert—with an overarching view of orchestration, and in the end, transformation of the organization by virtue of its integrated efforts. Those who employ such frames in managing the supply chain must be simultaneously coordinators, advisors, information brokers, relationship brokers, and knowledge and information managers. They must manage the organization's risks; collaborate with clinicians, suppliers, and intermediaries such as GPOs; and continually adjust the organization's supply design as new challenges arise.[22]

Many managers find it difficult to use frame analysis to change their view and actions for a set of issues that have long been defined as transactional. The health sector supply chain has been "viewed largely in buyer- and/or supplier-centric terms, with a transactional focus on distribution, logistics, and purchasing products into the user base."[23] The inadequacy of such a definition rests in the fact that, while everyone knows that healthcare providers cannot work without materials, the transaction frame does not easily let managers transcend questions regarding the price and quality of goods. However, if one begins to see the health sector supply chain as a "customer- and/or provider-centric model,"[24] it becomes possible to the view the supply chain as foundational to clinical services.

A more customer- and/or provider-centric view of SCM in hospitals and healthcare systems demands "a holistic approach to managing operations within collaborative inter-organizational networks allowing the formation and implementation of rational strategies for creating, stimulating, capturing and satisfying end customer demand through innovation of products, services, supply network structures and infrastructures in a global, dynamic environment."[25] As suggested in Chapter 1, required is a view of the supply chain within a set of inter- and intra-organizational networks, focusing on internal supply management (ISM), customer relationship management (CRM), SRM, and purchasing partner management (PPM). Critical for transformation is the ability of suppliers and purchasing partners to understand and meet the healthcare system's goals and expectations toward the creation of value in the broadest sense of the term. With such an understanding, it also becomes much easier to see supplies as assets for clinicians, the organization as a whole, and of course, patients.

In recognition of the potential for the supply chain to contribute to the organization's success, a few positive trends indicate the environment for SCM is changing. As previously mentioned, there has been an elevation of the supply chain leader to an executive-labeled role (e.g., vice president, chief supply chain officer). This alone is a shift in the recognition of strategic value of the supply chain. Yet, repositioning does not necessarily signal a full appreciation of the role. Assuming a more strategic role goes beyond being able to reduce the price of acquired goods and services to include: (a) total cost savings; (b) contribution to mission; (c) demonstration of the tie between business financials, and perhaps of greatest consequence; and (d) achievement of organizational objectives.[26]

10.3.1 No One Best Way to Manage an Organization

Executive search firms, charged by healthcare systems to recruit innovative leaders, including senior supply chain executives, report a

---

Side Bar 10.5

Talent Demands for the Next Generation of Leaders

Talent demands for the next generation of leaders must include:

- Deep domain knowledge and understanding of the space;
- Ability to think laterally;
- A "strong strategic sense of the inter-relationships of manufac-
  turers, distributors, providers, insurers, and patients";
- Ability to predict and drive the future;
- Ability to "see what can be";
- Understanding and utilization of data;
- Understanding that the MD component of leadership will grow;
- Skills for customer engagement;
- Understanding innovation for products/technologies;
- Ability/Courage to take risk;
- Toleration of failure; and
- Ability to entertain the disruptive.

Source: Herzlinger, R., & Schneller, E. Presentation at HMPI Meeting, University of Alabama, May 2015.

---

scarcity in talent with the ability to meet the challenges for managing in the quickly changing and diverse healthcare delivery environment (Sidebar 10.5). Scrutiny of these challenges will lead readers to question the ability to put together a portfolio of managerial skills to meet the requirements for success. However, it has been long recognized, by contingency theorists, that there are no universal prescriptions for management.[27] Contingency theory posits that the correct management principle or technique to be applied should be related to the existing set of circumstances or situation. The idea of strategic fit, as discussed in Chapter 8, recognizes the importance of aligning strategy, structure, and culture. The theory envisions good management as the ability to perceive the significant or limiting factors in a situation. This is especially important for managing in the complex healthcare environment we have described throughout this book. Thus, successful managers, recognizing the characteristics of circumstance, apply the multiple management frames[28] and develop consequential strategies for obtaining value from the supply chain. Therefore, a supply chain manager interested in understanding more fully how to satisfy physician demands might employ the service frame in seeking a solution. In contrast, when interested in working with physicians on standardization to improve outcomes and safety, as well as to reduce costs, the transformational frame might be a more powerful perspective. The need for orchestration,[29] as a management frame and as one sensitive to human resources and transformation, is evident in the efforts undertaken to work closely with physicians in standardization—as illustrated in the work to achieve product standardization in cardiology in the Plymouth Trust (Appendix 2).

Not only do organizations and people value different products in different ways, hospitals and systems have developed diverse strategies in solving their supply chain challenges. Some have decided to manage the entire process internally. Others outsource as many functions as possible. Many systems, as is discussed in Chapter 3, closely involve physicians and other clinicians in their purchasing deliberations, while others keep clinical staff at an arm's length. Among organizations that are considered progressive (effectively managing sourcing, information, and relationships), numerous combinations are observed.

Differences in supply chain organization design, in consideration of the strategic fit required to achieve alignment with the vision and values of a hospital or hospital system and its culture, is elaborated on in Chapter 8. Decisions must be made in consideration of the optimal course of action for a given organization or situation. Important decisions, such as centralization and decentralization, must consider a wide range of institutional and environmental factors. Designers and orchestrators of the supply chain must show agility and flexibility in their analysis.

An academic health center, in pursuit of its central mission to expose clinician learners to options, may demand a wider range of equivalent products than its non-academic counterparts. Consequently, outsourcing distribution "as a service" may be compatible with an academic health center's education and teaching goals—preferring to manage a relationship with a distributor versus taking on the responsibilities itself. Such a decision reflects on knowing one's culture and areas of expertise. The desire to not internally develop a specific supply chain competency reflects a deep understanding of strategic fit.

10.3.2 Future Leadership and Organization Design Considerations

Effective and efficient SCM represents an opportunity to add value and decrease costs in the U.S. healthcare system. To accomplish this end, it is necessary for top-level executives and supply chain managers to reframe their approach to the supply chain. In a market-based/commercial healthcare system, each hospital or healthcare system must determine what value can be achieved through the supply chain. This will vary, depending on the product, organization, and environment. As a result, few universalistic solutions, as suggested in the earlier discussion of contingency theory, can be provided.

Over two decades ago, Smeltzer and Ramanathan[30] questioned the extent to which the healthcare sector can learn from other industries. Their work suggested seven key areas for comparison between hospital and other industry supply chains, including differences associated with: (a) customer; (b) task, complexity, specialization, and professionalism; (c) organizational structure; (d) organization-employee relationship; (e) product; (f) markets; and (g) information management. Learned during the period of COVID-19 is that the health sector shares many vulnerabilities with other sectors. Reflecting on the disruptions and innovations that occurred during the COVID-19 pandemic, we believe that cross-sector learning is a key to the healthcare supply chain achieving excellence in every-day performance and longer-term resilience. Across sectors, organizations and their leaders are bringing their services and products closer to the customer. Business-to-customer (B2C) efforts take products and services to customers, on customer terms, leading to challenges for traditional "brick-and-mortar" venues. With the objective to maximize the overall value of the product or service, while reducing costs and delighting end users, supply chains are dynamic systems[31] that must be designed to fit the product or service involved.[32] Sidebar 10.6 discusses the concept of providing acute-level care in the home, which involves the movement of activities once performed only in the hospital "as the factory" to where the customer is. To ensure that the supply chain design fits the product, the processes integral to the industry must be considered. "The key is to choose the right advantage that the supply chain can provide, again and again."[33] As the care venue evolves, supply chain managers need to adapt and incorporate supply chain elements that have proven successful in other industries.[34]

Reflected in our discussion of clockspeed in Chapter 1 is a need for supply chain managers to consider rates of change for products and processes. Rapid innovation, or what can be described as rapid clockspeed, in cardiology and spine implants and medical imaging requires an agile supply chain and ability by supply chain managers to work closely with clinicians. Such attention is less critical in mental health services, where change is at a much slower pace. Indeed, the health sector is composed of a robust mix of supply chain demands. In areas where change is rapid, supply chain managers must be agile, assessing new products and venues of care and assuring that their past commitments (e.g., for sourcing, outsourcing, use of intermediaries, and

Side Bar 10.6

Bringing Care to the Patient—Acute-level Care at Home

Organizations in many sectors have long recognized the importance of bringing their services closer to the customer. Another major impact of the COVID-19 pandemic was the rapid conversion of care from within the hospital or doctor's office to the patient's home, ranging from a virtual televisit to the delivery of acute-level care in the home, the latter made possible in part by advances in remote patient monitoring.

The "hospital at home"—an acute-care model of particular value for older patients who run the risks of mental and physical decline resulting from long hospital stays—has been shown to reduce costs compared to in-hospital care, while increasing patient satisfaction and reducing readmissions. Use of the model grew exponentially during the pandemic, as the Centers for Medicare and Medicaid Services (CMS) extended waivers to allow reimbursement for more than 250 hospitals in 37 states. The Veterans Health Administration has operated a hospital-at-home program for more than a decade.

First conceived and implemented by Johns Hopkins School of Medicine in 1995, the program is highly dependent on the ability of the supply chain to orchestrate the scheduling and delivery of both trained personnel and necessary supplies and equipment to patients' homes. More recently, technology platforms have been developed that allow physicians and remote care teams to coordinate the care delivered by personnel on site.

Sources: Healthcare Purchasing News website. (2022, June 24). Conway, K. Supply chain delivers hospital-level care at home. Retrieved December 3, 2002, from https://www.hpnonline.com/sourcing-logistics/article/21271718/supply-chain-delivers-hospitallevel-care-at-home.

contracting) are appropriate to the respective pace of change within the industry.

Exhibit 10.2 provides insights into the complex terrain of SCM transformation over three-plus decades. This is a seismic shift—offering to future managers in the health sector supply chain a set of unprecedented challenges.

Exhibit 10.2: Supply chain management transformation over three-plus decades.

	1999 MATERIALS MANAGEMENT	2009 SUPPLY CHAIN 1.0	2023 SUPPLY CHAIN 2.0
Management focus	Product-focused	Process-focused	Clinical-focused
Governance	Finance	Operations	Clinical
Organization design	Decentralized	Centralized	Partnerships
Decision factors	Price	Total cost	Value chain
Decision-making sources	Silo-based	Information-based	Evidence-based
Processes	Inefficient processes	Efficient processes	Automated processes
Performance metrics	Operational expense	Outcome & revenue- focus	Cost, quality, outcomes, & readiness
Lead role	Material manager	Supply chain manager	Value chain manager
Information flows	Multiple touches	No touch, paperless	Integrated & cloud- based

10.3.3 Leading for Resilience

The COVID-19 pandemic exposed a wide range of vulnerabilities in supply chains across many sectors of the economy—but especially for healthcare provision. The critical nature of supply chain to support patient care and the well-being of those providing care and the public at large became part of everyday conversation. As mentioned above, to our knowledge, no hospitals or systems had "preparedness" as part of their mission statement, and disaster recovery plans, which should have been an essential part of their business continuity plans, were not designed to meet the challenges of such uncertainty. Many provider organizations believed that the manufacturers with which they contracted, the GPO supplier selection processes and distributor contracts were considering of such disruptions. Critical lessons learned have sparked more collaborative work between the public and private health sectors on resilience.[35]

In the wake of the COVID-19 pandemic, both the public and private sector organizations proffered strategies to recover and assure resilience for future disruptions—especially those with the uncertainties associated with a long-lasting event. At the national level, Presidential Directives were put forth to strengthen the domestic supply chain, including bringing manufacturing near or on-shore within the United States, establishing predictive models and information systems to increase visibility regarding the availability of critical supplies, expanding capacity through advanced manufacturing, and better procurement and inventory management of critical supplies.[36] Going forward, if we are to meet the challenges of likely future disruptions, it is important to build collaborative resources at both regional and community levels to account for the fragmentation in the healthcare system.[37]

To buffer their members from disruption, professional trade associations also assessed the supply chain environment.[38] Distributors,[39] GPOs,[40] and manufacturers of medical supplies[41] continue to be attentive to disruption-related risks. Importantly, collaborative efforts, frequently among competing supply chain participants, continue to evolve.[42]

Reliance on upstream entities carries its own risks. Thus, it is important for supply chain professionals to recognize the continued risks associated with pandemics and other kinds of disasters that pose challenges to the delivery of health and medical services.[43] They must assess their partners' adherence to plans to strengthen resilience, anticipate disruptions, and have plans in place to support their own organizations in times of disruption. In this regard, consideration should be given not just to the inevitability of another pandemic, but for all hazards. In short, the design of an operational, resilient, and prepared health sector supply chain is critical to both the short- and long-term well-being of provider organizations, their customers, and the communities they serve.

The widespread shortages of intravenous (IV) bags after Hurricane Maria provided a valuable lesson to healthcare supply chain professionals, creating awareness of the risks associated with natural or other disasters that can disrupt production of supplies centralized in a single location[44] (Sidebar 10.7).

Ensuring an operationally efficient and cost-conscious supply chain that also strengthens resilience and preparedness is not easy. Careful rethinking of supply chain operational decisions from this vantage point is especially important.

An unintended consequence of the COVID-19 pandemic has been stimulating supply chain academics, consultants, and managers to challenge their core beliefs and assumptions as to how strategies work—or fail to work. A good example, with origins in the 1970s, is the concept and practice of just-in-time (JIT) inventory, which gained traction as organizations began to view full warehouses and excess inventories as a disadvantage. During COVID-19, as manufacturers were cut off from their global suppliers,[45] distributors found that their sources could not deliver needed products in time. Many have since suggested that JIT inventory

Side Bar 10.7

Not All Hazards Are from Pandemics

When Hurricane Maria devastated Puerto Rico in late September 2018, hospitals across the mainland United States were already facing intermittent shortages of intravenous fluids. When the Category 4 hurricane severely damaged several manufacturing plants owned by Baxter International, one of the major manufacturers of the small IV bags used to deliver such fluids, it set in motion a major national shortage.

Nearly six months later, the scarcity of IV bags in the United States had reached crisis levels, illustrating what damage to a supply chain concentrated in a single location can do to one of the world's most advanced healthcare systems. This development underscores an inescapable reality: a strong sector may have great doctors, nurses, and hospitals, but if one link in the supply chain breaks, people suffer.

IV bags (simple plastic bags that are used to mix and deliver a liquid medication or salt water to patients through an intravenous line) are involved in nearly every facet of patient care in a hospital. Healthcare professionals use IV bags to administer drugs and to hydrate people who have difficulty swallowing liquids. They are one of the most basic medical items in a hospital; many people stay in hospitals because they are unable to self-administer medicine, and IV bags are often the easiest and safest way for those patients to ingest their drugs.

There have been intermittent IV bag and fluid shortages across the country since 2014, and the hurricane amplified the problem. Dr. O'Neil Britton, chief medical officer at Massachusetts General Hospital (MGH) in Boston, one of the country's top hospitals, told *The American Prospect* that while he'd seen other medical device or drug shortages, "they've never been this persistent or widespread, and it's never affected the entire industry on this scale."

Source: Ecker, Jordan. (2018, Feb. 20). How neglect of Puerto Rico sparked a national IV bag shortage: Hurricane Maria inflicted severe damage on Puerto Rican manufacturing plants that make the plastic bags that medical facilities need to administer drugs. *The American Prospect.* https://prospect.org/environment/neglect-puerto-rico-sparked-national-iv-bag-shortage.

(inventory arriving or being produced immediately before shipment or arriving near the next process for which it is needed) should be abandoned given that health systems have little redundancy or surge capacity for responding to pandemics or other widespread, long-lasting emergencies.

Others have suggested alternative approaches, such as having peer and even competing organizations share resources to act as regional buffers, not just stockpiles of inventory.[46] Use of distributed ledger technologies, such as blockchain (which is described in Chapter 9), and subscriptions to risk monitoring services organizations for more proactive alerts about potential and impending disruptions can support such buffering and inventory decisions.[47]

Going forward, those responsible for the continued success of their organizations should consider:

- Including in their system mission and vision statement (Chapter 2) an assertion regarding the importance of resilience and preparedness as critical to health organizations sustaining their core roles in patient care.
- Elevating the role of supply chain risk management to include consideration of manufacturers and intermediaries' attention to disruptions as part of their strategic sourcing and contracting activities.
- Increasing, where appropriate, standardization of product characteristics and proactive determination of equivalences to assure agility in meeting needs for patient care in times of disruption.
- Entering into collaborative relationships, including with competitors, to assure the viability of the healthcare ecosystem.
- Including discussions of resilience when engaging clinicians in the value analysis process. The result is an increased opportunity for supply chain leaders to collaborate and orchestrate change with clinicians.
- Participating in healthcare resilience collaboratives with a focus on the full ecosystem of provider organizations that serve the same communities.[48]

Innovation in the health sector is challenging.[49,50] COVID-19 accelerated the rate of innovation in many ways that continue to impact supply chain—challenging systems to take greater responsibility for their own supply chains.[51] For example, some healthcare systems have begun deploying 3D printing, a technology employed to produce needed products at the point of care.[52,53,54] Another example of providers taking responsibility for their own supply chains is the proliferation of consolidated service centers (CSCs). Those with CSCs in place before the pandemic have noted that their existence helped them better respond to critical shortages—providing another example of a strategic and supply chain design decision but not necessarily one that will be a good fit for all organizations.

Pre-pandemic, many supply chain departments, were seen as "merely" practical and operational organizations and cost centers securing products and assuring that care was not delayed. Associated with enhanced expectations for their role is the need to assess performance and develop plans for evolving into high-performing entities. Gartner, the supply chain consulting company, annually rates healthcare supply chain departments by their level of maturity.[55] The FISCO model, which has origins in the Gartner methodology for assessing healthcare system maturity, provides a framework for assessing maturity. The importance of performance and system maturation (covered in Chapter 7) provides further insight into the value of benchmarking the relative performance of one's own supply chain functions compared to peers and provides direction for moving forward.

Throughout this book, we have emphasized the diversity in healthcare systems with attention to their size, mix of services, geographic spread, and mission. No one design appears to be dominant. Supply chain managers are now tasked with orchestrating the complex factors that go into their supply chain efforts. Without a thoughtful and purposeful design, accomplishing one's mission and enacting a strategy is not possible.

The maturation and proliferation of information technologies has changed the world of supply chain practice in healthcare systems. Free from the manual tasks required a decade ago to process a purchasing order and receive and pay for supplies, supply chain managers can focus on monitoring and fine-tuning supply chain processes. And the value of data, as analytics are employed, provides an opportunity for further developing a clinically integrated supply chain.

10.4 Summary

The four overarching themes throughout this book: (a) excellence in supply chain design; (b) the need for integration between supply chain and clinical care; (c) the achievement of value through investments in and through supplies and supply management; and (d) leadership and managerial challenges in a resource dependent and complex network requires careful attention to resilience and preparedness. Purchasing for care refers to the process through which healthcare providers select, contract, and manage relationships with suppliers of clinical and non-clinical inputs.[56] Significant is recognition that supply chain disruptions could not "merely" lead to a postponement of care; such disruptions could create risks over the long term, even threatening the viability of individual integrated delivery networks and healthcare systems. Value-based purchasing, from the perspective of the health sector, "holds healthcare providers accountable for both the cost and quality of care they provide. It attempts to reduce inappropriate care and to identify and reward the best-performing providers."[57] Armed with an understanding of myriad stakeholders, strategic alternatives, design options, and the value of technology, supply chain managers will be prepared to guide their organizations' journey to become a FISCO, bringing value to provider organizations, and ultimately, their patients.

Notes

1. Begun, J. W., Zimmerman, B., & Dooley, K. (2003). Health care organizations as complex adaptive systems. *Advances in health care organization theory*, *253*, 288.
2. Ramos, G., & Schneller, E. S. (2022). Smoothing it out: Military health care supply chain in transition. *Hospital Topics*, *100*(3), 132–139.
3. Montgomery, K., & Schneller, E. S. (2007). Hospitals' strategies for orchestrating selection of physician preference items. *The Milbank Quarterly*, *85*(2), 307–335.
4. CAPS. Research. (2006, Oct.). Critical Issues Report: Hot Topics in Today's Supply Chain Management.
5. AHRMM. (2013, Dec. 19). AHRMM Supports Healthcare Industry in Addressing Costs, Quality, and Outcomes through Release of New Guidance Document. https://www.ahrmm.org/resource-repository-ahrmm/pr-ahrmm-cqo-metrics-guidance-document-121913-1
6. Institute for Health Improvement, Overview: What is the triple aim. https://www.ihi.org/Topics/TripleAim/Pages/Overview.aspxhttps://www.ihi.org/Topics/TripleAim/Pages/Overview.aspx
7. AHRMM. CQO & the triple aim: Supply chain's strategic connection report. https://www.ahrmm.org/resource-repository-ahrmm/cqo-the-triple-aim-supply-chains-strategic-connection-report-1
8. Rau, J. (2022, Oct. 31). Look up your hospital: Is it being penalized by Medicare? *Kaiser Health News*. https://khn.org/news/hospital-penalties/
9. Cohen, J., & van der Meulen Rodgers, Y. (2020). Contributing factors to personal protective equipment shortages during the COVID-19 pandemic. *Preventive Medicine*, *141*, 106263.
10. Handfield, R., Finkenstadt, D. J., Schneller, E. S., Godfrey, A. B., & Guinto, P. (2020). A commons for a supply chain in the post-COVID-19 era: The case for a reformed strategic national stockpile. *The Milbank Quarterly*, *98*(4), 1058–1090.
11. Ibid., 141.
12. Cohen, op. cit.
13. CAPS Research: Extent of and Experiences with Centers of Excellence (COEs). (2008, April 3). And CAPS Research, Extent of and Experiences with Centers of Excellence (COEs). https://capsresearch.org/blog/posts/2020-caps-blog-posts/march/caps-stats-centers-of-excellence/
14. Handfield et al., op. cit.

15. Industrial Automation Asia. (2022, Sept.). The Clinically Integrated Supply Chain, Industrial Automation. https://www.iaasiaonline.com/the-clinically-integrated-supply-chain-2

16. VanLare, J. M., & Conway, P. H. (2012). Value-based purchasing—National programs to move from volume to value. *New England Journal of Medicine*, *367*(4), 292–295.

17. Bethke, M, Giest, D, Lowry, A, Bailey, R., Fleisher, D, & Weger, J. (2020, Dec.). Value based health care models in a shifting economy., What is value based care? Deloitte. https://www2.deloitte.com/content/dam/Deloitte/be/Documents/strategy/Value%20based%20procurement%20-%20Deloite%20Belgium.pdf

18. Lee (2014). Bundled payments. Give surgeons a powerful new incentive to reduce costs. *Modern Healthcare*, *44*(9), 15–0015.

19. Fink, J. (2015). Mandatory bundled payment getting into formation for value-based care. Healthcare Financial Management, 69(10), 54–63. http://login.ezproxy1.lib.asu.edu/login?url=https://www-proquest-com.ezproxy1.lib.asu.edu/trade-journals/mandatory-bundled-payment-getting-into-formation/docview/1726463495/se-2

20. Bulens, J., Segers, K, Reynthens, N, & Desmet, B. (2018). How to eat the value-based procurement elephant? A Deloitte point of view. https://www2.deloitte.com/content/dam/Deloitte/be/Documents/strategy/Value%20based%20procurement%20-%20Deloite%20Belgium.pdf

21. Ellram, L. M., Tate, W. L., & Billington, C. (2004). Understanding and managing the services supply chain. *Journal of Supply Chain Management*, *40*(3), 17–32.

22. Schneller, E., & Harland, C. (2013). Systems of exchange: Cooperative purchasing in the. *The SAGE Handbook of Strategic Supply Management*, 214.

23. Saunders, C., quoted in Werner, C. (2004, July). The supply chain beast: Hospitals slowly coming to grips with importance of supply chain strategies that work. *First Moves*.

24. Saunders, op. cit.

25. Harland, Lamming, Richard, & Cousins, op. cit.

26. Zwemke, G. (2019, Aug.). Prove your value with key metrics. CAPS Research. https://www.capsresearch.org/library?tag=&phrase=proof%20of%20impact&conjunct=and&type=&status=&start=1/1/1988&end=10/24/2022&searchlimit=25&sort=2

27. Luthans, F., & Stewart, T. I. (1977). A general contingency theory of management. *Academy of Management Review*, *2*(2), 181–195.

28. Bolman, L. G., & Deal, T. E. (1977). *Reframing Organizations: Artistry, Choice, and Leadership*. Jossey-Bass.

29. Wallace, M., Fertig, M., & Schneller, E. (ed.) (2009). *Managing change in the public services*. John Wiley & Sons.

30. Smeltzer, L., & Ramanathan, V., 2002. Supply chain processes that lead to a competitive advantage for a manufacturer compared to a health care provider. Decision Sciences Institute, 2002 Annual Meeting Proceedings.

31. Simchi-Levi, D., Kaminsky, P., & Simchi-Levi, E. (2000). *Designing and Managing the Supply Chain: Concepts, Strategies, and Case Studies.* Irwin/McGraw-Hill.
32. Lee, H. L. The Triple-A Supply Chain. Harvard Case 8096, 2004.
33. Fine, C. (1998). *Clockspeed.* HarperCollins Publishers.
34. Miller, D., & Whitney, J. O. (1999). Beyond strategy: Configuration as a pillar of competitive advantage. *Business Horizons, 42*(3), 5–19.
35. Healthcare and public health sector. Public Health Emergency website. Retrieved December 3, 2022, from https://www.phe.gov/Preparedness/planning/cip/HPH/Pages/default.aspx
36. Biden, Joseph. (2021, Feb. 24). Executive Order on America's Supply Chains.
37. Bohnett, E., Vacca, R., Hu, Y., Hulse, D., & Varda, D. (2022). Resilience and fragmentation in healthcare coalitions: The link between resource contributions and centrality in health-related interorganizational networks. *Social Networks, 71*, 87–95.
38. Association for Healthcare Resources and Materials Management. AHRMM Recommended Initiatives for the Healthcare Supply Chain. https://www.ahrmm.org/ahrmm-recommended-initiatives-health-care-supply-chain
39. Health industry Distributors Association. (2021, Oct. 20). The U.S. must adopt a policy to diversify manufacturing and sourcing of critical medical supplies. *Repertoire Magazine.* http://repertoiremag.com/the-u-s-must-adopt-a-policy-to-diversify-manufacturing-and-sourcing-of-critical-medical-supplies.html https://supplychainassociation.org/covid-19
40. Healthcare Supply Chain Association (HSCA), Covid–19 Recommendations: Principles and Recommendations to Further Strengthen Supply Chain Resiliency and Support Effective Response to Public Health Crises.
41. Advanced Medical Technology Association. (2022, June 6). New AdvaMed, Deloitte Semiconductor Chip Study looks at impact of shortages on medtech. https://www.advamed.org/industry-updates/news/new-advamed-deloitte-semiconductor-chip-study-looks-at-impact-of-shortages-on-medtech
42. Healthcare Industry Resilience Collaborative. https://hircstrong.com
43. Penta, S., Kendra, J., Marlowe, V., & Gill, K. (2021 Sep). A disaster by any other name?: COVID-19 and support for an all-hazards approach. Risk hazards crisis. *Public Policy, 12*(3), 240–265. http://dx.doi.org/10.1002/rhc3.12213. Epub 2021 Apr 7. PMID: 34230843; PMCID: PMC8251020
44. Harvard T.H. Chan School of Public Health. How Hurricane Maria caused U.S. IV bag shortage. *In the News.* https://www.hsph.harvard.edu/news/hsph-in-the-news/hurricane-maria-u-s-iv-bag-shortage
45. Yu, K. D. S., & Aviso, K. B. (2020). Modelling the economic impact and ripple effects of disease outbreaks. *Process Integration and Optimization for Sustainability, 4*, 183–186. https://doi.org/10.1007/s41660-020-00113-y

46. Sodhi, M., & Choi, T. (2022). Don't abandon your just-in-time supply chain, revamp it. *Harvard Business Review.* https://hbr.org/2022/10/dont-abandon-your-just-in-time-supply-chain-revamp-it

47. Linton, T, & Vakil, B. (2020, Mar. 5). Coronavirus is proving we need more resilient supply chains. *Harvard Business Review.*

48. Eckler, J., Polyviou, M., & Schneller, E. (2022, June). Building supply chain resilience in the Arizona healthcare system: ASU-AzCHER Study of the Needs of the Arizona Ecosystem.

49. Herzlinger, R. E. (2006). Why innovation in health care is so hard. *Harvard Business Review, 84*(5), 58.

50. Wutzke, S., Benton, M., & Verma, R. (2016). Towards the implementation of large scale innovations in complex health care systems: Views of managers and frontline personnel. *BMC Research Notes, 9*(1), 1–5.

51. Liu, Z., Shi, Y., & Yang, B. (2022). Open innovation in times of crisis: An overview of the healthcare sector in response to the COVID-19 pandemic. *Journal of Open Innovation: Technology, Market, and Complexity, 8*(1), 21.

52. Bluewave Consulting. Global 3D printing medical devices market to grow at a CAGR of 15.4% until 2028.

53. Tan, Z., Khoo, D. W. S., Zeng, L. A., Tien, J. C. C., Lee, A. K. Y., Ong, Y. Y., Teo, M. M., & Abdullah, H. R. (2020). Protecting health care workers in the front line: Innovation in COVID-19 pandemic. *Journal of Globalization and Health, 10*(1).

54. Bag, S., Gupta, S., Choi, T. M., & Kumar, A. (2021). Roles of innovation leadership on using big data analytics to establish resilient healthcare supply chains to combat the COVID-19 pandemic: A multimethodological study. *IEEE Transactions on Engineering Management.*

55. Gartner. (2022, Nov. 19). Announces rankings of the Gartner Healthcare Supply Chain Top 25 for 2022. https://www.gartner.com/en/newsroom/press-releases/2022-11-09-gartner-announces-ranking-of-the-gartner-healthcare-supply-chain-top-25-for-2022

56. van Raaij, E. (2016). *Purchasing value: Purchasing and supply management's contribution to health service performance.* file:///C:/Users/cinnabar/Downloads/EIA2016068LIS.pdf

57. Centers for Medicare & Medicaid Services. Value-based purchasing (VBP). https://www.healthcare.gov/glossary/value-based-purchasing-vbp/#:~:text=Linking%20provider%20payments%20to%20improved,reward%20the%20best%2Dperforming%20providers

Appendix 1: Best Practices within the Context of Non-Governmental Fully Integrated Supply Chain Organization (FISCO)

Prepared by:

Arizona State University

W.P. Carey School of Business

Department of Supply Chain Management

P.O. Box 874706

Tempe, AZ 85287-4706

Origin for this report, including Attachments A through G, was conducted under contract number W81XWH-15-9-0001and submitted to the Defense Health Agency and Advanced Technology International on March 7, 2019. This version does not include assessment of the FISCO levels of development for the Defense Health Agency. For more information, please contact: Eugene S. Schneller, Ph.D., W.P. Carey School of Business Gene.Schneller@asu.edu

This document is the result of research and analysis by a number of investigators including Jim Eckler/Co-Principal Investigator (Eckler Associates), Carol Fraser (Expression Networks), Michael Gillespie (GHX), Mikaella Polyviou (ASU), George Ramos (ASU), Richard Perrin (Active Innovations), Dale Rogers (ASU), Eugene Schneller/Principal Investigator(ASU) and, Michael Gillespie (GHX). The administration of the project was supported by Amanda Koeller and David Winkle.

I. ENTERPRISE SYSTEMS

A. THE IDEA OF AN ENTERPRISE AND ITS ARCHITECTURE

In academic literature and in practice within industry, an enterprise system is seen as a support entity that brings together information, processes, and human resources to facilitate decision making at the operational, tactical, and strategic levels. As depicted in Exhibit A.1.1, an enterprise solution, with its information, process, and human resource components has value beyond everyday operations by monitoring and supporting the goals, strategy, vision, and mission of the organization.

Our characterization is not "merely" an enterprise resource planning (ERP) IT solutions, but depicts a systemic integrator of the people, processes, and technology a health care system utilizes. We take a broad view of enterprise activity by considering organizational alignments (both internal and external) and the resources and governance needed to support and enhance cross-organizational decision-making and, ultimately, enhanced performance. In this instance, performance is

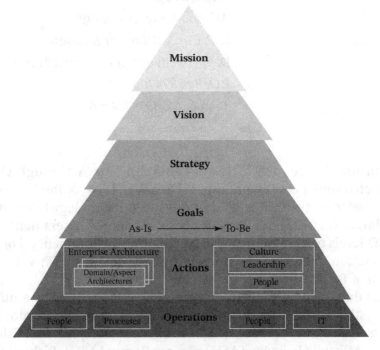

Exhibit A.1.1: Enterprise architecture positioned within an organization's context.[1]

considered within and across the branches and the multitude of settings supported that characterize a modern health care delivery system.

An important goal is to reduce the complexity emanating from the individual entities comprising a health care system. Enterprise architecture (EA), as elaborated below, refers to the structure of the system. Our concern is not merely on information systems, but a comprehensive solution involving business processes, technologies, and related governance.

Exhibit A.1.2 depicts a series of stages depicting an organization's information technology evolution from holding information to an architecture that can support advanced analytics and decision-making. It was estimated in 2012[3] that most hospitals in the US were in the early stages of such enterprise architecture (EA) development, meaning that they had not yet developed an EA to facilitate long range planning, strategic value assessment, IT infrastructure flexibility platform independence, application modularity, and the strategic agility, enterprise- wide governance and application beyond organization boundaries. Not all organizations achieve excellence in the same manner. Some organizations successfully put into place processes to assess and compare products to carry out supply base reduction, standardize product identification for carrying out product tracking and tracing, employ technologies for point of use, and consider the use of virtual product capture (voice and vision recognition) at the bedside. Others have developed advanced analytics, machine learning, and artificial intelligence to reduce their supply base and to assess product utilization and impact. And yet others are using outsourced risk identification tools to alert them to relevant disruptions that affect their product supply.

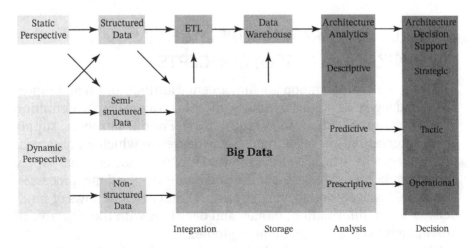

Exhibit A.1.2: Enterprise architecture analytics.[2]

Gosselt[4] has written extensively about enterprise architecture. He states:

> *Good architectural practice helps a company innovate and change by providing both stability and flexibility. The insights provided by an enterprise architecture are needed on the one hand in determining the needs and priorities for change from a business perspective, and on the other hand in assessing how the company may benefit from technological innovations.*

The architecture ideally sells an organization's vision to leaders and IT management, helps to align the use of technology with strategic goals and objectives, facilitates communication of plans, helps to manage the increasing complexity of the organization's vision. This provides guidance for adapting the architecture that packaged solutions brings to the architectural vision. In this report we focus on the architecture and technologies that currently exist and assess them against external practices. In a subsequent report we will consider evolving technologies and their strategic fit in meeting supply chain integration goals and objectives.

As discussed throughout this document, achieving a high level of performance is not merely about information system architecture and its contribution to outcomes. It also encompasses organizational processes and support. The idea of a maturity model, such as the highly recognized Gartner five stage maturity model,[5] is adapted for analysis throughout this report, with its focus on outcomes, metrics, processes, technology, and organization. The resultant stages reflect the organization's ability to *react, anticipate, integrate, collaborate and orchestrate*. See Attachment B.

B. FULLY INTEGRATED SUPPLY CHAIN ORGANIZATION (FISCO) CONCEPTS

While the idea of integration is a fundamental attribute of EA and supply chain and logistic s maturity models, there is no agreed upon definition of the term supply chain integration (SCI). For our purposes, supply chain integration can be defined as the degree to which an organization strategically brings together internal functions and external supply chain members to manage the intra- and inter-organizational processes. Robust SCI is necessary to achieve effective and efficient flows of products, services, information, money and decisions with the objective of providing maximum value to the customer.[6]

We put forth the idea of a Fully Integrated Supply Chain Organization (FISCO) to depict a robust effort to gain control over related organizational processes and to meet critical operational and strategic goals. A FISCO evolves from decisions enabling control and alignment of internal, external and outsourced functions. The hallmark of a FISCO is the reduction of complexity. The most progressive healthcare systems are truly integrated delivery systems where supply chain management makes significant contributions to the success of the enterprise. Current trends in industry are to integrate clinical requirements, patient outcomes and supply chain performance. Our characterization is based on our knowledge of integrated health systems and their consolidated service centers[7] as well as learnings from a variety of non-health sector organizations. FISCOs are characterized by the following processes, technology and organization characteristics (Exhibit A.1.3):

The consequences of a FISCO include:

- Cost – reduction of expenses through:
  - Leverage
  - Standardization
  - Innovation
  - Quality management

Exhibit A.1.3: Key FISCO functions.

SCM Processes	Technology Tools	Organization Support
Product Sourcing	System Integrational Architecture	Organization Structure
Product Selection & Standardization	Key Performance Indicators & Metrics	System Training
Contracting	Item Master Management	Governance of the Supply Chain
Supplier Relationship Management	Electronic Health Record Integration Preparedness	
Accounts Payable (AP)		
Order Processing		
Inventory Management		
Receiving		
Asset Management		
Supply Chain Risk Management		

- Risk – management of risks
- Predictability – creation of defined support services budgets
- Capacity – increased capacity for healthcare system growth
- Opportunity – identified opportunities for systemic improvement

The idea of a FISCO was developed from an ASU Department of Supply Chain Management effort in the process of scrutinizing healthcare systems that had successfully implemented a shared service organization and implemented a wide-range of supply chain management and integration functions to bring high quality healthcare services to war fighters and their dependents.

1. CHARACTERIZATION MEASURES

The scale we have adapted for this work has its genesis in the maturity model developed by Gartner, the premier consulting firm that scrutinizes health sector and private sector supply chains across industries. The scoring scheme has a five-point scale consisting of the markers (1) react, (2) anticipate, (3) integrate, (4) collaborate and for the most mature organizations, and (5) orchestrate (Exhibit A.1.4).[8] This allows us to locate each FISCO feature and characterize gaps between a system's practices and best practice organizations. The complete Gartner table is presented in Attachment B.

The FISCO framework characterizes the maturity of an organization's supply chain based on levels of maturity against FISCO categories. There are five FISCO levels of maturity that relate very closely to the Gartner Group Capability Maturity Model Integration (CMMI) stages for "Technology" (Attachment C). While FISCO level one organizations are the

Exhibit A.1.4: Gartner levels of maturity for technology.

Level 1 React	Level 2 Anticipate	Level 3 Integrate	Level 4 Collaborate	Level 5 Orchestrate
Disparate transactional systems of record with limited functional support	Push for integration of systems of record; siloed functional solutions	Technologies to support end-to-end supply chain processes; improved data rationalization and integration capability	Technology that enables trading partner connectivity and supports mature processes in the extended supply chain	Innovative technology tools to enable network-wide value creation, risk management and scenario analysis for profitable trade-offs

least integrated supply chain systems, FISCO level five organizations are fully integrated supply chain systems.

Attachment C provides the complete FISCO characterization roadmap used for this project and provides definitions for each category.

In assessing each of the dimensions, it is important to examine:

- Best Practices: Consideration of industry best practice for this supply chain management function as compared to other organizations
- Capability: The extent to which an organization supports this function and how well support is provided.
- Bridging the Gap: The steps that can be taken to bridge the gap between to achieve industry best practice.

A. HEALTHCARE SCM PROCESSES

FISCO categorizes SCM processes into 10 distinct dimensions:

1. Product Sourcing
2. Product Selection and Standardization
3. Contracting and Purchasing
4. Supplier Relationship Management
5. Accounts Payable
6. Order Processing
7. Inventory Management
8. Receiving
9. Asset Management
10. Supply Chain Risk Management

Each of these dimensions are assessed below. Additional information about the characterization of dimensions 1 through 5 are in Attachment C.

1. PRODUCT SOURCING

Product sourcing is the supply chain process involved in identification, investigation, and decision to acquire products to fulfill a clinical or business need. In the healthcare field the sourcing process is led by experienced managers with industry and product knowledge of the specific branches of medicine such as cardiac, orthopedics, neuro, and oncology.

A description of Product Sourcing maturity levels is provided in the following table.

Level	Product Sourcing - Description
1 React	▨ Use of purchasing agents that lack product knowledge and do not provide added value; they simply source products that users demand
2 Anticipate	▨ Use of purchasing agents organized by clinical specialty but without clinical experience or product knowledge
3 Integrate	▨ Use of purchasing agents organized by clinical specialty and given access to clinical experts; experts not integrated within the organization's processes ▨ Heavy reliance on GPOs for sourcing decisions
4 Collaborate	▨ Use of highly specialized sourcing managers with some clinical experience ▨ Moderate reliance on GPOs for sourcing decisions
5 Orchestrate	▨ Use of specialized sourcing managers with direct clinical experience focused by specialty; organization by product categories at the sub-specialty level ▨ GPO use limited to commodity products

Notably, few organizations operate at Level 5 today. However, there are many healthcare systems in the US which currently operate at Levels 2 through 4.

Bridging the Gap
Some examples of technologies, processes, and/or organization tools that are used by IBP organizations include:

- Automating the RFP processes.
- Developing governance and protocols to create an automated purchasing system in which a web service or other technology and interface may display pricing from multiple pre-approved vendors for the convenience of purchasers.
- IBP product sourcing employs risk management technologies by balancing supplier reduction with risk reduction.

2. PRODUCT SELECTION AND STANDARDIZATION
The product selection and standardization processes are carefully orchestrated supply chain processes that ensure that the best and most appropriate products are chosen for use in the healthcare system.

A description of Product Selection and Standardization maturity levels is provided in the following table.

Level	Product Selection and Standardization
1 React	▪ Little attention to product standardization, leading to an exceptionally large product base for the clinical services provided ▪ Formulary of frequently ordered items which lack accompanying standardization
2 Anticipate	▪ Limited or sporadic product standardization programs ▪ Standardization working groups and evaluation of vendor products, product selection decisions, and contracting processes as applicable ▪ Compliance metrics gathered and reported
3 Integrate	▪ Promotion of product standardization programs, although broad-based clinical engagement may not be achieved ▪ Standardization working groups; market research; evaluation of vendors/sources, vendor products, product decisions, and contracting processes as applicable; risk management review ▪ Compliance metrics gathered and reported
4 Collaborate	▪ Formalized product standardization programs with clinical staff appreciating the value of standardization, but not fully engaged ▪ Standardization working groups and standardized clinical pathways (including equipment, supplies, and quantity to be used, not just clinical procedure) ▪ Standardization determined by the working group and based on the clinical pathway and market research; evaluation of vendors/sources, vendor products, product decisions, and contracting processes as applicable; risk management review ▪ Compliance metrics gathered and reported
5 Orchestrate	▪ Similar to Level 4 but adding: ▪ Standardization programs that are part of the culture – all clinical and administrative staff are fully aware, appreciate, and are committed to the process ▪ Standardization working groups and standardized clinical pathways ▪ Patient outcomes also monitored, and compliance or deviation form clinical pathway is determined; re-evaluation of the clinical pathway is for potential modification

3. CONTRACTING AND PURCHASING

The contracting process establishes formal arrangements for the ongoing acquisition of products and services at pre-determined terms and prices. The purchasing process describes the steps involved in conveying a demand for a product to the supplier of the goods. It may be electronically or manually communicated; and it may be through a central purchasing department or by individual users.

A description of Contracting and Purchasing maturity levels is provided the following table.

Level	Contracting and Purchasing
1 React	▪ The very early stage of development in purchasing ▪ Almost all acquisitions done on the spot with no contractual commitments
2 Anticipate	▪ Limited contracts with vendors ▪ Reliance on GPOs and distributors for contracted products
3 Integrate	▪ Recognition of the value of contracted commitments but yet to achieve a high percent of purchases that comply with contracts
4 Collaborate	▪ Commitment to contracted purchases; contract compliance level of 50% to 85% ▪ Less dependent on general distributors such as Cardinal and Owens & Minor
5 Orchestrate	▪ Full commitment to contracted purchases; contract compliance level >85%

We have identified best practice organizations that operate at Level 5.

Bridging the Gap

Examples of technologies, processes, and/or organization tools that are used by IBP organizations include:

- Using enterprise analytics to assure suppliers real time insight into demand and utilization.
- Assuring that distributors and prime vendors have significant utilization data and observability into the operating units. This creates a significant ability for the Prime Vendor to provide efficiency.

4. SUPPLIER RELATIONSHIP MANAGEMENT/VENDOR PERFORMANCE MANAGEMENT

Supplier Relationship Management (SRM) is the business process involved in bilateral communications between suppliers and buyers to ensure that each side understands its role and best meets its obligations.

Scorecards are often prepared to track the performance of the relationship and each party's contribution to the relationship.

A description of Supplier Relationship Management/Vendor Performance Management maturity levels is provided the following table.

Level	Supplier Relationship/Vendor Performance Management
1 React	▪ No relationship with supplier aside from standard purchase orders ▪ No supplier performance tracking
2 Anticipate	▪ Periodic (quarterly) reviews of supplier performance (based on self-reporting) and subsequent review with the supplier
3 Integrate	▪ Formal supplier performance reporting process ▪ Collect and analyze supplier performance KPIs that affect supplier behavior and future relationships
4 Collaborate	▪ Sophisticated supplier scorecards and scorecard review with suppliers ▪ Collect and analyze supplier performance KPIs that affect supplier behavior and future relationships ▪ More frequent reviews with the supplier executive team and the healthcare system
5 Orchestrate	▪ Sophisticated supplier scorecards and scorecard review with suppliers ▪ Collect and analyze supplier performance KPIs that affect supplier behavior and future relationships ▪ More frequent reviews with the supplier executive team and the healthcare system ▪ Link vendor performance directly to patient outcomes and adjust purchases accordingly

We have identified best practice organizations which operate at Level 5, however, many healthcare systems in the US currently operate at Level 4.

Bridging the Gap
Examples of technologies, processes, and/or organization tools that are used by IBP organizations include:

- Providing vendors with visibility into utilization and demand.
- Involving suppliers in product selection.
- Best practice organizations have strong relationships with both their distributors as well as with direct suppliers. Technologies, such as smart cabinetry, can transmit data to upstream partners.

5. ACCOUNTS PAYABLE

Accounts Payable is the business process of paying a supplier for the delivery of their products in accordance with the agreed upon commercial terms. Typically, before a payment is made a three-way match (physically or virtually) of purchase, receiving, and invoice is required.

A description of Accounts Payable maturity levels is provided in the following table.

Level	Description
1 React	■ SCM has no direct control of accounts payable, which is typically managed by the finance department ■ Product vendors can be established and paid without SCM approval
2 Anticipate	■ Same as Level 1
3 Integrate	■ Accounts payable managed by the finance department, but specific criteria are established to restrict the approval of a vendor without adhering to SCM acceptance criteria
4 Collaborate	■ Sophisticated vendor scorecards and scorecard review with vendors ■ SCM controls and operates the accounts payable process ■ All vendor payments managed in an integrated manner along with other SCM processes (such as sourcing and contracting) to mitigate unauthorized 'pirate' purchasing of non-standard products
5 Orchestrate	■ Same as Level 4

We have identified best practice organizations which operate at Level 5.

6. ORDER PROCESSING

Moving requisitions to purchase orders and transmitting those orders to the suppliers is of utmost importance. Failure to complete this process efficiently can result in duplicate supply requests, stockpiled supplies with requestors due to lack of faith in the process as well as not having enough suppliers on hand to support the needs of the organization. As such, there are some key leading practices that need to be implemented to support a highly functioning, modern supply chain.

This is achieved through a combination of systems and procedures that work in concert to support the supply chain resources and requesting departments.

A description of Order Processing maturity levels is provided in the following table.[9]

Level	Order Processing
1 React	▪ Lack of a true electronic exchange ▪ Disparate systems in a highly manual environment (e.g., phone, fax, and email)
2 Anticipate	▪ Utilization of electronic orders with select suppliers using a limited EDI transaction set via direct connections with those suppliers purchase orders (EDI850)
3 Integrate	▪ Maximized number of trading partners and EDI transactions sets ▪ Purchase Order Acknowledgement (EDI855) ▪ Daily reconciliation of 885 exceptions ▪ Strong exception management processes
4 Collaborate	▪ Real time contract 3-way price validation to ensure accurate pricing ▪ Automated reconciliation between purchase orders and acknowledgements resulting in discrepancy identification and line status updates ▪ Utilization of 810s for automated invoice reconciliation and payment processing
5 Orchestrate	▪ Use of process codes to segregate POs ▪ Feedback loop to ensure item source detail is updated to reduce future exception ▪ Predictive analytics around usage needs ▪ Automatic order creation based on consumption events

A civilian highly integrated system would be at 4 to 5 on such a scale.

Bridging the Gap

Examples of technologies, processes, and/or organization tools that are used by IBP organizations include:

- ▪ Utilization of an electronic data interchange to transact electronic business documents with trading partners.
- ▪ Continuous efforts to maximize the amount of trading partners and the transaction sets utilized within the exchange to expand upon further automation.
- ▪ Developing governance, protocols, metrics for assessment and enforcement of templates, communication channels and frequency, as well as feedback and quote management.

7. INVENTORY MANAGEMENT

Inventory management and distribution encompasses the process of moving sourced and purchased products from the supplier to the intended recipient within the healthcare organization. This movement of product also encompasses the management of fixed inventories. Management in this context is further defined as the planning of inventory levels to ensure that the products stocked are appropriate for the type of location and customer.

A description of Inventory Management maturity levels is provided in the following table.

Level	Description
1 React	▪ Inventory managed through manual intervention and based on ordering par levels ▪ Lack of system automation and integration
2 Anticipate	▪ Utilization of inventory management technology, but still reliant on manual counts and reconciliation ▪ Inability to fully utilize the technology functionality
3 Integrate	▪ Centralized inventory and purchasing management ▪ Strong inventory and demand planning team with a strong demand and planning process. ▪ Planners divided by purchasing groups ▪ Utilization of point of use systems for medical/surgical supplies to reduce annual spend for tracked items
4 Collaborate	▪ Implementation of a formal approach to manage excess inventory and shelf life aging ▪ Full implementation of bar code technology to track inventory ▪ Inventory function linked to master data maintenance group
5 Orchestrate	▪ Product expiration management ▪ Full implementation of barcode technology for accurate cost, usage tracking, predictive analytics, and demand forecasting ▪ Clinically integrated barcode technology to provide accurate patient records and associated cost detail

Mature distribution processes incorporate their ability to use big data into their processes and leverage their information in relationships with distributors and, consequently, distributors leverage their acquisitions from suppliers.

A civilian highly integrated system would be at Level 4 to 5.

Bridging the Gap

Examples of technologies, processes, and/or organization tools that are used by IBP organizations include:

- RFID, auto-replenishment systems, artificial intelligence and predictive analytics are all examples of technologies being utilized by industry leaders.
- Optimization of existing technology investments to ensure integration between technologies are realizing true automation and value.
- Strong inventory management processes and governance structures are deployed to ensure the realization of value these technologies bring are achieved.

8. RECEIVING

Receiving is an essential function in warehouse and inventory management. When done correctly, it systematically enables high efficiencies for all downstream processes. If done incorrectly, the negative impacts can be far reaching and result in lost products, overstocks, and mistakes when fulfilling orders. Leveraging automation and clear procedures will drive efficiencies into your organization resulting in cleaner data and knowledge of what items are contained in the warehouses.

A description of Receiving maturity levels is provided in the following table.

Level	Receiving
1 React	- Manual receiving processes with little use of technology - Single warehousing location, limited controls
2 Anticipate	- Receiving processes ensure all stock purchase order receipts come through the dock - Ability to cross dock - Manual recordkeeping of goods recipients
3 Integrate	- Fully automated receiving process and technology module using advance shipment notifications (856) as the receiver - High volume, dependable vendors bypass the receiving process - Low Unit of Measure process deployed to manage inventory costs, reduce stock on hand and the reduction of waste

Level	Receiving
4 Collaborate	■ Robust return goods process ■ Utilization of delivery tracking (bar code) with status capability ■ Scanning software to track delivery of products to end-users ■ Extensive use of advanced shipment notifications (EDI856) and unit load labels (MH10)
5 Orchestrate	■ Automated adjustments ■ Electronic item tracking (bar code or RFID) ■ Staggered supplier delivery management ■ Expedited delivery process to the unit location

A civilian highly integrated system would be at Level 4 to 5.

Bridging the Gap

Examples of technologies, processes, and/or organization tools that are used by IBP organizations include:

- Process compliance.
- Use of EDI 856 (advance shipment notice) in conjunction with MH-10 labels on packaging to enable direct receipt to putaway.
- Strategic use of barcoding to identify receiving effectiveness, efficiency and planning.

9. ASSET MANAGEMENT

Asset management is the process of identifying requirements for nonexpendable moveable property, procuring it, assigning accountability and responsibility for it, maintaining it throughout its life cycle and planning for its replacement.

A description of Asset Management maturity levels is provided in the following table.

Level	ASSET MANAGEMENT
1 React	■ Manual tracking of equipment (fixed capital equipment and patient care mobile equipment) ■ Reactive response to downed equipment
2 Anticipate	■ Automated property tracking/management system with barcode labels applied to equipment for tracking and physical inventory using HHT devices ■ Use of another automated system for service of equipment, store, order, tracking of repair parts. ■ Use of service contracts to manage scheduled and unscheduled maintenance

Level	ASSET MANAGEMENT

3
Integrate
	▪ Use of passive RFID system for:
	  ▪ Automated property tracking, management, and maintenance
	  ▪ Storage, ordering, and tracking of repair parts
	  ▪ Maintenance (scheduled and unscheduled) management, with resource certifications and predictive budget needs for basic life cycle management
	  ▪ Tracking of personnel training and certification

4
Collaborate
	▪ Use of passive and active RFID system for:
	  ▪ Automated property tracking, management, and maintenance
	  ▪ Storage, ordering, and tracking of repair parts
	  ▪ Maintenance (scheduled and unscheduled) management, with resource certifications and predictive budget needs for basic life cycle management
	  ▪ Tracking of personnel training and certification

5 Orchestrate	▪ Use of passive and active RFID system as in Level 4, but added integrated life cycle process for biomedical equipment ▪ Use of ECRI recall data for automated generation of quality control (QC) messages ▪ System support for recall closure processes (e.g., recall results, cost, impact of cancelled procedures, etc.) ▪ Support technology assessment for future needs with ability to access EHR and asset management data.

Best practice organizations also use a comprehensive work-order and repair parts management system. They are moving towards the capture of usage data by machine in order to determine maintenance activities based on usage. Best practice organizations are assessed at Level 5.

Additional detail regarding best practices for asset management is provided in Attachment G.

Bridging the Gap

Examples of technologies, processes, and/or organization tools that are used by IBP organizations include:

▪ Automated system for tracking equipment with passive and active RFID or alternate real time location system tracking capabilities (e.g., infrared), and comprehensive life cycle management processes.

▪ IBP use predictive budgeting and comprehensive maintenance scheduling.

▪ Recall data with auto generated QC messages.

▪ Recall notice processing is coupled with QC closures (recall outcomes, costs, procedure impacts, etc.).

10. SUPPLY CHAIN RISK MANAGEMENT

Supply chain risk management (SCRM) is a cross-functional process to identify, assess, mitigate, and monitor relevant risks (e.g., natural disasters, accidents, sabotage, or production problems) that can disrupt an organization's supply chain operations. Best practices on recall management identified from healthcare and other industry sectors are provided in Attachment D.

In healthcare supply chains, a recall refers to the removal or correction of a marketed product (e.g., pharmaceutical or medical device) to address a problem with that product that violates the laws administered by the U.S. Food and Drug Administration.

A description of Supply Chain Risk Management[10] maturity levels is provided in the following table.

Level	Supply Chain Risk Management
1 React	▪ No SCRM resources ▪ Lack of risk identification, assessment ▪ Ad hoc reaction when an event is triggered
2 Anticipate	▪ Informal and functional risk identification, assessment, and mitigation program but none to limited cross-functional coordination ▪ Informal supply chain mapping ▪ Ad hoc reaction when an event is triggered
3 Integrate	▪ Formal but functional risk identification, assessment, and risk mitigation program ▪ Proactive risk mitigation strategies ▪ Formal supply chain mapping
4 Collaborate	▪ Formal and cross-functional risk identification, assessment, and mitigation program ▪ Collaboration with key supply chain partners ▪ Formal supply chain mapping across all critical products
5 Orchestrate	▪ Formal and cross-functional risk identification, assessment, and mitigation program ▪ Collaboration with supply chain partners ▪ Continuous improvement of SCRM programs ▪ Risk metrics included in scorecards ▪ SCRM aligned with organization's objectives and embedded in the culture

Bridging the Gap

Examples of technologies, processes, and/or organization tools that are used by IBP organizations include:

▪ Providing information to end-users in formats that are conducive to efficient tracking and tracking of products – including serial numbers, lot numbers and/or unique identification.

- Having a "full court press" with a focus on a broad range of supply disruptions. The feed for such information is frequently a commercially available technology.
- Utilizing machine learning/artificial intelligence for early identification of defective products.
- Utilize 3rd party provider to engage in the monitoring and providing alerts regarding disruptions due to natural disasters and other events by providing supply node mapping, event monitoring, supplier monitoring, etc.

B. TECHNOLOGY TOOLS

In this section we assess four dimensions of technology for a FISCO:

1. System Integration/Architecture
2. KPIs and Metrics
3. Item Master Management
4. EHR Integration Preparedness

1. SYSTEM INTEGRATION/ARCHITECTURE

System Integration & Architecture is a FISCO concept that evaluates the supply chain information technology systems to determine their level of integration. Enterprises with Disparate systems are inefficient while those with tightly coupled or highly integrated systems are more efficient.

A description of System Integration/Architecture maturity levels is provided in the following table.

Level	SYSTEM INTEGRATION ARCHITECTURE
1 React	▪ Disparate systems requiring duplicate entry/processes
2 Anticipate	▪ Client-server technology that is interfaced with other logistics systems or support systems and with the General Ledger ▪ Standalone capabilities that can pass data to another system using designated formats for required operations
3 Integrate	▪ Integrated end-to-end logistics IT system, cloud based with one item master file and visible for both hospital and enterprise use ▪ Systems designed to share data within a common set of data bases and do not require separate transfers of data to other systems to complete actions

Level	SYSTEM INTEGRATION ARCHITECTURE
4 Collaborate	▪ IT Logistics systems are fully integrated POU, 70% scan rate, location aware inventory management, auto generate replenishment based on location decrements, and charge at point of issue.
5 Orchestrate	▪ Clinically Integrated Supply Chain (Logistics suite interfaced to EHR and General Ledger) ▪ Usage captured, outcomes captured, supply expense per episode of care ▪ Predictive analytics are used to determine if changes to a clinical pathway will reduce expenses, risk, or negative outcomes

Best practice organizations perform at FISCO Level 4 and one organization that we interviewed has made strides toward Level 5.

Bridging the Gap

Examples of technologies, processes, and/or organization tools that are used by IBP organizations include:

- Logistics suite interfaced to EHR and General Ledger.
- Predictive analytics to anticipate clinical outcomes (e.g., expenses, risk, etc.) and assist with clinical decision making.
- Fully integrated with POU systems.
- Employment of metrics to track compliance with enterprise wide policies and performance characteristics.
- Continuously assessing stakeholder satisfaction with enterprise-wide supply chain and logistics tools.
- Have in place change management tools to reduce disruptions as innovations enter the enterprise architecture.

2. KPI/METRICS

KPI/Metrics are a FISCO concept that evaluates the enterprises use of metrics to determine the health of the supply chain. Using the correct metrics/KPIs allows an enterprise to anticipate and resolve issues before they occur.

A description of KPI/Metrics maturity levels is provided in the following table.

Level	KPI/METRICS
1 React	▪ Only tracks basic supply performance KPIs for individual facilities
2 Anticipate	▪ Manages, tracks, and reports supply performance KPIs ▪ KPIs are tracked at facility and at an enterprise organization level

Level	KPI/METRICS
3 Integrate	▓ Composite metrics correlate actionable steps ▓ For example, if demand satisfaction is below goal then possible influencing data is also displayed in order to quickly ascertain why the KPI goal was missed (e.g. zero balance rate over the period)
4 Collaborate	▓ Composite metrics are prescriptive ▓ System observes, reacts, and guides/advises
5 Orchestrate	▓ Composite metrics driven by clinical pathways and outcomes

Industry Best Practice organizations use "composite" Metrics. For example, Best Practice Organizations capture "Average Cost per Case" combining the: 1) total cost per case, 2) total cost amount, 3) labor and overhead, 4) supply cost used, 5) supply cost wasted, and 6) case count.

Best Practice Organizations prioritize their metrics with a set of finite and specific measurements at Tier 1 and drill in to greater detail at different Tiers. Best practice organizations interviewed are rated at Level 4.

Bridging the Gap

IBP organizations use machine learning in order to leverage forensic models and predictive analytics to create complex/composite KPIs and dashboards. This gives these organizations actionable metrics. To bridge this gap:

▓ Incorporate machine learning tools and visualization techniques.
▓ Add data scientist to the mix of SMEs.
▓ Develop complex Key Performance Indicator rules to prescribe actions or possible actions.
▓ Incorporate "cost avoidance" KPIs and associated composite metric displays.

3. ITEM MANAGEMENT STRATEGY

Developing a Modern Item Data Strategy that drives the integrity of supplies and implant data is critical, yet often overlooked in many organizations. Many hospitals traditionally address the individual "pieces" of master file maintenance (purchasing, standardization, agreements) but do not align the individual functions to interact collaboratively. High functioning organizations maintain current product data integrity through integration across various systems enabled by a Master Data Maintenance Group and a strong governance model. As enterprise systems grow in size and complexity, industry leaders embrace the importance of data as the life blood of their organizations to provide valuable insights across a clinically integrated supply chain.

A description of Item Management Strategy maturity levels is provided in the following table.

Level	Item Management Strategy
1 React	▪ Disparate systems with highly manual processes of item management ▪ Lack of clear process around master data management
2 Anticipate	▪ Utilization of ERP item master, centralized supply chain team, no clear item additions, update, inactivation process ▪ Lacks strong item management processes or automation
3 Integrate	▪ Fully integrated and centralized item master ▪ Utilization of data cleansing and enrichment tools to assist with standardized product part information ▪ Item add process defined and controlled by select group of administrators to ensure quality control
4 Collaborate	▪ Normalized Item Master to remove generalized items, enumerate manufacturer name, part number for every active item, applying United Nations Standard Products and Services Code (UNSPSC) classification, and building vendor hierarchy per item ▪ Strong governance model established around master data with defined key performance indicators that are routinely tracked
5 Orchestrate	▪ Clinically integrated item master, strong value analysis collaboration, feedback loop from electronic exchange for updates to item detail and pricing ▪ Clinically friendly descriptions and nomenclature developed to ensure clinician satisfaction is high

A civilian highly integrated system would be at Level 3 to 4 on such a scale.

Bridging the Gap
Electronic Health Record (EHR) Integration Preparedness

With the rapid expansion and use of the EHR across the healthcare continuum, supply chain data, or more specifically, the item master, is evolving to become a strategic asset. As the single source of truth for item information, this data is being leveraged to support clinical documentation and patient billing, including supply and implant capture at the point of use. With this increased use of the data, a new set of challenges arise that the supply chain team is faced with solving. Accuracy, breadth, and consistency, to name a few, are all critically important, and the EHR is leading to an exponential growth of the item master and associated maintenance.

As healthcare systems have shifted their focus to value-based care, product content information has become critical in enabling the promise of their EHR investments. In developing a clinically integrated enterprise, the importance of a strong data core provides the fundamental building blocks to support the objectives of EHR functionality, such as Total Cost of Care, Reimbursement, Risk Exposure, Quality of Care, Minimization of Clinical Variation, and Compliance.

A description of EHR Integration Preparedness maturity levels is provided in the following table.

Level	Electronic Health Record
1 React	■ Manual item master entry to the electronic health record with no item master integration ■ Lack of strong data entry controls or automation
2 Anticipate	■ Utilization of supply chain item master data, manual upload of product detail, supply chain item description nomenclature, static preference cards and correlating data set ■ Data is more supply chain focused without automated integration
3 Integrate	■ Daily item master integration, item updates, additions, pricing changes remain reactive, strong process with Charge Description Master for item additions as needed ■ Direct automated integration from ERP to EHR
4 Collaborate	■ Enhanced item core that incorporates accurate charge and categorization codes ■ Barcode detail passed to or maintain within the electronic health record to ensure higher scan rates at the bed side during documentation and accurate patient records and billing
5 Orchestrate	■ Clinically Integrated Supply Chain ■ Usage and outcomes captured, supply expense per episode of care, predictive analytics ■ Supply decisions based on clinical pathway standards and usage (receipt, POU issue, inventory with lot number)

A best practice civilian highly integrated system preparedness would be at Level 4.

Bridging the Gap

Examples of technologies, processes, and/or organization tools that are used by IBP organizations include:

■ Utilization of the ERP Item Master combined with partnerships with established data integrity 3rd party software services to ensure a continuous review, cleansing, and enrichment of item data and clinical data attributes (e.g. Revenue Code, HCPCS Code, Charge Code, Implantable Flag, Chargeable Flag, GTIN's,

UOM, Vendor/Manufacture Part Numbers, UNSPSC categorization, descriptions, and price).

- Strong governance structure with the creation of a master data management group to apply rigor and focus around the complexities of authoritative data.
- Focus on driving towards a clinically integrated supply chain and full realization of the EHR investment.

C. ORGANIZATION SUPPORT

In this section we assess three dimensions of organization support for an enterprise system including:

1. Organization structure considerations
2. System training
3. Governance

In addition to the assessment below, Attachment D provides more detailed descriptions of best practices and capabilities.

1. ORGANIZATION STRUCTURE

The organization structure defines the design of the organization relationships and the roles of the leaders of each of the entities. It also portrays and defines the relationships between the multiple entities within the enterprise.

A description of Organization Structure maturity levels is provided the following table.

Level	Organization Structure
1 React	■ Discrete supply chain teams with limited interaction focused on transactional services
2 Anticipate	■ Mid-level supply chain leadership focused on transactional services with responsibility for some strategic initiatives
3 Integrate	■ SCM team led by manager reporting to member of the corporate leadership team but with limited visibility ■ Focus on SCM KPIs
4 Collaborate	■ Senior executive led SCM organization driving shared services targeting corporate and strategic mission of organization
5 Orchestrate	■ Clinically driven SCM team led by senior executive with non-core operations outsourced or through shared services

We have identified best practice organizations that operate at Level 5. These are fully integrated supply chain organizations (FISCOs).

Bridging the Gap

Examples of technologies, processes, and/or organization tools that are used by IBP organizations include:

- Implementing an organization structure for system that has resilience flexibility and deals with exceptions that supports supply chain efficiencies.
- Designing an organization structure with single chain of command with clear accountability and full line of sight to supply chain management decisions.
- Designing an organization that supports a clinically driven supply chain.
- Migrating to one enterprise system across the services with a single database for a single source of truth.

2. SYSTEM TRAINING

The process for training users of the information systems and the supply chain business processes how to fully use the systems to gain the maximum value from their use. The training should help the users understand not only how to use the systems but why the system and related business processes are important for fulfilling the mission.

A description of System Training maturity levels is provided below.

Level	System Training
1 React	<ul><li>Organization that has On-the-Job Training (OJT) only</li><li>No formal training on the logistics systems is available</li></ul>
2 Anticipate	<ul><li>Organization that has OJT, formal classroom, and as needed self-paced tutorial training (how to)</li></ul>
3 Integrate	<ul><li>Organization that has OJT, formal classroom, and as needed self-paced CBT or Client Server tutorial training (how to)</li></ul>
4 Collaborate	<ul><li>Organization that has OJT, formal classroom, and web-based training available for the convenience of the user (how to)</li></ul>
5 Orchestrate	<ul><li>Organization that has OJT, classroom, tutorial web-based training (how to), integrates functional logistics training (why, when), and provides a context sensitive help and training capability to limit the amount of searching required by the user</li></ul>

It appears that Industry Best Practice performs at a Level 4.

Bridging the Gap

Examples of technologies, processes, and/or organization tools that are used by IBP organizations include:

- Training programs that build knowledge and skills necessary to achieve enterprise wide integration.
- Programs that incorporate strong change management skills into training modules.
- Training programs that bring together clinical and supply chain leadership modules to assure linking-pin roles to create and sustain a clinically focused supply chain.
- Modules that focus on business analytics training.

3. GOVERNANCE OF THE SUPPLY CHAIN

The structures and rules for governing supply chain business processes and systems. Key to the governance is specifying the levels of authority for decisions and in complex situations where multiple organization entities are involved, the decision-making processes.

A description of Governance of the Supply Chain maturity levels is provided below.

Level	Governance
1 React	- Leadership of disparate SCM functions by disconnected, transactional managers - Reacts to procurement needs rather than the organization's mission
2 Anticipate	- Multiple SCM functions/entities directed by policies but each controlled distinctly
3 Integrate	- Single SCM organization in the early stages of integrated management led and controlled by manager reporting to non-executive - Not strategically focused nor possessing authority to influence dispersed operations
4 Collaborate	- Single SCM organization led, controlled and measured by manager reporting to executive team - Recognizes the value of integrated SCM but has not given it full authority and visibility within the organization to focus across the organization
5 Orchestrate	- Single SCM organization led, controlled and measured by manager at executive team level - Recognizes that SCM is of strategic importance and provides the authority to align and control the supply chain at the highest level of the organization

We have identified best practice organizations which operate at Level 5, however, there are many healthcare systems in the US which currently operate at Levels 2 through 4.

Bridging the Gap

Some examples of technologies, processes, and/or organization tools that are used by IBP organizations include:

- Clear and straightforward decision-making process for all SCM decisions where decisions are accessible to all key SCM staff.
- A decision-making process that supports a clinically driven supply chain.
- A decision-making process that is held accountable to the objectives of the supply chain and which drives compliance to SCM goals.

II. CONCLUSIONS

As supply chain management practitioners seek to deliver maximum value, they now focus on meeting clinical needs while respecting administrative obligations. Consequently, in the world of civilian healthcare, Industry standards and policy are driving the supply chain to develop what is referred as a clinically focused supply chain strategy. Just as clinicians are patient focused, SCM practitioners and systems must start with the patient and work backwards as they develop solutions.

Logistics and purchasing are no longer considered as arms-length to the point of use. This means that system processes have been adopted that allow for data analytics and outcome analysis, down to the procedure, patient, doctor, and supply and equipment utilization. Further, clinician involvement in supply chain management decision-making has expanded greatly in the past few years. Supply chains processes and structures today are designed from the perspective of a *clinically driven supply chain* which incorporates more than cost to include quality and patient outcome goals.

This differs from the past when supply chains were designed mainly from an *efficiency* perspective. The Drug Supply Chain Serialization Act, for example, will challenge health care systems to put into place systems that facilitate track and trace for pharmaceuticals.[11] Now is the time to bring such changes into discussions regarding enterprise system competencies and capabilities.

The FISCO concept has been proffered as a means to depict the most progressive supply chain organizations in the health sector. FISCOs are characterized by a centralized sourcing and purchasing platform–including purchasing, standardized value analysis process, integrated order and inventory management systems, centralized distribution, FISCO managed materials attendants throughout all settings, integrated quality management and standardization programs, centralized accounts payable, and other financial systems managed by supply chain.

The FISCO assessment is summarized below (Exhibit A.1.5). For each dimension we practice organizations along a five-point scale adapted from the Gartner Maturity Model. A recurring observation that we discovered in our investigation has been the unusually high degree of variation of practice and compliance in various parts of the medical logistics system. This is likely due to the significant transformation underway as systems integrate new technology into their information systems. The system is very large. It is very complex. Its scope is global and its operating environment is often harsh. Such variation during transformation can be expected.

III. ATTACHMENTS

Attachment A

A. LIS T OF ACRONYMS

AED	Authoritative Equipment Data
AMEDDPAS	Army Medical Department Property Accounting System
AP	Accounts Payable
ASU	Arizona State University
CAIM	Customer Area Inventory Management
CMMI	Capability Maturity Model Integration
EA	Enterprise Architecture
EAF	Enterprise Architecture Framework
ECAT	Electronic Catalogue
EDI	Electronic Data Interchange
EHR	Electronic Health Record
FISCO	Fully Integrated Supply Chain Organization
GPO	Group Purchasing Order
HHT	Hand Held Terminal
IAB	Industry Advisory Board
KPI	Key Performance Indicator
MEDLOG	Medical Logistics

OJT	On-the-Job Training
P-card	Purchase Card
POU	Point of use
PVM	Prime Vendor Med Surg
PVP	Prime Vendor Pharmacy
RFID	Radio Frequency Identification
SCDM	Supply Chain Disruption Management
SCI	Supply Chain Integration
SCM	Supply Chain Management
SCRM	Supply Chain Risk Management
SKU	Stock Keeping Unit
SLA	Service Level Agreement
SME	Subject Matter Expert

Exhibit A.1.5: Assessment summary.

SCM Business Processes / FISCO Functions	Level 1 React	Level 2 Anticipate	Level 3 Integrate	Level 4 Collaborate	Level 5 Orchestrate
(1) Product Sourcing				IBP	
(2) Product Selection and Standardization				IBP ▲	
(3) Contracting and Purchasing					IBP
(4) Supplier Relationship Management/ Vendor Performance Management					IBP
(5) Accounts Payable					IBP
(6) Order Processing				IBP ▲	
(7) Inventory Management				IBP ▲	
(8) Receiving				IBP ▲	
(9) Asset Management				IBP	
(10) Supply Chain Risk Management					IBP

FISCO Functions	Level 1 React	Level 2 Anticipate	Level 3 Integrate	Level 4 Collaborate	Level 5 Orchestrate
(11) System Integration/Architecture				IBP	
(12) Key Performance Indicator (KPI)/Metrics				IBP	
(13) Item Master Management Strategy			IBP▪▶		
(14) Electronic Health Record Integration Preparedness				IBP	
(15) Organization Structure					IBP
(16) System Training			IBP▪▶		
(17) Governance of the Supply Chain					IBP

Technology Tools (functions 11–14)

Organization Support (functions 15–17)

Attachment B

B. GARTNER MATURITY MODEL

DDVN 5-Stage Maturity Model	Stage 1 React	Stage 2 Anticipate	Stage 3 Integrate	Stage 4 Collaborate	Stage 5 Orchestrate
Outcome	Business unit revenue focus, but achieving misaligned and/or siloed objectives	Supply chain functional performance improvements	Integrated supply chain decision making, with early connections to product and/or sales	Profitable demand-driven fulfillment through internal collaboration, as well as with customers and suppliers	Profitable shared value creation through innovation across internal and external networks
Metrics	Business-unit-specific	Functionally specific, competing metrics	Integrated supply chain metrics used to manage trade-offs	Outside-in metrics across the extended value chain	Value-based metrics aligned across the ecosystem
Process Focus	Revenue focus; firefighting with no centralized analysis	Scaling and cost-efficiency within each function	Functional excellence; integration across core supply chain processes	Integration across the extended value chain to make profit-driven decisions	Network- and solution-centric decisions; translating innovation into execution
Technology	Disparate transactional systems of record with limited functional support	Push for integration of systems of record; siloed functional solutions	Technologies to support end-to-end supply chain processes; improved data rationalization and integration capability	Technology that enables trading partner connectivity and supports mature processes in the extended supply chain	Innovative technology tools to enable networkwide value creation, risk management and scenario analysis for profitable trade-offs
Organization	Dominance of the sales or manufacturing groups in Organization decision making	Functional leaders within business units, regions or manufacturing; emergence of Centers Of Excellence (COEs)	Cross-functional decision making across internal supply chain; process-focused COEs to enable the business	Head of supply chain participates in corporate strategy as end-to-end process owner	Head of supply chain shapes corporate strategy

Attachment C

C. FISCO CHARACTERIZATION ROADMAP

FISCOCategory	Level 1 React	Level 2 Anticipate	Level 3 Integrate	Level 4 Collaborate	Level 5 Orchestrate
1. Product Sourcing	Basic purchasing agents with no particular product knowledge.	Purchasing agents organized by clinical specialty but without clinical experience.	Purchasing agents organized by clinical specialty but with access to clinical experts. Heavy reliance on GPOs.	Specialized sourcing managers with limited clinical experience. Moderate reliance on GPOs.	Sourcing managers with direct clinical experience focused by clinical specialty. GPO use limited to commodity products.
2. Product Selection/ Standardization	Formulary of frequently ordered items. (No standardization review).	Standardization working groups. Evaluation of vendor products, decision-making, contracting if applicable compliance metrics gathered and reported.	Standardization working groups. Market research, evaluation of vendor, vendor products, RMF review, decision, contracting if applicable; compliance metrics gathered and reported.	Standardization working groups. Standardized clinical pathway ▪ includes equipment to be used, supplies and quantity to be used ▪ not just clinical procedure.	Standardization working groups. Evaluate Impact on patient outcomes and compliance or deviation from clinical pathway. Re- evaluate clinical pathways and modify as necessary.
3. Contracting & Purchasing	Limited use of contracts for purchasing. Typically purchased as spot deals.	Some contracts negotiated with vendors.	Contracts in place but limited compliance to contracts.	Contract compliance at 50% or better.	Almost all products procured through contracted arrangements. Contract compliance level >85%
4. Supplier Relationship Management/ Vendor Performance Management	No vendor performance tracking.	Quarterly Business Reviews where vendor self- reports.	Organization that collects and analyzes vendor performance KPIs.	Organization that collects and analyzes vendor performance KPIs and also evaluates performance with composite Vendor Report Card.	Organization that has composite vendor report card and analyzes vendor performance as an effect on productivity and patient outcome.

FISCO Category	Level 1 React	Level 2 Anticipate	Level 3 Integrate	Level 4 Collaborate	Level 5 Orchestrate
5. Accounts Payable (AP)	Invoices paid through finance managed AP.	Invoices paid through finance managed AP.	Finance driven AP subject to supply chain acceptance criteria.	AP tied to supply chain controlling buyer access to non-standard products.	AP tied to supply chain controlling buyer access to non-standard products.
6. Order Processing (EDI Transaction Codes)	Disparate systems requiring duplicate manual entry/ processes such as phone, fax, and email.	Electronic ordering with select group of preferred vendors. Utilization of basic transaction codes for purchasing (850).	Maximize electronic transmission of purchase orders to vendors (850), purchase order acknowledgement (855), and reconciliation of exceptions (885) daily. Exception management.	Real time 3-way contract price validation, automated reconciliation between purchase orders, and acknowledgements resulting in discrepancy identification and line status updates. Automated invoice reconciliation (810) and payment processing.	Use of process codes to segregate purchase orders, feedback loop for exception management to item master for reduction of exceptions by correcting source detail, predictive analytics around usage needs, automatic order creation based on consumption events.
7. Inventory Management	Manual inventory counts based on par levels. Lack of system automation and integration.	Utilization of inventory management technology. Reliant on manual counts and reconciliation.	Centralized inventory and purchasing management. Strong inventory and demand planning. Planners divided by purchasing groups and usage reports. Point-of-use (POU) systems for medical/ surgical supplies to reduce annual spend for tracked items.	Repeatable approach to excess inventory management and shelf life product management. Utilization of Barcode technology to track inventory. Inventory function linked to master data maintenance group.	Product expiration management with defined process around excess inventory and shelf life management. All products have barcodes for accurate cost and usage tracking. Predictive analytics for demand forecasting.

FISCO Category	Level 1 React	Level 2 Anticipate	Level 3 Integrate	Level 4 Collaborate	Level 5 Orchestrate
8. Receiving	Manual processes with little use of technology, single warehousing location, and limited controls.	Stock purchase order receipts come through the dock, and a manual record keeping of goods and recipients is logged.	Automated receiving process using the EDI (856) Advanced Shipment Notification as the receiver and bypassing the receiving process (for high volume, dependable vendors). Low Unit of Measure.	Robust returned goods process. Utilization of a delivery tracking bar-code with status capability, and scanning/ tracking software to track delivery of products to end-users.	Automated adjustments, electronic item tracking (Barcode or RFID). Staggered supplier delivery management. Expedited delivery process to the unit location.
9. Asset / Equipment Management	Manual tracking of equipment and reactive response to downed equipment.	Two different automated systems; property tracking using Barcode labels and hand held terminals (HHTs). Separate system for servicing equipment. Service contracts primarily used to manage maintenance.	Automated System using passive RFID to locate and service equipment and manage needs for maintenance significant items with resource certifications and predictive budget needs for basic life cycle management.	Automated System using passive and active RFID for tracking and managing service needs for equipment maintenance. Tracks resource certifications and predicts budget and schedule needs for life cycle equipment management.	Automated system provides tracking equipment with passive and active RFID, and comprehensive life cycle management processes for bio- medical and asset management. Uses predictive budgeting and comprehensive maintenance and scheduling. Uses ECRI recall data with auto generation of QC messages and supports QC closures (recall results, costs, procedure impacts, etc.) and future needs assessment.

FISCO Category	Level 1 React	Level 2 Anticipate	Level 3 Integrate	Level 4 Collaborate	Level 5 Orchestrate
10. Supply Chain Risk Management (SCRM)/ Recall Management	Reactive: No SCRM resources. Lack of risk identification and assessment. Ad hoc reaction when an event is triggered.	Aware: No SCRM resources. Lack of risk identification and assessment. Ad hoc reaction when an event is triggered.	Proactive: Formal but functional risk identification, assessment, and risk mitigation program. Proactive risk mitigation strategies. Formal supply chain mapping.	Integrated: Formal and cross-functional risk identification, assessment, and mitigation program. Collaboration with key supply chain partners. Formal supply chain mapping across all critical products.	Resilient: Formal and cross-functional risk identification, assessment, and mitigation program. Collaboration with supply chain partners. Continuous improvement of SCRM programs. Risk metrics included in scorecards. SCRM aligned with organization's objectives and embedded in the culture.
11. System Integration & Architecture	Disparate systems requiring duplicate entry/ processes.	Client-server technology that is interfaced with other logistics systems or support systems and with the General Ledger.	Integrated end-to-end logistics IT system, cloud based with one item master file and visible for both hospital and enterprise use.	IT Logistics systems are fully integrated with POU 70% scan rate. Location aware inventory management will auto generate replenishment based on location decrements and charge at point of issue.	Clinically Integrated Supply Chain (Logistics suite interfaced to EHR and General Ledger). Captures usage, outcomes, supply expense per episode of care, predictive analytics, supply decisions based on clinical pathway standards, and usage (receipt, POU issue, inventory with lot number).
12. KPI / Metrics	Basic supply performance KPIs.	Basic supply performance KPIs managed and tracked/ reported at Enterprise.	Composite metric - combining KPI with correlating/actionable influences.	Composite metric - prescriptive- system observes, reacts, guides and advises.	Composite metrics driven by clinical pathways.

FISCO Category	Level 1 React	Level 2 Anticipate	Level 3 Integrate	Level 4 Collaborate	Level 5 Orchestrate
13. Item Master Management Strategy	Disparate systems requiring duplicate entry/processes, manual item review, and overall lack of automation.	Utilization of ERP item master, and centralized supply chain team. No clear item add, update, or inactivation process in place.	Fully integrated and centralized item master. Utilization of data cleansing and enrichment tools to assist with standardized product part information. Item add process defined and controlled by select group of administrators to ensure quality control.	Normalized item master to remove generalized items, enumerate manufacturer name and part # for active items, and apply UNSPSC classification, and building vendor hierarchy. Key performance indicators are defined and tracked. Strong governance model is established around master data.	Clinically integrated item master, clinically driven description nomenclature, strong value analysis collaboration, and feedback loop from electronic exchange for updates to item detail and pricing.
14. EHR Integration	Manual item master entry to the electronic health record. No item master integration. Lack of strong data entry controls.	Utilization of supply chain item master data, manual upload of product detail, supply chain item description nomenclature, static preference cards and correlating data set.	Daily item master integration, item updates, additions, pricing changes remain reactive, strong process with CDM for item additions as needed.	Enhanced item core that incorporates accurate charge and categorization codes. Barcode detail passed to or maintained within the electronic health record to ensure higher scan rates at the bed side during documentation and accurate patient records.	Clinically Integrated Supply Chain. Usage captured, outcomes captured per episode of care, predictive analytics, supply decisions based on clinical pathway standards and usage (receipt, POU issue, inventory with lot number).
15. Organization Structure	Discrete supply chain teams with limited interaction focused on transactional services.	Mid level supply chain leadership focused on transactional services with responsibility for some strategic initiatives.	SCM team led by manager reporting to member of the corporate leadership team. Focus is on SCM KPIs.	Senior executive led SCM organization driving shared services that are targeting corporate mission.	Clinically driven SCM team led by senior executive with non-core operations outsourced.

FISCO Category		Level 1 React	Level 2 Anticipate	Level 3 Integrate	Level 4 Collaborate	Level 5 Orchestrate
16. System Training		OJT	OJT, Classroom, tutorial training database available, providing how.	OJT, Classroom, tutorial web-based training, providing how.	OJT, Classroom, tutorial web-based training, and integrate functional logistics training, providing how, why and when.	OJT, Classroom, tutorial web-based training, and integrate functional logistics training, providing how, why and when. Prescriptive context sensitive training for actions in user's dashboard.
17. Governance of the Supply Chain		Leadership of disparate SCM functions by disconnected, transactional managers.	Multiple SCM organizations directed by policies but each controlled distinctly.	Single SCM organization led and controlled by manager reporting to non-executive.	Single SCM organization led, controlled and measured by manager reporting to executive team.	Single SCM organization led, controlled and measured by manager at executive team level.

Attachment D

D. PROCUREMENT PROCESSES

The beginning of all supply chain processes is the procurement stage. The exhibit below provides a useful overview of the elements of the procurement process.

The Procurement Process

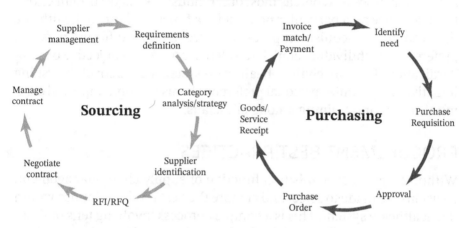

For purposes of this study on procurement in the healthcare field, we will include the following processes within this section. See the exhibit for the processes and their relationships:

- Sourcing
- Product Selection & Standardization
- Contracting
- Supplier Relationship Management
- Accounts Payable

Procurement Processes

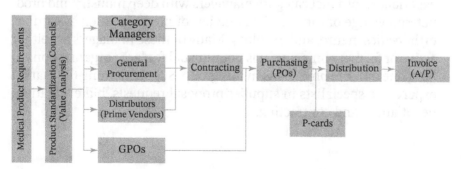

For many supply chain management organizations in the healthcare field this is deemed as the most important and most visible supply chain function. It is through this function that decisions are made regarding which products are to be made available and which are not. For clinicians, who rely on these products to practice their trade, this is a mission impacting decision. In most healthcare organizations, this SCM activity garners the most attention from clinicians.In the healthcare field, perhaps more distinct than any other industries, the personal preferences of products used by professionals (i.e., clinicians) is a major focus of the acquisition process. Whereas most other industries make strident efforts to standardize on a particular product for a functional use, in healthcare the need for the acquisition process to accede to the differing personal preferences of individual clinicians often overrides the objective of standardization. Leading civilian healthcare systems are actively pursuing initiatives to minimize personal preference items through improved communications and training among clinicians.

PROCUREMENT BEST PRACTICES

Within the product acquisition function of supply chain management, decisions are made to select and acquire the best products for use within the healthcare system. This is a complex process involving tens of thousands of products that require both a technical clinic al assessment as well as administrative process oversight. The goal of oversight is to ensure that fairness and compliance are achieved. The target for most best in class healthcare organizations is to have the maximum number of products sourced and purchased through this process. For best practice healthcare organizations, this same process applies for the full range of products sourced including med/surg supplies, medical devices, medical equipment, pharmaceutical, and office supplies.

1. Sourcing

   In best practice organizations, the Sourcing process is led by highly experienced product category managers with deep industry and product knowledge of the specific branches of medicine such as cardiac, orthopedics, neuro, and oncology. Many of these managers are either active or former clinicians. It is not unusual for large organizations to have one or more physicians in this group. Supplementing the market experts are specialists in supplier proposal requests, bid evaluation, negotiating, and contracting.

Sourcing Processes

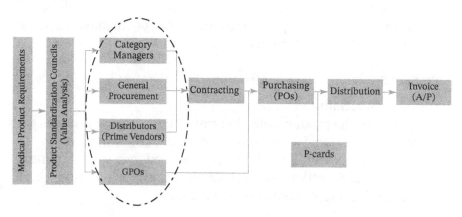

In today's world of careful compliance to international and national regulatory requirements as well as local corporate standards, the assurance of fairness and compliance in the process is supreme. Best practice organizations invest considerable time and effort to ensure that all sourcing activities comply with these standards. The cost of non-compliance can be very high. Sourcing initiatives that are challenged by disgruntled bidders can lead to litigation, civil penalties, and considerable rework.

* *Group Purchasing Organizations*
  Many if not all healthcare organizations outsource some (and sometimes all) of the sourcing function to a Group Purchasing Organization (GPO).[12,13] There are various reasons for this ranging from access to highly specialized resources to sharing volumes with others to garner market leverage. There is also a regulatory rationale in that GPOs have been afforded a safe harbor provision enabling them to receive rebates from suppliers, a capability not available to individual hospital systems due to anti-kickback regulations. GPOs:
  * carryout market assessments
  * assessing supplier competencies and capabilities
  * engage in strategic sourcing efforts,
  * support supplier evaluation and supply base reduction efforts
  * support product standardization a and efforts through clinical councils

  A number of healthcare systems have realized the benefit of establishing their own internal GPOs, which offer them greater direct control over the products sourced and the retention of margins.[14]

When conducting sourcing programs within best practice organizations, leaders have access to information systems that control the process as well as providing a rich data pool to make informed product selection decisions.

2. Product Selection & Standardization

* *Selection & Standardization*
  As part of the product selection process, healthcare is characterized by an extensive internal process to <u>standardize</u> and rationalize the number of products that are used for a specific clinical procedure. Supplier base reduction is a characteristic of high performing supply chain organizations.

  Standardization Processes

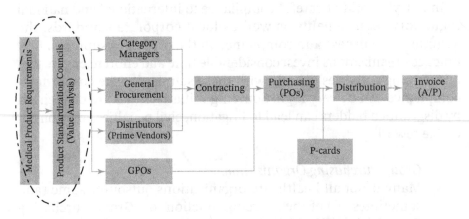

The process employed to assess products has several names within the civilian healthcare field. Sometimes referred to as 'value analysis' or 'product standardization', best practice programs convene on a regular basis a team of clinicians (physicians, nurses, and technologists) and clinic al program staff, and administrative staff. This team reviews all proposals for the introduction of new products to assure that they provide benefit to both medical practice and financial objectives. Their recommendations have a direct impact on the decisions regarding product use. For pharmaceuticals, pharmacy and therapeutics committees (P&T) serve this role.

We note, however, that the term 'standardization' has different meanings to different people. Within the healthcare supply chain management field, we often use the term 'product standardization' when we actually mean 'product rationalization'. *Rationalization is the process of <u>limiting</u> the number of products that are used in* *order to focus more on the products that deliver the most value.* This is an important endeavor designed to maximize the value from the choice and use of medical products. Yet in some organizations, the product standardization process is simply endorsing the use of a particular product within the healthcare system based on its market suitability – and doing nothing to limit product proliferation. Standardization is not "merely" about limiting SKUs – but about supplier base reduction, operational efficiencies, and trust gained as we limit the number of companies with which we do business.

Product standardization is simply the process of developing and implementing <u>acceptability</u> standards based on the consensus of all stakeholders. Ultimately, it is the test of market suitability for a product. We have many examples of such usage of standardization including the infamous, "Good Housekeeping Seal of Approval." This just means that a product is technically acceptable for use as intended. The FDA does this; medical professional associations do this; as do manufacturers.

Important is the effort to manage the proliferation of similar products that may yield varying medical outcomes. Endemic in medicine, however, is the acceptance of a clinician's personal preference for a particular product (and manufacturer) that may differ from the consensus of his or her colleagues. Too often such preference, while not justified, is tolerated. Supply chain managers point out that such proliferation leads to quality issues. Excessive products in use lead to the following:

- Added complexity in supply chain and clinical services
- More product use errors
- Reduced contract leverage
- Reduced service levels from suppliers
- Additional cost for sourcing, ordering, and storing

Through the efforts of value analysis teams and other similar programs, leading hospital systems limit product proliferation. In addition to examining new product introductions, these teams also review the appropriateness of all products in use. Given the thousands of products in use within a hospital setting, such reviews of products already in use can be overwhelming. Policies are established to manage the extent of such reviews to balance resource efforts.

Standardization efforts for both new and existing products are intended to result in several positive outcomes for the healthcare system including:

- Assurance that the best products are used in clinical practice
- Optimization of the number of products sourced and inventoried according to financial and clinical needs
- Increased leverage when negotiating contracts with suppliers
- New Technology Assessment

* *New Technology Assessment*
  Given the large number of new medical products approved and introduced to the market each year, some control measures are needed to ensure that the best and most appropriate products are used. This is done through a <u>New Technology Assessment</u> process. Without such controls the number of products within an organization's product master could expand exponentially. Consequently, leading organizations as part of the standardization process conduct a special assessment for new technology. Often the review process is separated into two streams:

  - Transformative new products
  - Minor new products

  Best practice organizations have formal business processes for conducting these standardization/value analysis programs as well as information tools for controlling the process, providing product rigorous objective databases, and assisting with the decision-making.

3. Contracting and Purchasing

   Once that the decision is made to source a particular product and a vendor has been chosen to provide the product, the sourcing team addresses its attention to formalizing the business relationship in a contract. Such contracts specify terms such as:

   - Contract term and renewal process
   - Product specifications
   - Service and delivery expectations
   - Purchase volume commitments
   - Pricing
   - Supplier and Buyer obligations
   - Dispute resolution processes

Contracting & Purchasing Processes

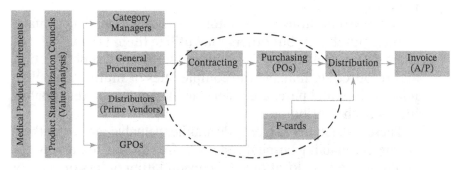

These contracts form the basis of the supply chain management relationship between the supplier and the hospital system. Details of the contractual terms are typically uploaded into a special contract management module of the ERP system used by the hospital. This module is used to track all activity between the supplier and the buying organization pertaining to the products under contract. Importantly, it is key to assuring that the pricing provided in supplier invoices is aligned to the terms stipulated in the contract. In essence it provides a complete history of the intent as well as the actual activity between the supplier and the buying organization.

With a contract in place the next step in the process is to affect the purchase of the product through an order to the supplier. Based on demands determined either by inventory requirements set through the ERP or an immediate direct demand from an authorized buyer within the hospital, a formal purchase order is transmitted to the supplier. This is a standard process within most ERP systems. In best practice organizations such orders are transmitted electronically between the buyer and supplier. Well established e-commerce procedures are typically in place to control and monitor the order process. For best practice organizations, over 95% of purchase orders are issued electronically with no paper documents created in the process.

* Distributors (Prime Vendors)
Many healthcare systems will rely on distributors (such as Cardinal, Owens & Minor, and Medline) to consolidate their orders acting as intermediary in the process. On behalf of the healthcare system, they supply a broad range of products from a broad range of suppliers. Distributors enable one-stop shopping. In addition, they supplement the product array with privately branded products

that compete with major global brands, although typically for commodity type products.

Some systems utilize distributor services for a small percentage of their purchases, but others may utilize them for a very large share. Often smaller systems, without the internal sophistication and resources to manage the complexities of multiple supplier relationships and purchase orders, are dependent on the capabilities of such distributors.

These distributors also provide another valuable service for their customers enabling hospital systems to free up on-site warehouses and other storage locations. By consolidating orders on a daily basis and directing them to specific areas of the hospital, they create a just in time (JIT) solution that saves facility space and inventory costs but comes at a marked up premium.

* *Self-Distribution*

Large healthcare systems often source and purchase directly from manufacturers thus eliminating the expenses of a distributor. Through their internal processes and staff resources, they place purchase orders and receive products in centralized warehouses for self-distribution within their operations. They may order full container loads of products (often low value commodity products) directly from factories around the world. This type of scale and direct purchasing achieves significant net savings to the system budget by elimination or replacement of distribution fees by internally managing these activities

* *Purchasing Cards (P-Cards)*

An alternative to this organized contracted process is ad hoc purchasing at the discretion of individual clinicians and others. Often purchasing cards (p- cards) provided by the hospital are used to conduct these purchases. P-Cards provide far fewer controls and assurances of quality results. They provide simplicity and ease to quickly purchase products through B2C (business to consumer) on-line websites such as Amazon or through any vendor without a purchase order. Personnel can purchase items quickly without going through the established procurement procedures. While providing ease of use the lack of controls greatly limits the quality outcomes available from an effective supply chain management organization. Most leading healthcare organizations would prefer to reduce the use of p-cards in favor of formal contracted relationships with suppliers.

4. Supplier Relationship Management and Quality Assurance

A hospital system will typically have thousands of suppliers. All are important. Some, however, are more critical than others in strategic activities of the healthcare system. Often the largest 100 suppliers may account for over 90% of the total purchase spend. These suppliers need special attention and oversight. Leading organizations establish a formal Supplier Relationship Management system for this purpose. For a supplier to be an effective supplier to a hospital and for a hospital to be an effective buyer for a supplier, there must be effective communication and understanding between them. To achieve this, best practice organizations provide suppliers with limited access to the organization's ERP system and conduct review meetings with suppliers. These supplier management meetings allow suppliers to provide feedback to hospital staff about market developments while hospital staff share their strategic and operational plans. The information sharing that comes from these review meetings leads to products and services that are better designed for the hospital's needs and service performance that generates higher quality performance.

Within ERP and supplier purchasing systems, supplier relationship management tools are available to support this requirement. These systems enable suppliers to directly update product catalogs resulting in faster and more accurate information.

As part of supplier management in these procurement systems are processes to ensure product quality that meets the needs of clinicians. With thousands and thousands of sourced products from global manufacturing sites, control of quality cannot be left to suppliers alone. Leading hospital systems have established quality assurance teams to ascertain that products arriving from suppliers meet all contracted specifications. This includes not only the products themselves but compliance with quality manufacturing practices such as hygiene, child labor law adherence, and others.

5. Accounts Payable

Many organizations will place the accounts payable function within the finance department. However, in healthcare given that the vast majority of payables are in reference to product purchases, one of the best tools for supply chain management practitioners to control the spend is to also have control of the payables. This provides a logical and powerful tool to drive compliance with contractual spending and reduce maverick spending.

Accounts Payable Process

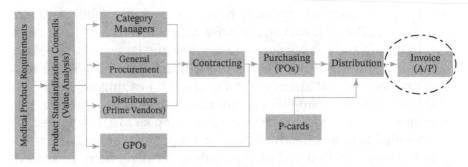

Through this process alignment SCM staff will have direct view of those in compliance and those who are not. This provides a more effective means of influencing change. As well, with a direct connection to the payment terms of the supplier contracts, SCM staff can manage strategies for early payment of invoices to gain maximum discounts.

While the finance department has overall governance for the financial affairs of the corporation, they can still have control of the overall accounts payable spend through approvals for global payments, it is the SCM staff that can best manage the individual payable transactions.

Attachment E

E. BEST PRACTICE ASSET MANAGEMENT CRITERIA

In our evaluation of Asset Management, we have found that:

- An asset management organization that manages the life cycle of nonexpendable moveable property designated by price threshold or policy.
- Asset database is managed by equipment experts and updates the financial database.
- Every managed item is assigned a standard nomenclature.
- An individual is assigned accountability and responsibility for every item.
- Every item has an assigned a location (may be general location for lesser items).
- A means is in place to investigate and assess pecuniary liability to persons who damage or lose assets due to gross negligence.
- Scheduled and unscheduled checks/inventories are conducted to validate accountability of assets.

- A procedure is in effect to identify people having accountability and/or responsibility for equipment prior to their departure from the organization and to ensure that accountability is transferred.
- All accountable assets are identified with a readable/scannable unique identifier that relates to the asset database. Identifier may be Barcode or RFID depending on the characteristics of the item.
- Leased or borrowed assets are included in the asset database with a code to identify the owner.
- Assets are categorized as maintenance significant or non-maintenance significant. Maintenance significant items identify the source of maintenance, e.g. biomedical maintenance, contract maintenance etc.
- A user's manual and maintenance manual is available for every maintenance significant item.
- All scheduled and unscheduled maintenance is done on a work order. The asset record for maintenance significant items includes or accesses the maintenance history of each item.
- All new maintenance significant equipment is given an acceptance inspection when received. Users are trained in the use of new equipment as appropriate.
- All maintenance whether in-house or by contract is performed by personnel certified and trained to work on the asset.
- A means is in place to gather recalls or corrective maintenance requirements which leads to a work order for appropriate action. All suspended items are clearly marked to prevent use.
- Common repair parts are identified for each maintenance significant item and stocked based on criteria and number of similar assets.
- Criteria are in place for each maintenance significant item to plan for replacement based on obsolescence, time in service, loss/damage, or excessive maintenance cost.
- A collaborate effort is established including logistics and clinical personnel to identify new technologies, methodologies and the state of the art of medical equipment.
- Existing and required equipment are evaluated for IT interoperability requirements and patient record interface.
- New equipment requirements are identified by a formal process. Level of approval, and financing options may be dependent of cost thresholds.
- A formal process is in place to prioritize new equipment requirements, based on cost thresholds, so that the most important requirements are procured within budget constraints.

Attachment F

F. BEST PRACTICES FOR RECALL MANAGEMENT

Based on interviews with leading organizations in the healthcare industry, academic literature , and industry reports, we have identified best practices that organizations can use to improve their readiness for potential recalls and the effectiveness of the recall management process:

- Understand the recall standards and regulations governing the industry.
- Understand the organization's product portfolio and a product's potential for future recall:
  - Understand the characteristics of products in the product portfolio and classify them based on low versus high risk. Risk may be based on complexity of specifications, quality, number of suppliers, supply complexity, availability of substitutes, etc.
  - Assess the likelihood and severity of a potential product recall for a given product.
  - Identify and maintain a registry of alternative products for a given product, particularly for the high-risk products.
- Develop traceability in the supply chain.
- Ability to identify the root cause of a problem.
- Tracking of lots, batches, and link to specific suppliers and distributors/customers.
- Collect information about the likely destination for products that have already been provided to end-users, who may reside outside of the organization's walls,
- Set early warning signals through, for example, consumer complaints and reporting, routine quality control on problematic products, or trend analysis on problematic products, and monitor trends.
- Develop a recall plan for a given organizational division.
  - Identify recall management team or committee (members, departments).
  - Define each member's roles and responsibilities.
  - Include contact information of each team member and backup personnel for each team member.

- Communication:
    - Communicate with consumers. Document communication.
    - Communicate with vendors, distributors, retailers, and logistics service providers. Document communication.
    - Communicate with FDA. Document communication.
- Determine, set, and execute the reverse logistics process to retrieve the product.
- Determine, set, and execute the product disposal process (e.g., incineration).
- Conduct mock recalls to assess the effectiveness of the recall management process in place.
- Provide documented recall management process to legal team.
- Set metrics to evaluate the recall management process, such as: number of days to report to manufacturer, number of days to report to the FDA, response rate from customers, percentage of recalled product, time from notification to full recall, or number of days to complete recall.

Attachment G

G. ORGANIZATION SUPPORT, DESIGN AND GOVERNANCE FOR FISCO

An enterprise characterization is insufficient without reference to the processes for commanding and controlling its activities. These processes have three requisites: an organization structure designed to facilitate effective decision-making across the enterprise, a governance model to dictate how, when and by whom decisions are made affecting the enterprise, and thirdly, access to qualified staff to do the work. Without all three components the enterprise cannot function effectively.

These three requisite dimensions of an enterprise are embodied in FISCO organizations that we have studied. While these characteristics do not deviate from best practice organization design principles, surprisingly many healthcare organizations have not yet reached the best practice. We recognize, however, that such organization and governance shifts are evolutionary. Such changes cannot be imposed too quickly or without careful preparation. The key point to ensure is that the organizational decision makers have a clear vision for the future organization design and its governance and that they communicate it effectively.

1. ORGANIZATION BEST PRACTICES

Organization design (i.e., structure) has a direct impact on the effectiveness of an enterprise to carry out its mission. The required design must comprise the full set of supply chain management functions together with the relationships that connect them. This does not mean that all SCM functions need to be performed within the same organization. There are variants to design that may be most appropriate to the extended organization. These variants are tied to the different types of connecting relationships as shown in the exhibit below.

- Direct line control
- Indirect staff control
- Outsource to a third party
- Shared corporate service
- Independent functions with policies to guide management

Organization Design Options

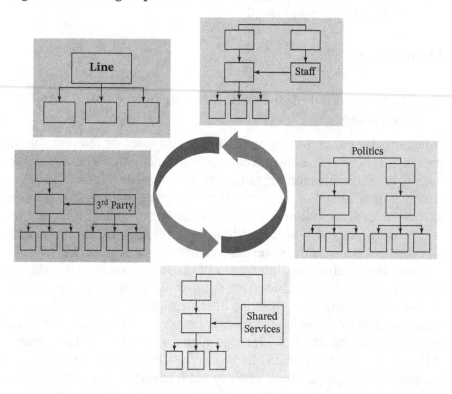

Governance is the management process of commanding and controlling the actions of organizational units. Governance styles may range from oversight of performance such as done through management boards through to minute functional control of all decisions by a supervising superior. Good governance considers many factors.

In the following sections we describe the best practices in organization design and governance in the healthcare supply chain field.

2. ORGANIZATION DESIGN

Our studies of FISCO organizations have shown that there is not a standard organization design. Some organizations utilize a shared services organization, others through a conventional line organization, yet others through a staff organization.

In all cases, the organization design is successful when combined with strong executive support from within the organization. This requires explicit commitments from either CEO or Board level leaders endorsing the role of the FISCO and commanding full support from all other parts of the organization. This expression of commitment is an absolute necessity for the FISCO to effectively conduct its mission that will regularly cross organizational boundaries and responsibilities.

Line organization structures are typically used in small to mid-sized healthcare systems. They offer a straightforward solution where conventional command and control practices apply. Often such organizations would report directly to the organization CEO or to another executive that reports to the CEO. This provides a high level of executive oversight enabling influence over a broad set of medical programs.

Generally, in the larger healthcare systems, the preferred organization structure is a form of shared services.[15] This provides the ability of the FISCO to tailor its services for a broad and diverse set of users. A shared services organization operates like an arms-length services provider such as IBM or Accenture with the capability to meet a wide variety of client needs. These providers can be expected to operate successfully in different geographic regions with different service requirement profiles.

Best practice shared services providers establish formalized service level agreements (SLAs) with their clients. These SLAs specify the type of services provided and their organizational scope along with appropriate performance targets. In healthcare supply chain management, the services are typically defined according to the business processes with the shared services organization undertaking some or all of the SCM processes.

The key to success that best practice systems have discovered in whichever organization design is chosen is to include as many of the SCM business processes under a single management structure. In supply chain management value increases as the number of business functions are managed by a single party in an integrated manner. This is the underlying premise of the FISCO concept.

3. GOVERNANCE

Governance and organization design go hand in hand in driving the performance of best practice supply chain management enterprises. Good governance is a skill and capability that leading organizations, no matter what industry, strive to achieve. It leads to responsiveness, fairness, and ultimately effective management of large complex organizations. This applies to large publicly traded corporations, governments, and international organizations. Consequently, even great organization designs without effective governance will fail.

Good governance requires leadership. In best practice organizations, and in particular supply chain management organizations, the leaders must act as orchestrators who oversee and direct the operations. The orchestra leader must intimately know all aspects of the enterprise and just as a musical orchestra leader can detect when one section is out of tune or off the beat, the SCM orchestrator must be sensitive to disconnects and respond to them.

Experts in the governance field will often characterize good governance as having the following characteristics:

- Adheres to the rule of law
- Transparent
- Responsive
- Accountable
- Participative

In best practice healthcare supply chain management organizations these good governance practices apply. In particular, when dealing with physician needs, best practice organizations carefully balance the needs of individual physicians with the broader needs of the organization as a whole, which seeks standardization to achieve quality and fiscal goals.

To achieve this balance, best practice organizations ensure that physicians and other clinicians are directly involved in the leadership structure of the supply chain management organization. Decisions regarding product choice and use should always have significant clinical involvement. Some supply chain management organizations appoint clinicians to senior leadership positions. Others establish standing committees with significant clinical involvement that make recommendations to support SCM decision-making. Best practice organizations establish formal processes for these regular value analysis reviews.

Notes

1. Gosselt, R.W. (2012). A Maturity Model Roadmap for Implementing TOGAF. In Proceedings of the 17th Twente Student Conference on IT.

2 Adapted from "Towards a framework for enterprise architecture analytics," by Schmidt, R., Wißotzki, M., Jugel, D., Möhring, M., Sandkuhl, K., & Zimmermann, A. (2014, September). *2014 IEEE 18th International Enterprise Distributed Object Computing Conference Workshops and Demonstrations* (pp. 266–275). IEE.

3 Bradley, R. V., Pratt, R. M., Byrd, T. A., Outlay, C. N., & Wynn, D. E., Jr. (2012). Enterprise architecture, IT effectiveness and the mediating role of IT alignment in US hospitals. *Information Systems Journal.*, *22*(2), 97–127.

4 Gosselt, R.W. (2012). A Maturity Model Roadmap for Implementing TOGAF. In Proceedings of the 17th Twente Student Conference on IT. (p. 2).

5 Rob van der Meulen. (2017). 5 Stages of Logistics Maturity. Retrieved from `https://www.gartner.com/smarterwithgartner/5-stages-of-logistics-maturity/`

6 Qi, Y., Huo, B., Wang, Z., & Yeung, H. Y. J. (2017, March). The impact of operations and supply chain strategies on integration and performance. *International Journal of Production Economics*, *185*, 162–174. `https://doi.org/10.1016/j.ijpe.2016.12.028`

7 Abdulsalam, Y., Gopalakrishnan, M., Maltz, A., & Schneller, E. (2015). The emergence of consolidated service centers in health care. *Journal of Business Logistics*, *36*(4), 321–334.

8 Rob van der Meulen. (2017). Op. Cit.

9 These number signify EDI transaction types: 850 = Purchase Order, 855 = Purchase Order Acknowledgment, and 810 = Invoice

10 The maturity model for Supply Chain Risk Management was adapted from the Supply Chain Risk Leadership Council's SCRM Maturity Model and is aligned with Gartner's Maturity Model.

11 GS1 US. (2015, October 28). Drug Supply Chain Security Act (DSCSA)—for Pharmaceutical Manufacturers: Who Can Help?

12 Burns, L. R., & Lee, J. A. (2008). Hospital purchasing alliances: Utilization, services, and performance. *Health Care Manage Rev*, *33*(3), 203–215.

13 Schneller, E. S., & Scmeltzer, L. R. (2006). *Strategic management of the health care aupply chain*. Jossey-Bass.

14 Abdulsalam, Y., Gopalakrishnan, M., Maltz, A., & Schneller, E. (2015). The emergence of consolidated service centers in health care. *Journal of Business Logistics*, *36*(4), 321–334.

15 Ibid.

Appendix 2: Clinician, Supplier, and Buyer Working as One to Improve Patient Outcomes

A Case Study by Ian B. Shepherd*
MCIPS
Plymouth Hospitals NHS Trust

The benefits described within this case study have been delivered because of excellent working relationships based on trust, openness and sustained mutual commitment. With our suppliers in the cardiothoracic market we have demonstrated that we truly are working together in partnership. This is the second edition of the case study "Clinician, Supplier, and Buyer Working as One to Improve Patient Outcomes" which was presented at the Ministerial Conference on 14 May 2002.

Clinician, Supplier and Buyer Working as One to Improve Patient Outcomes

---

*Ian Shepherd was Lead of Procurement & Logistics at Plymouth Hospital NHS Trust at the time this case was written. Ian led a groundbreaking process, documented in this case, that set the foundation for stakeholder engagement for the health sector. The revealed strategy, processes and thinking provide insights into the continued dynamic relationships between and among stakeholders. Provided is insight for the development of a robust supply management program. The orchestration lens for a health sector supply chain manager is revealed. The challenge remains – across organizations and their systems and across nations.

Executive Summary

This case study highlights the significant benefits derived from the implementation of a patient focussed purchasing strategy. The traditional approach to purchasing in the NHS is to either utilise national framework agreements or invite tenders for a specified volume of a single commodity. The approach adopted at Plymouth Hospitals NHS Trust was to analyse and segment the market by patient activity, supplier sales value and expenditure category – maximising synergies for consolidation and aggregation of demand. This was undertaken with support of clinical colleagues, as their role was vital in ensuring commitment to the procurement process from exploring conceptual ideals through to the award and subsequent monitoring of contracts. Having gained an understanding of clinical need and market opportunity, our primary aim was to influence expenditure to enable 10-15% more patients to be treated within the existing budget. Our success in exceeding our objectives in meeting this challenge is described here.

1 Background

Plymouth Hospitals, NHS Trust ("the Trust") provides general hospital services to a local population of 430,000 in Plymouth, West Devon, South Hams and East Cornwall. At Derriford Hospital, the Trust also provides a number of specialist hospital services to more than 1.6 million people in Devon and Cornwall and in some cases to bordering areas of Dorset and Somerset. The main specialist or tertiary services provided are:

- Cardiothoracic surgery and cardiology
- Neurosurgery and neurology
- Renal transplant surgery
- Some specialist cancer treatments
- Plastic surgery and burns

The Trust's vision for the next 5 years is to be recognised as a leading centre of excellence for a wide range of general hospital services and complex specialist services for people living within the South West Peninsula. The Trust has established an agenda to work with its health partners to ensure that services are planned and delivered around the needs of the patient.

Of the Trust's specialist services, the South West Cardiothoracic Centre represented the biggest commercial challenge given its growth potential and the opportunity to influence significant expenditure. Colleagues described it as the Trust's hotspot!

The South West Cardiothoracic Centre opened late 1997 treating 274 patients as finished consultant episodes (FCE's). Since then the center centre has increased the number of patients treated each year to 2,105 (FCE's), during 2001. More patients have been able to benefit from coronary artery bypass grafts and other heart operations. In addition, the centre is leading on the introduction of a new day-case technique for performing coronary angioplasty and stenting on patients with heart disease. The standard approach is to gain access to the coronary artery from the groin (femoral artery), which involved an overnight stay for the patient. The new procedure involves introducing a tube through the wrist (radial artery) – a procedure known as Transradial Intervention. The risk of bleeding is reduced, patients can regain movement earlier and they can often go home the same day, helping to reduce waiting times for other patients. "The first patient sat up and read a newspaper within 30 minutes of the procedure and he was discharged without complication in less than 4 hours" says Dr Joe Motwani, Consultant Cardiologist. "I now use this route of access in over 90% of patients and we are using the procedure more extensively than any other centre in the UK".

In the most recent survey, November, (2003/2004) the centre was rated as the top hospital in the UK on its combined results for all heart operations, according to the Society of Cardiac Surgeons. The mortality rate for the period April 1998 – March 2000 was the lowest at just 2.3%. This compares with a national average of 4.0%.

In the last year we have implanted 430 pacemakers for bradycardia indications (new implant rate about 700 per million). The centre prescribes using the British Pacing and Electrophysiological Group guidelines. Many patients have additional arrhythmia; particularly atrial fibrillation and we have actively developed a programme of using new devices with anti-atrial fibrillation therapy.

As part of our collaboration with our suppliers we have had a productive research programme and are about to publish a study into onset mechanisms of atrial fibrillation and flutter after coronary bypass graft surgery. For this, the centre used an advanced dual chamber pacemaker with excellent Holter functions. In addition, we are now pacing for heart failure with bi-ventricular pacing systems.

Dr Marshall and Dr Haywood, Consultant Cardiologists, both participated in the Multi Site Stimulation in Cardiomyopathy (MUSTIC) trial, making Plymouth one of the 17 European Centres at the forefront of this clinical development. Exhibit A.2.1 shows that expenditure has been brought in line with budget while treating more patients.

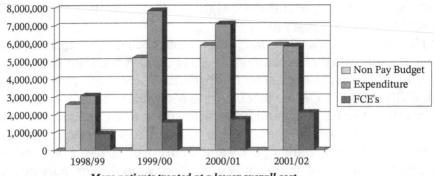

More patients treated at a lower overall cost

Exhibit A.2.1: Budget Expenditure, And Patient Activity, Cardiothoracic Center (In Pounds Sterling).

2 The Perennial Challenge

The perennial challenge facing most Trusts is to treat more patients, sooner, while improving clinical outcomes, within a finite budget. Increasingly, the vast array of products required to meet this demand are subjected to dynamic market forces where the introduction of innovative devices attracts premium prices. Commercial aims to meet this challenge were to:

- Widen purchasing influence over core expenditure with increased commitment to contracts
- Improve supply chain operational efficiency
- Reduce our supplier base
- Rationalise catalogue line items
- Manage the introduction of new technologies
- Reduce inventory value and associated replenishment costs
- Ensure 100% stock availability
- Generate savings of at least £800,000 per annum

In consideration of these primary aims, we set ourselves the overall goal of treating 10-15% more patients within the existing budget. Subsequently, the Trust's Purchasing and Logistics Strategy was developed as a by-product of taking this approach.

3 Purchasing Strategy

In support of realising our aims, the Trust Board endorsed our vision and mission statements as:

- Vision
  "Development and management of an integrated supply chain optimising total costs of acquisition, possession and use"

■ Mission

"To provide all customers with the timely delivery of the right quality and quantity of products and services at the lowest overall cost"

Recognising that we did not have the skills or resources available to influence all of the Trust's non-pay expenditure, our initial focus was to meet the needs of the South West Cardiothoracic Centre. Demand for treatment of coronary heart disease was growing at a rate in excess of 30% per year and the centre's budget would need to increase to approximately 10% of the Trust's annual revenue, to meet this need. Furthermore, following a pareto analysis of expenditure, just 180 key products and eight of the Trust's top twenty suppliers accounted for 60% of the Cardiothoracic Centre's budget.

Exhibit A.2.2 represents an analysis of the Trust's supplier portfolio. It links expenditure of each operating division within a corporate entity, by aggregating sales values. This revised and validated data were then used to identify the Trust's top fifty suppliers. However, compiling this list highlighted that 150 suppliers represented 79% of expenditure and 10% of transactional volume. At the other end of the spectrum 1,500 suppliers represented 10% of expenditure and 70% of transactional volume. In developing objectives in pursuit of partnership relationships it was essential to determine our starting point and understand the relative strategic significance of existing and prospective suppliers. Our objective was to develop partnerships with a number of category 'A' suppliers ensuring sales growth, while consolidating transactional activity and significantly reducing the number of category 'D' suppliers.

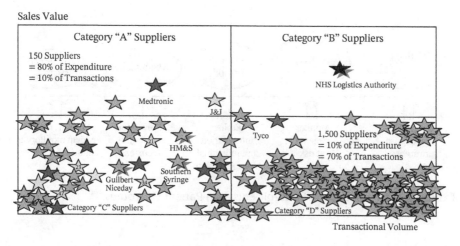

Exhibit A.2.2: Analysis of the Trust's supplier portfolio.

The added advantage of pursuing a different approach with the Cardiothoracic Centre was that suppliers in this market were few and therefore potentially more manageable and in most cases suppliers were able to meet the majority of the Trust's demand for key categories of products from within their corporate portfolios. In addition, niche suppliers were already known to the Trust and we had a good understanding of their potential for growth.

Our overriding strategic aim was to test and develop the concept of partnership working from both the clinical and commercial perspective. Our criteria for appointing suppliers to this programme were:

- Year on year commitment to improve clinical outcomes
- Sound research and development track record with innovative product improvement programmes for the future
- Robust communication and information links
- Willingness to share information on costs
- Commitment to training, education and development of clinical and managerial staff
- Consistent high quality customer service
- Process efficiency and cost containment in working towards e-business solutions
- Shared risk and benefits associated with market growth

Exhibit A.2.3 is a summary of how one of our key supplier's strategic focus influences patient outcomes, maximising the use of new technologies and therapies as the enabler. By working together with our clinical colleagues and suppliers, we hoped to influence and improve the quality of life for patients with coronary heart disease and reduce the overall cost of each finished consultant episode.

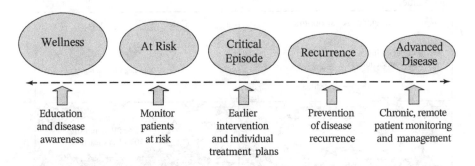

Exhibit A.2.3: Influence of Strategic Focus on Patient Outcomes.

4 Market Analysis and Segmentation

Continuous monitoring of market dynamics is essential for products that have continued growth or have yet to reach maturity, given that new entrants are launched at premium prices and in a competitive market, mature products are priced to protect or grow market share. Exhibit A.2.4 shows the dynamic nature of the Cardiothoracic market. This serves to further illustrate the point that new product launches or additional features to existing products, dependant upon there positioning within the lifecycle, are often priced at premium rates. The challenge for the buyer is to work with clinical staff to determine whether these new devices provide differentiated clinical outcomes and therefore represent value for money. We are currently working on two business cases to determine the benefits of drug eluting stents and cardiac resynchronisation therapies. If these are proven to be cost effective we will then have the added challenge of convincing commissioners of health care and budget holders of the need to change their outlook by focussing holistically on budget provision, to meet these new treatment regimes.

By working closer with our clinical colleagues we not only gained a better understanding of their needs but also used this opportunity to improve our knowledge of the products and suppliers within the cardiovascular market. Examples of the level of detail we believed was required in understanding product usage and the stability and growth in demand for products, is demonstrated in Exhibits A.2.4 and A.2.5:

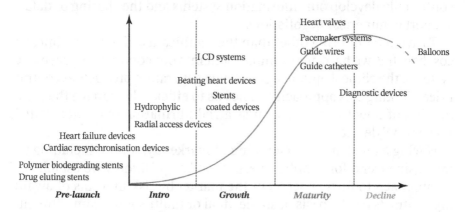

Exhibit A.2.4: Product lifecycle.

The interesting dynamic here is that clinical staff are pioneering transradial intervention. This change in clinical practice utilises niche products where technological advancements are producing smaller lumen sizes in the hope that this will improve patient outcomes. Products are increasingly being coated with hydrophilic agents to improve speed of access and reduce the risk of infection. As the market develops these products should see sustained growth and this commercial opportunity is not lost in our relationships with niche suppliers. The challenge we have set them is to provide product improvements with pricing to match established equivalent items.

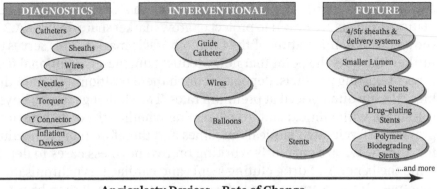

Angioplasty Devices – Rate of Change

Exhibit A.2.5: Angioplasty Devices – Rate of Change.

At the opposite end of the spectrum we have a decreasing need for balloon catheters given that interventional cardiologists are continuing to increasingly use direct stenting to reduce overall procedure costs. Managing market share and leveraging these commercial opportunities for maximum benefit is not possible without accurate up to date information. In recognising this need we have implemented plans to continually develop our information systems and the sharing of data to support commercial negotiations.

To avoid monitoring other than the significant differential clinical or cost benefits, we have, for example, built into our contract for pacemaker systems, the clinical option to select next generation products at contract prices. Taking this approach enables us to efficiently manage the introduction of new therapies, such as atrial fibrillation with Medtronic's Prevent AF device.

Having gained an understanding of market dynamics, including the increasing trend for supplier mergers and acquisitions, we established an approach to further segment the market by risk in terms of awarding contracts on the basis of single, dual or multi-source commitments. Duration of contract term was an added consideration given our desire to reduce administrative costs and to develop longer-term commitments based on partnership relationships.

Following this detailed analysis of market conditions our conclusions were to award;

■ a seven year single source contract for the supply of generic commodity items (cardiology diagnostic devices). Items in this category would not be influenced by technological change (stable market). Given strong competition in the NHS market this represented minimal risk. Price would be easily managed by benchmarking and cost analysis, with performance reviewed annually;

■ a twelve month contract for the supply of catheter mounted stents, in the first instance, given that this was considered to be a highly volatile market in terms of falling prices, growth in demand and technological advancement. There was a prior agreement with clinical colleagues that as the market matured, we would increasingly commit larger volumes to a primary supplier and ultimately move to a dual source contract. This has recently been honoured with the award of contracts for a three year commitment. The added complication in managing this market in the future, is around the introduction of premium priced drug eluting and coated stents.

Exhibit A.2.6 shows the considerable change in demand for stents, with future growth anticipated at 30% per year. The added dynamic in managing products in this category of expenditure is the variance in clinical preference as to whether to pre-dilate vessels with a balloon or to direct stent the lesion. Sustained monitoring and annual negotiation has seen unit prices fall from £800 to £250 per stent. Moving forward we awarded:

■ a five-year multi-source contract for the supply of mechanical and tissue heart valves. The overriding dynamic in this contract was that products are in a stable market, but there was a desire within the Centre to undertake a comprehensive randomised research project. This was agreed as part of the procurement process with the award of contracts, including the provision of significant research funding coterminous with contract expiry. It was believed that by taking this approach we would develop increasingly closer relationships with our core suppliers
■ a two-year dual-source contract for pacemaker systems. The primary supplier had previously acquired the secondary supplier

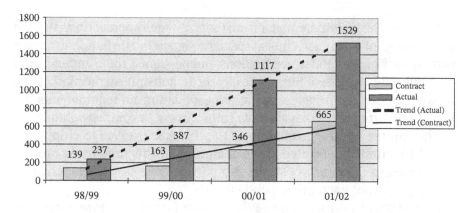

Exhibit A.2.6: Contract vs. actual procedure volumes for stents—March 2002.

and risk was considered to be minimal given that separate research and development platforms and manufacturing processes were retained. Following successful completion of the initial term, the option to extend the contract period by a further three to five years was recently granted

In taking this approach we have significantly reduced the number of primary suppliers serving the Cardiothoracic Centre and further rationalisation is to continue given sustained performance monitoring leading to partnership status. However, in recognising this change there was still a need to provide access to new and/or innovative enhancements to products. Evaluation of items in this category were conducted within a maximum 10% of total sales value. This flexibility in the evaluation of products was easily accommodated given the growth in demand for interventional angioplasty and cardiac rhythm management therapies.

5 The Procurement Process

The procurement process was not unlike any other invitation to tender, except for real emphasis on:

- Clinical outcomes and growth in demand for specific treatment regimes
- Commitment for the long term with mutual benefits
- Product quality and reliability of performance in use
- After sales support services
- Added value services e.g. training, education and research
- Performance management
- Information sharing
- Reducing costs and of course price

However, the key differentiator from the traditional approach was that the lead consultant from each clinical specialty signed the invitation to tender, participated in pre-tender negotiations and co-signed the contract award schedule. The purpose of this was to clearly demonstrate to the market that we were serious about aggregating and consolidating our requirements and would support this through absolute commitment to contract volumes.

The sample contract schedule at Exhibit A.2.7 serves to emphasise that the commitment stated at the beginning of the purchasing process is reflected in the contract award. All parties have signed the schedule in recognition of each other's obligations.

Postcontract performance reviews have further demonstrated our sustained commitment to contract volumes and growth. For pacemaker

CONTRACT FOR: IMPLANTABLE PACEMAKER SYSTEMS.	BUYER: IAN B SHEPHERD MCIPS SUPPLIER CONTACT: STEWART WOOD LEAD CLINICIAN: ANDREW MARSHALL	DATE OF ISSUE: 5th May 1999 DATE LAST REVISED: 31st March 2001 SUPPLIER CATEGORY: 'A'
CONTRACTOR: MEDTRONIC LTD SUITE ONE SHERBOURNE HOUSE CROXLEY BUSINESS CENTRE WATFORD HERTS WD1 8YE TEL: 01923 212213 FAX: 01923 241004 MOBILE: 0802 160935 EMAIL: stewart.wood@medtronic.com	TERMS OF CONTRACT: NHS Standard Terms and Conditions of Contract apply, with formal annual review to take place in April each year. In addition, quarterly review meetings will be held in July, October and January each year, throughout the contract term. TYPE OF CONTRACT Alliance agreement as the primary supplier for the single and dual sourcing of products at reference. Preferred supplier status.	REFERENCE NO: 98/S247-169988/EN CONTRACT NUMBER: IBS/001/A/T/PAD PERIOD OF CONTRACT: 1st April 1999 to 31st March 2001, with options to extend to 31st March 2004 and 31st March 2006. 36 month maximum price agreement. ACCOUNT MANAGEMENT: Pacing product specialist - Stephen Allen (Medtronic) - David Todd (Vitatron) Technical Support - David Rowley (Medtronic) - David Todd (Vitatron)
This contract covers the terms and conditions relating to the supply of implantable pacemaker systems by Medtronic and Vitatron to the Trust and will form part of the overall 'Partnership Agreement' between Medtronic Corporation and Plymouth Hospitals NHS Trust.		

APPROVED BY:	APPROVED BY:	APPROVED BY:	APPROVED BY:
DR ANDREW MARSHALL Consultant Cardiologist	IAN B SHEPHERD MCIPS Head of Procurement and Logistics	GEOFF MORRIS Country Manager, UK & Ireland Medtronic Limited	GARY SLACK Country Manager Vitatron Ltd
01 March 2001	01 March 2001	01 March 2001	01 March 2001

Exhibit A.2.7: Plymouth Hospitals NHS Trust contract schedule.

systems 99.9% of volume is shared with two manufacturers. Exhibit A.2.8 is an example of this approach as applied to monitoring the commitment given to our preferred supplier of surgeons' gloves. Exhibit A.2.8 clearly demonstrates commitment to primary supplier 'B', as changes introduced October 1998 have resulted in sustained erosion in usage of alternative suppliers' products.

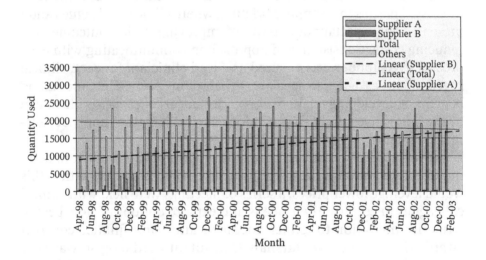

Exhibit A.2.8: Product use comparison.

Instead of inviting tenders for each category of expenditure, a notice was published in the Official Journal of European Communities (OJEC) inviting tenders for devices to meet the Cardiothoracic Centre's entire needs. We believe that this approach to aggregating expenditure is unique within public sector procurement and it is interesting to note that this approach was well received by participating suppliers due in part, to its significant reduction in tender administration costs.

The core product categories representing 80% of expenditure included in the invitation to tender were:

- Pacemaker systems
- Implantable cardioverter defibrillator systems
- Heart valves (mechanical and tissue)
- Coronary artery bypass graft (procedure packs)
- Coronary stents
- Diagnostic cardiology devices
- Interventional cardiology devices
- Perfusion devices for bypass surgery
- Electrophysiology devices

Key items used within these core product categories are summarised in Exhibit A.2.9. The price comparator in Exhibit A.2.9 shows that effective price management has been sustained throughout the contract term. The cumulative total saving, as a result of this approach, currently stands at £1.4 million.

Invitation to tender pre-qualifying criteria determined a shortlist of suppliers from whom tenders were invited. Our next step was to invite all interested parties to a supplier briefing, where clinical colleagues and I presented our expectations in terms of improving clinical outcomes and reducing costs. Consistency of approach in communicating with each prospective supplier was ensured as a lead clinician, for each clinical specialty was assigned to speak on behalf of his peers. The process and benefits of developing relationships with clinical colleagues is illustrated by the innovative purchasing solution developed for the supply of pacemaker systems.

Having gained senior management support of the concept to commit absolute volumes to longer term contracts, in the hope that this would leverage lower prices, a series of meetings were held with clinical colleagues to confirm their needs and explore options of how best to structure invitation to tender documentation and finalise contract award criteria. Andrew Marshall, Consultant Cardiologist, was very receptive to the concept of a longer-term commitment but wished to ensure his team received the appropriate level of training and education required to keep them at the forefront of pacing technology. His primary concerns were to improve clinical outcomes, have freedom of choice in selecting a therapy to treat patient need and to share risk, should there be an unfortunate future occurrence of a manufacturer's product being recalled.

Exhibit A.2.9: Price Comparator for Cardiothoracic Core Products.

	1997/98	1998/99	1999/00	2000/01	2001/02
Coronary Stents	£800	£700	£427	£350	£315
Pacemaker Systems (average price)	£2,370	£1,800	£1,570	£1,450	£1,400
ICD Systems (average price)	£22,000	£18,500	£14,500	£13,000	£12,000
Heart Valves (mechanical)	£1,930	£1,650	£1,405	£1,405	£1,350
Heart Valves (Tissue)	£1,700	£1,650	£1,350	£1,350	£1,300
Angioplasty Balloons	£275	£200	£140	£125	£100
Blood Cardioplaegia	£54	£49	£47	£45	£45
Guide Catheters	£60	£50	£35	£32	£25
Guide Wires (average price)	£80	£60	£49	£42	£39
Thoracic Cannulae		£8.48	£6.00	£5.83	£5.83
CABG Procedure Pack (increased components)		£218.08	£218.08	£175.38	£175.38
Angiography Pack (increased components)			£64.20	£34.23	£32.50

Invitation to tender documentation made reference to these primary concerns and specifically forewarned prospective suppliers that addressing these key elements would feature in our pre-tender negotiations. During these meetings suppliers were asked to demonstrate their track record and, subject to non-disclosure agreement, advise us of their upcoming product launches and future research and development plans. An essential feature of their response to this criterion was how they demonstrated their corporate philosophy in terms of ability to work in partnership. It is worth noting that at this stage price was not a factor.

Subsequent pre-tender negotiations ensured that there was no ambiguity about the clinical and commercial expectations of the Trust. During these meetings it was reiterated that we would honour absolute commitment to current and projected future contract volumes.

Following analysis of tenders received, Andrew Marshall and I together with representatives of senior management and the Finance Department, invited short listed suppliers to formally present their tender submission. This aided clarification of technical aspects of product detail and ensured parity of approach in respect of commercial comparisons.

Because of the ongoing openness between all parties, it was a relatively straightforward final analysis in selecting our preferred partners.

Engaging suppliers early on in the process met a primary objective of the Trust's purchasing strategy, in respect of developing partnership relationships. Parity of approach ensured open discussion on how suppliers could play a part in this process. Indeed, they were invited to comment on draft documents prior to their inclusion within the invitation to tender. I am sure this approach enabled prospective suppliers to focus on meeting our needs, within their tender submission, by highlighting key differentiators that would impact on clinical outcomes and cost.

5.1 Benefits

The benefits from taking this innovative approach are as follows:

Clinical Benefits

The benefits for clinical staff and patients is the ability to access leading edge therapies with device selection based on the need of each patient. Price is no longer a consideration given the introduction of average pricing, within a capped budget.

Continued training and development ensures clinical staff have access to supplier networks with a high level of technical support. This is supported by sustained provision of genuine added value.

The opportunity to work with a market-leading suppliers on the introduction of new technologies with whom there is potential to conduct clinical studies and research. One example of this is to evaluate the potential of devices that may be upgraded by software downloads as a patient's disease progresses. The benefit of this for the patient is that no further invasive treatment is required.

British Pacing and Electrophysiology Guidelines are adhered to in prescribing the mode and type of device suitable for each patient. However, the unknown is whether future patient demand would be skewed towards the higher cost, more complex modes. By adopting an average price, for all therapies, the supplier shares the risk associated with unknown patient demand, as all patients' needs are met from a finite budget. Annual reconciliation of the account, if skewed to less complex modes, would result in a rebate to the Trust, if the total value of sales, at unit prices, is less than the total expenditure based on the agreed average price per pacemaker system.

Exhibit A.2.10 illustrates actual activity during the last two years. The adoption of average pricing with risk transfer, compared to mode and lowest benchmark equivalent prices is proven to be of benefit. However, the real significance of using this review model is the benchmarking intelligence it provides in negotiating revised prices for the coming year.

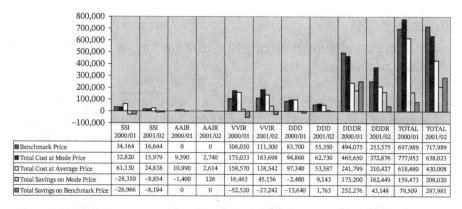

	SSI 2000/01	SSI 2001/02	AAIR 2000/01	AAIR 2001/02	VVIR 2000/01	VVIR 2001/02	DDD 2000/01	DDD 2001/02	DDDR 2000/01	DDDR 2001/02	TOTAL 2000/01	TOTAL 2001/02
Benchmark Price	34,164	16,644	0	0	106,050	111,300	83,700	55,350	494,075	253,575	697,989	717,989
Total Cost at Mode Price	32,820	15,979	9,590	2,740	175,033	183,698	94,860	62,730	465,650	372,876	777,953	638,023
Total Cost at Average Price	61,130	24,838	10,990	2,614	158,570	138,542	97,340	53,587	241,799	210,427	618,480	430,008
Total Savings on Mode Price	−28,310	−8,854	−1,400	126	16,463	45,156	−2,480	9,143	175,200	162,449	159,473	208,020
Total Savings on Benchmark Price	−26,966	−8,194	0	0	−52,520	−27,242	−13,640	1,763	252,276	43,148	79,509	287,981

Exhibit A.2.10: Risk transfer—pacemaker systems.

Supplier Benefits

Our primary suppliers have been successful in developing our relationship due to their:

- Aggressive pricing
- Service excellence
- Quality products
- Education and support infrastructure
- Mutual desire to work towards long term goals
- Open and consistent communication
- Belief and realisation that mutual commitment will and has been honoured

Being able to demonstrate we are in it for the long term has meant that we have worked together in an environment where the supplier's business is not at risk, save acceptable performance. This has allowed all parties the ability to focus on continuous improvement, improved clinical outcomes and have a trusted partner with whom to pioneer new ideas and technologies. Development of our relationship is based on shared objectives and a mutual belief that we are playing on the same side. Additional benefits for the supplier are:

- Long term absolute commitment
- Prompt payment and in some cases, pre-payment
- Reduced sales, marketing and associated administrative costs
- Opportunities to test new ideas
- Ongoing education of how the NHS functions
- Better mutual support mechanisms

Buyer Benefits

In addition to preferential pricing in return for long-term commitment are these commercial benefits:

- All expenditure is visible therefore, off contract creep, if any, is kept to a minimum (during financial year 2001/02 just £61,000 of the centre's £6million expenditure was not influenced by the Purchasing Department)
- Continued development of our product knowledge and under-standing of market dynamics provides intelligence to be used in a non threatening way when reviewing the market, costs and prices annually
- Continuous improvement in transforming supply chain processes has led to improved efficiency in managing:
  - Receipting and quality control
  - Product catalogue data conversion
  - Business protocols and policies
  - New product introduction protocols
  - Invoice matching and payment performance
  - Compliance in the use of a standard (agreed) product range
  - Inventory levels and associated acquisition costs
  - E-commerce solutions

The most important benefit is the collective energy of clinician, industry and buyer working together as a team to provide the best possible outcomes for patients at the lowest overall cost.

5.2 Continuous Improvement

The iterative process of ongoing performance monitoring has led to the development of the performance management schedule in Exhibit A.2.11.

Exhibit A.2.11: Supplier performance monitoring.

Supplier Name:		Reviewed with:		Reviewed by:		
Date: From:	Period of review: To					
	100	90	80	60	40	20
Price: supplier's prices have:	exceeded expected reduction	been reduced	stayed constant	increased by < inflation	increased at inflation	increased by > inflation
Delivery: % on time	100%	99%	> 98%	> 96%	> 94%	> 90%
% complete	100%	99%	> 98%	> 96%	> 94%	> 90%
% Packaging Damage	0.1%	0.2%	0.3%	0.4%	0.5%	0.6%
Invoicing: 0% matched zero tolerance	100%	99%	> 95%	> 99%	> 85%	> 80%

In addition to assessment of supplier performance in completing Exhibit A.2.11 we review service provision with customers in consideration of less objective criteria:

1. Has sincere desire to serve customer needs
2. Supplies all necessary information on demand
3. Consistently provides agreed level of support to meet our business aims
4. Willingly helps in emergencies
5. Answers all communications within defined time
6. Advises on progress or trouble
7. Keeps promises
8. Maintains good usable records in support of data exchange targets
9. Reacts well to adverse incidents/criticisms/rejections
10. Proactively offers efficiency gains/service improvements/cost reductions
11. Has well trained/courteous staff
12. Able to make prompt decisions

The objectivity in assessing performance by using the criteria at Exhibit A.2.11 has meant that complacency by either party is avoided. Indeed, the opposite applies as performance management has enable the relationship to be increasingly more challenging than would have been the case without its introduction.

Beyond ensuring the right products are available to meet clinical need at the lowest price, our performance review with suppliers has increasingly become focussed on continuous improvement of supply chain processes – for example the average invoice settlement period of Trusts throughout the NHS with our primary supplier is 70 days. This is at odds with the public sector payment policy of 30 days (PSPP). In Plymouth we have done much to improve our payment performance with all suppliers and this is reflected in Exhibit A.2.12:

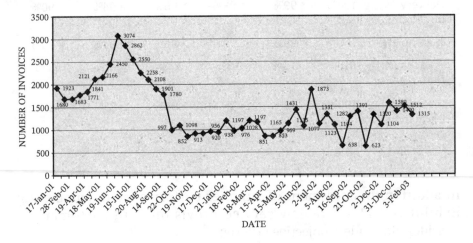

Exhibit A.2.12: Unit of Purchase Price Invoice Rate Versus Variance Report.

Exhibit A.2.12 illustrates the transformation in payment performance from a position in 1999 where 60% of the Trust's invoices were unmatched with a tolerance of £10 or 2% whichever was the greater. Current performance stands at more than 90% of invoices are matched with zero tolerance. In the early part of 2001 we believed we had performance under control but, failed to recognise process change was not embedded. However, we have learnt from this and now have greater understanding of what is required to improve further.

Taking ownership of the entire process of purchase to payment has helped to build stronger relationships with our top 50 suppliers. Increasingly, we are able to pinpoint root cause of errors that if undetected, would result in significant upstream corrective action. Transformation of our payment performance has not been just about validating item catalogues and unit prices to enable an invoice match, but has had more to do with continuous improvement of core tasks and managing the whole process to drive greater efficiency throughout the supply chain. For example, if items are not correctly reconciled to match goods receipted as invoiced, in a timely manner then poor payment performance could result. Our approach to improving management of this function has been the creation of a central goods receipting facility and if required, for technical purposes, to adopt second stage receipting as close to the point of use as is practicable. This proves a quantitative and technical assurance, as opposed to a first-stage quantitative acceptance. Further improvements are in hand as we explore the use of manufacturer's barcodes to facilitate an end-to-end match of data ultimately, enabling point of receipt self-billing.

Our e-trading capability will increase following the introduction of system–to-system data transfer using the Global Healthcare Exchange from May 2002. GHX provides a fully integrated solution for business-to-business transactions. Information is converted to the standard GHXml™ language for transmission. The Trust's EROS catalogue is maintained by the suppliers via the internet. Prices which we put on orders are automatically compared with those held by our suppliers in their price files – making error free trading realisable for the first time in the NHS. Orders are raised in EROS itself – not in a browser – and are then forwarded directly into the supplier's order processing system, the system then sends an order acknowledgement back to the Trust confirming product availability and the date of delivery. Working in partnership with our suppliers and GHX we will continue to develop these new technologies to further improve and automate our transactional processes as shown in Exhibit A.2.13. This diagram shows the full extent of our processes. Every greyed out activity above can be eliminated or simplified significantly using GHX technology.

The ability to place orders directly into our supplier's systems within seconds and send and receive real time information is just the start. GHX will be constantly adding to the functionality of its product and features such as electronic invoicing will soon be available. Additional mutual benefits will accrue as we implement the next phase of our e-commerce strategy, with our top 20 suppliers. This phase is to integrate the products required to meet predictable patient demand into our suppliers' production forecasting. It is hoped that this approach to sharing data will lead to increased operational efficiency, reduced inventory and ensure 100% availability to match patient demand.

6 Lessons Learned

The iterative strategic approach adopted in managing aggregated revenue expenditure has without doubt proven to be a success. The benefits as stated are significant however, the experience in itself and application of lessons learned are of equal importance.

By refining our thinking, reviewing actions and occasionally taking time out for a reality check we have maintained our focus to enable

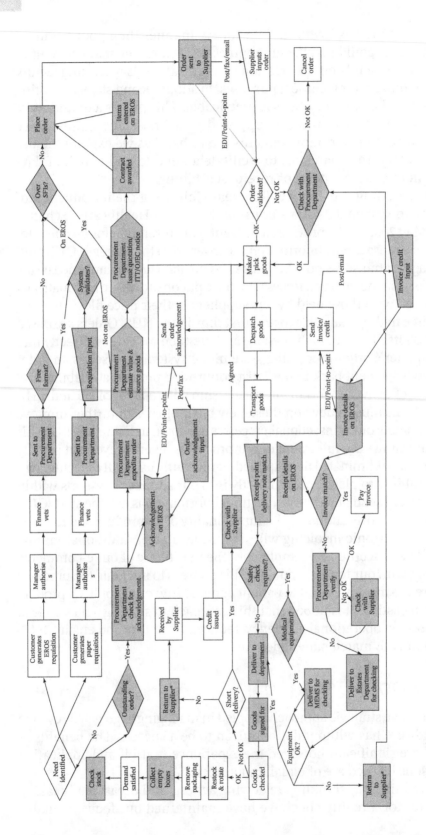

Exhibit A.2.13: Purchasing cycle.

sustained continuous improvement. This systematic appraisal of what is really going on, together with an eye on the future, has resulted in our ability to maintain influence over expenditures and ensure compliance in the use of specialised high value core products.

Sustained use of Trust item catalogues is essential in controlling expenditure of generic commodity items. Our approach in managing these less contentious products was to adopt a policy of 'commodity item best value denominator', defined as: the evaluation of a lowest price generic product and the next lowest and so on until a standard item is agreed by a representative customer group. Initially, this approach was applied to non contentious commodity items and then extended to all other products residing within validated supplier catalogues, subject to clinical or end user specific evaluations. Not only has this approach enabled rationalisation and standardisation but, has aided the promotion and compliance 'in use' of a Trust wide catalogue across clinical specialties.

Our key to success has been ongoing performance management. An example of where this has led to a practical operational improvement is the introduction of a policy for suppliers visiting the Trust to evaluate new products. Previously suppliers would cold-call or pre-book time with clinical staff to use products and then submit their invoice for payment. In effect, this unmanaged approach was eroding preferred suppliers market share, often at premium prices. Ongoing performance monitoring enabled identification of this off-contract activity. Given its significance, a revised policy has now established an agreed price, lower than contract price. This price is applied with absolute parity to all visiting suppliers, for a stated generic product e.g. stent. Prices are reviewed annually in line with contract renewals. The major difference in taking this approach is that instead of the supplier just presenting an invoice, as was previously the case, the supplier is now required to submit their item catalogue to the Purchasing Department so that we may preload this prior to the goods being presented to clinical staff. Failure to adhere to this policy will result in the invoice being returned to the supplier, advising that retrospectively presenting an invoice is not acceptable and the goods used are considered to have been donated 'free of charge'. Implementation and compliance with this policy was not possible without maintaining excellent working relationships with clinical staff and supplier's sales representatives.

Sustained benefits realisation has required tenacity, strong management and effective communication to ensure our focus is not eroded. This has required dedicated resource with the skills and knowledge to lead the change. Commodity specialisation to support ongoing development is an essential requirement in a dynamic market, such as the continued innovation in cardiac rhythm management. In addition to developing product knowledge we have learned that success requires one to:

- Focus on wants and needs to identify what clinicians and key stakeholders are really interested in and then develop an innovative solution to meet their needs, which also maximises the commercial opportunity
- Develop robust plans and stick to them, ensuring change is embedded
- Validate data and if comparing this with information provided by your supplier, make sure you are looking at the same reference period. We were surprised at the magnitude of difference caused by not agreeing the same cut off date against which to compare data. Do not assume their data is any more accurate than your own
- Benchmark what you have achieved and then devise plans to 'leap frog' better performers
- Be selfish about maintaining and further developing relationships. Resist the temptation to apply what you have learnt elsewhere, too soon, as this could erode or destroy the good work thus far. Relationships of the type described have taken longer to achieve than anticipated. We under estimated the skill shift and resources required by a factor of at least three
- Recognise that realising the big prize takes longer than expected but, when reached avoid complacency, strive for further improvements as they are achievable
- Promote your ability to add value, beyond price, by making life easier for your stakeholders. This helps build individual relationships and has ultimately broadened commitment, as awareness increases our role to genuinely add value
- Celebrate your mistakes as well as your successes. By trying to make a difference and occasionally failing, we have learnt much more about what is required to further improve that which has not worked
- Keep it simple. We have explored numerous approaches to managing price and the application of discounts and rebates for growth. In the light of this experience we now believe that the best approach is 'keep it simple' and apply validated prices to each line of a supplier specific catalogue. The benefit of this is less administration to monitor and validate pricing and provides easy assimilation of data matching on presentation of invoices
- Embrace relationships. Albeit that we have modified our organisational structure to embrace customer and supplier relationship management and associated category management, we have recognised that rigid organisational structures restrict our collective

ability to affectively influence all expenditure within a corporate entity. A virtual organisation with the ability to augment established policies and essential practices with innovative business solutions is what we now aspire to

- Challenge values and status quo. We have challenged cherished values and the status quo but attempting this without credibility or a well thought out plan is likely to result in alienating those stakeholders without whom change would be impossible. Finding common ground, on occasions through compromise to build a platform for success has worked

Partnership is not about cosy relationships or complacency. Our experience is that to deliver short, medium and long-term benefits of the magnitude described here, all parties must have mutual commitment to continually challenge the current. Without the right relationships and a passion to make a difference, sustained improvement is not possible.

7 The Future

During the progressive development of our approach in managing cardiothoracic expenditure, we transferred the principles of our strategy and applied them to other key categories of products within the Trust. Parallel procurement initiatives have resulted in the realisation of savings totalling £4.7million during the past three and a half years. However, relationships in other market sectors are not as clearly defined and efficiently managed as in the cardiothoracic market and to ensure sustained performance, improvement plans are in place so that we continue to develop our skills, knowledge and experience and apply these to maximise our influence over expenditure and outcomes. To achieve this will require transformation of the existing purchasing and supply organisational structure and the continued development of the team to focus on new skills as commodity and customer relationship management increasingly become core competencies.

The recent appointment of a Clinical Nurse Advisor to the purchasing team has already enhanced the department's capabilities. All staff as well as conducting traditional operational tasks are increasingly taking on a new role as resource managers, monitoring product utilisation and taking a holistic approach in understanding how products perform in use. Focussed product management at an operational level however is just the start. As skills and knowledge increase staff will proactively influence buying decisions in support of an overall strategic sourcing agenda. In some markets change will be incremental, in others a more radical and rapid transformation is likely. Exhibit A.2.14 shows the resource impact of this change.

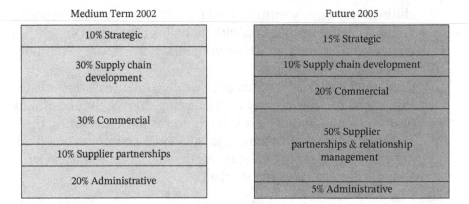

Exhibit A.2.14: The changing role of purchasing and supply.

This new role was considered essential to sustain the development of commodity buyers in gaining an in-depth appreciation of medical products and their performance in use. Having someone in the team from a clinical background will also aid further rationalisation and standardisation of user-specific and Trust-wide catalogues. The ability to liaise with clinical colleagues from a position of knowledge and experience will enable focussed product evaluation of new products and support determination of best value when evaluating variances in use from existing standard catalogue items. The ability to be more responsive to customer needs and to pro-actively support the introduction of new clinical legislation and policies is an additional significant advantage of this dynamic role.

As an enabler of our strategic direction, Exhibit A.2.15 highlights the resource shift needed to develop our e-trading systems and supporting

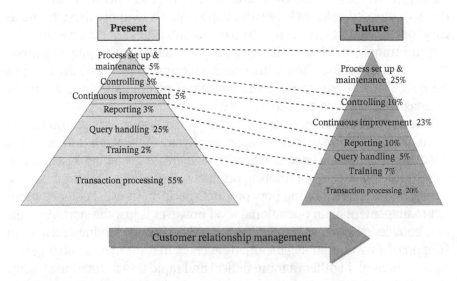

Exhibit A.2.15: Potential Resource Shifts.

processes to enhance our performance management capability, freeing up operational time so that this may be more productively utilised.

Future changes in respect of modernising the NHS and shifting the balance of power need to be better understood in respect of the challenges and opportunities that this presents to the purchasing and supply profession. Our strategic focus in developing commodity and customer relationship management must embrace and support the development of clinical networks. This extended role will augment an even greater understanding of clinical need and associated economic drivers so that our influence of market dynamics provides further added value benefits to a broader customer base. This holistic approach of meeting patient needs is to review the total cost of the clinical care pathway and explore the introduction of new therapies such as cardiac resynchronisation and atrial fibrillation management for the life of the patient, rather than comparing the price of a specific clinical intervention with current budget provision. We must engage commissioners of health care, within the local economy, to explore alternative funding arrangements and recognise that short-term levels of higher investment will reap medium to long-term cost reduction benefits. Working together on evidenced based outcomes supported by robust cost models is where purchasing in the future must demonstrate its ability to add real value. This collaborative activity is to be prioritised to match effort with potential benefits.

In taking a more holistic view of the market by cutting across existing purchasing and supply operational boundaries, we must analyse current practices, supporting treatment regimes, and develop innovative solutions that provide efficient process redesign. In addition to having the right skills, knowledge and experience available to meet this challenge, our future is also about recognising the value of investing to save, for strategic advantage, rather than expending disproportionate time managing marginal price improvement.

We must establish a strong relationship with the clinical lead of the South West Cardiac network, once established. It is anticipated that by becoming an active member of this network we would be in a position to manage the extension or creation of new contracts on behalf of the wider health economy and influence the range of products used. Given that the number of locations where patients may be treated with interventional therapies is likely to increase, it is essential that we manage the logistics infrastructure to provide this service and ensure optimum inventory controls are applied.

8 Conclusion

The Cardiothoracic Centre has developed a reputation for clinical excellence and it has expanded enormously to catch up with unmet demand.

By working together clinicians, suppliers and the purchasing team, have exceeded the initial aim of treating 10-15% more patients within the same budget. A saving of £1.2million has been achieved, this represents 19% of existing expenditure but has in reality resulted in the Trust's ability to treat an additional 400 heart disease patients who may have otherwise had to wait longer for their treatment. We must now extend our influence to all clinical activities by developing strategies to optimise products, services and operational costs.

Index